Essential
Cardiac
Electrophysiology
With Self Assessment

In loving memory of my brother Husainali
and
To my wife Karuna whose patience and understanding made this project possible
and
To my children Moeen, Sakena and Zameer

Zainul Abedin

To all the students of cardiac electrophysiology

Robert Conner

Essential Cardiac Electrophysiology

With Self Assessment

Zainul Abedin, MD, FRCP(C)
Associate Professor of Clinical Medicine
Texas Tech University Health Sciences Center
El Paso, TX
Adjunct Associate Professor of Electrical Engineering and Computer Science
University of Texas at El Paso

Robert Conner, RN

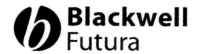

© 2007 Zainul Abedin & Robert Conner
Published by Blackwell Publishing
Blackwell Futura is an imprint of Blackwell Publishing

Blackwell Publishing, Inc., 350 Main Street, Malden, Massachusetts 02148-5020, USA
Blackwell Publishing Ltd, 9600 Garsington Road, Oxford OX4 2DQ, UK
Blackwell Publishing Asia Pty Ltd, 550 Swanston Street, Carlton, Victoria 3053, Australia

First published 2007

4   2010

Library of Congress Cataloging-in-Publication Data

Abedin, Zainul, MD.
Essential cardiac electrophysiology : self assessment/by
   Zainul Abedin and Robert Conner.
      p. ; cm.
   Includes bibliographical references and index.
   ISBN 978-1-4051-5108-5 (pbk. : alk. paper)
      1. Heart–Electric properties–Handbooks, manuals, etc.
2. Arrhythmia–Pathophysiology–Handbooks, manuals, etc.
3. Electrophysiology–Handbooks, manuals, etc. 4. Heart conduction system–Handbooks, manuals, etc. I. Conner, Robert P.   II. Title.
      [DNLM: 1. Arrhythmia–physiopathology–Handbooks.
2. Arrhythmia–therapy–Handbooks. 3. Electrophysiologic Techniques, Cardiac–Handbooks.
WG 39 A138e 2007]
QP112.5.E46A24 2007
612.1'71–dc22

                                                                    2006015740

ISBN 978-1-4051-5108-5

A catalogue record for this title is available from the British Library

Acquisitions Editor: Gina Almond
Development Editor: Lauren Brindley
Editorial Assistant: Victoria Pittman
Production Controller: Debbie Wyer

Set in 9/12pt Meridien by Newgen Imaging Systems (P) Ltd., Chennai, India
Printed and bound in Malaysia by Vivar Printing Sdn Bhd.

For further information on Blackwell Publishing, visit our website:
www.blackwellfutura.com
Address comments to essentialep@gmail.com

The publisher's policy is to use permanent paper from mills that operate a sustainable forestry policy, and which has been manufactured from pulp processed using acid-free and elementary chlorine-free practices. Furthermore, the publisher ensures that the text paper and cover board used have met acceptable environmental accreditation standards.

Contents

Foreword

Medical texts are written with the goal of disseminating knowledge. However, the approaches used to achieve this goal vary widely. There are comprehensive textbooks that cover a wide variety of topics in moderate detail, more focused textbooks that provide a great deal of detail on a single topic, and succinct texts that review the basics, providing quick and practical access to information that may assist in patient care.

Essential Cardiac Electrophysiology belongs in this last category. The first sections of the book provide a review of basic electrophysiology, providing essential facts in a fashion suitable for those studying for the Clinical Cardiac Electrophysiology board certification examination. Material that is relevant to patient care is emphasized, with a healthy dose of basic concepts. For example, the book provides a quick and simple way to look up a basic electrophysiology fact such as the gene mutation that causes catecholaminergic polymorphic ventricular tachycardia. The liberal use of tables and illustrations effectively supplements the concise text. The later chapters review all major areas of arrhythmia management in a succinct fashion. The chapters on supraventricular and ventricular tachycardia stand out as being particularly useful as a reference for those seeking a quick review. Other strengths include the self-assessment questions at the beginning of each chapter and references to key review articles published in 2001–2006. However, the book was not intended to be a "how-to" manual, and therefore provides no instructions on procedures such as catheter ablation or device implantation.

Dr Abedin has succeeded admirably in producing a concise review of both basic and clinical electrophysiology that complements but does not replace larger electrophysiology textbooks. This book should serve as an excellent resource for students of cardiac electrophysiology at all levels.

Fred Morady, MD

Preface

"Everything should be made as simple as possible, but not one bit simpler"
Albert Einstein

The subject of cardiac electrophysiology is vast and rapidly evolving at a basic, clinical, and therapeutic level. There are many excellent textbooks and monographs on basic and clinical aspects of Electrophysiology. This book is presented as a concise summary of electrophysiologic facts, with an emphasis on basic electrophysiologic concepts as applied to clinical syndromes. Each sentence or paragraph could be construed as an answer to a question. In keeping with the idea that repetition reinforces the subject matter, some topics are reiterated. An attempt has been made to answer clinical questions using basic electrophysiologic information.

The self-assessment questions at the beginning of each chapter allow the reader to assess his or her knowledge of the material presented in that related chapter. Having reviewed the chapter, the reader should be able to answer all the self-assessment questions correctly. References, provided at the end of each chapter, are a collection of review articles from the English literature.

This book will be an excellent resource for students, residents, cardiologists, cardiac electrophysiologists, nurses and anyone who is interested in management of cardiac arrhythmias. It presupposes some prior knowledge of electrophysiology.

Acknowledgements

We gratefully acknowledge the generous help of Professor Fred Morady, a true scholar and a superb teacher, in reviewing the manuscript and in providing many valuable suggestions.

We owe a debt of gratitude to Dr Christopher Wyndham, a skillful clinician and a great mentor, for reviewing the manuscript. We are greatful to Dr Prasrd Palakurthy for reviewing the manuscript.

We are grateful to Ms Susan Fernandez for secretarial assistance; and to Ms Gina Almond, Ms Lauren Brindley, Mr John Normansell and other members of the Blackwell editorial, publishing and marketing team.

Zainul Abedin and *Robert Conner*

List of Abbreviations

4-AP	4-Amino pyridine	CX	Connexion
AAG	Alpha1 acid glycoprotein	CYP	Cytochrome P
ABC	ATP binding cassette protein	DAD	Delayed after depolarization
Ach	Acetylcholine	DCM	Dilated cardiomyopathy
Ado	Adenosine	DFT	Defibrillation threshold
AF	Atrial fibrillation	EAD	Early after depolarization
AIVR	Accelerated idioventricular rhythm	EF	Ejection fraction
		EHL	Elimination half life
AJT	Automatic junctional tachycardia	ER	Eustachian ridge
AP	Action potential	ERP	Effective refractory period
AP	Accessory pathway	HCM	Hypertrophic cardiomyopathy
APD	Action potential duration	HCN	Hyperpolarization activated cyclic nucleotide gated
ARVD/C	Arrhythmogenic right ventricular dysplasia/cardiomyopathy	HERG	Human ether related a-go-go gene protein
AT	Atrial tachycardia	HPS	His Purkinje system
ATP	Adenosine triphosphate	HRV	Heart rate variability
ATP	Anti tachycardia pacing	I_{CaT}	Ca current transient or short acting
ATS	Andersen–Tawil syndrome		
AVD	AV dissociation	I_{CaL}	Ca current long acting
AVN	Atrio-ventricular node	ICD	Implantable cardioverter defibrillator
AVNRT	AVN reentry tachycardia		
AVRT	AV reentrant tachycardia	I_f	Hyperpolarizing cation current
BBB	Bundle branch block	I_K	Potassium current
BBRVT	Bundle branch reentry VT	I_{K1}	Inward rectifying potassium current
BRS	Baroreflex sensitivity		
Ca	Calcium	I_{Kach}	Acetylcholine mediated potassium current
CAD	Coronary artery disease		
cAMP	Cyclic adenosine monophosphate	I_{Katp}	ATP dependent potassium current
CHF	Congestive heart failure		
CICR	Calcium induced calcium release	I_{Kp}	Time independent background plateau current
CL	Cycle length		
Cl^-	Chloride	I_{Kr}	Rapidly activating potassium current
CS	Coronary sinus		
CSF	Cerebrospinal fluid	I_{Ks}	Slowly activating potassium current
CSNRT	Corrected sinus node recovery time		

I_{Kur}	Ultra rapid potassium current	PKA	Protein kinase A
I_{Na}	Sodium current	PPI	Post pacing interval
IP3	Innositol triphosphate	PVC	Premature ventricular
IST	Inappropriate sinus tachycardia		contractions
I_{to}	Transient outward current	QT_c	Corrected QT interval
IVC	Inferior vena cava	RA	Right atrium
K	Potassium	RB	Right bundle
KvLQT1	Voltage dependent potassium	RF	Radiofrequency
	controlling protein	RNA	Ribonucleic acid
LA	Left atrium	RSPV	Right superior pulmonary vein
LAFB	Left anterior fascicular block	RV	Right ventricle
LIPV	Left inferior pulmonary vein	RVOT	Right ventricular outflow tract
LOC	Loss of consciousness	SACT	Sino atrial conduction time
LQTS	Long QT syndrome	SAEKG	Signal average ECG
LSPV	Left superior pulmonary vein	SAN	Sino atrial node
LV	Left ventricle	SCD	Sudden cardiac death
LVH	Left ventricular hypertrophy	SCRC	Sarcoplasmic Ca release
LVOT	Left ventricular outflow tract		channel
M	Muscarinic	SND	Sinus node dysfunction
MHC	Myosin heavy chain	SNRT	Sinus node recovery time
MDP	Maximum diastolic potential	SR	Sarcoplasmic reticulum
MI	Myocardial infarction	SUR	Sulfonylurea receptor
MinK	Minimal potassium current	SVC	Superior vena cava
	controlling protein	SVT	Supraventricular tachycardia
$MnCl_2$	Manganese chloride	TA	Tricuspid annulus
MVT	Monomorphic VT	TCL	Tachycardia cycle length
Na	Sodium	TDP	Torsade de pointes
NAPA	N-acetylprocainamide	TEE	Trans-esophageal
NAT	N acetyltransferase		echocardiography
NSVT	Nonsustain VT	TIA	Transient ischemic attack
P	Purinergic	TWA	T wave alternans
PAC	Premature atrial contractions	ULV	Upper limit of vulnerability
PCA	Pulseless cardiac electrical activity	VA	Ventriculo atrial
PES	Programmed electrical	VF	Ventricular fibrillation
	stimulation	VT	Ventricular tachycardia
PG	P glycoprotein	WCT	Wide complex tachycardia
PJRT	Permanent form of junctional	WPW	Wolf Parkinson white
	reciprocating tachycardia		syndrome

1 Ions, Channels, and Currents

Self-Assessment Questions

1.1 POTASSIUM CHANNELS AND CURRENTS

1 In a diagram of AP shown below, which one of the following currents is active where arrow is pointing?

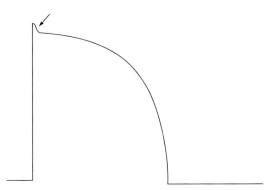

  A I_{to}
  B I_{K1}
  C I_{Na}
  D I_{Ca}

2 Which one of the following genes controls the expression of I_{Kr}?
  A KCNQ1 (KvLQT1)
  B KCNH2 (HERG)
  C SCN5A
  D MinK

3 Which one of the following actions is likely to activate I_{Katp} current?
  A Rise in intracellular ATP
  B Rise in intracellular calcium
  C Fall of intracellular ATP
  D Fall of intracellular calcium

4 How does congestive heart failure affect depolarizing/repolarizing currents?
  A Outward repolarizing currents are reduced
  B Inward depolarizing currents are reduced
  C Outward repolarizing currents are increased
  D APD is decreased

5 Which one of the following is least likely to occur with prolongation of the plateau phase of the AP?
  A Increase in strength of contraction
  B Increase in conduction velocity
  C Increase in the duration of contraction
  D Increase in refractoriness

6 Which one of the following is likely to increase the activity of I_{Kr}?
  A Increased extracellular potassium
  B Exposure to Sotalol
  C Decreased extracellular potassium
  D Increase in chloride current

7 Which one of the following agents is likely to block I_{Ks}?
  A Aminophylline
  B Indapamide
  C Activation of protein Kinase C
  D Erythromycin

8 When does the reverse use dependent block occur?
  A It occurs with repeated activation of the channel
  B It occurs when the sodium channel is blocked
  C It occurs at a slow heart rate but not at a fast heart rate
  D It occurs in the presence of catecholamines

9 Which one of the following is the least likely attribute of I_{to}?
  A It is present in ventricular epicardium but not in endocardium
  B It is responsible for the spike and dome characteristic
  C It is a chloride current
  D It is also present in the human atrium

10 Which one of the following is associated with Brugada syndrome?
  A Defect in the SCN5A gene
  B Loss of I_{Kr}
  C ST segment depression in precordial leads
  D Deafness

1.2 SODIUM CHANNELS AND CURRENTS

1 Which one of the following currents is likely to occur when the Na moves across the cell membrane and into the cell?
   A Inward current
   B Outward current
   C Repolarizing current
   D No change in current

2 A patient receiving a Na channel blocker develops AF with rapid ventricular response. What changes on ECG can be anticipated to occur?
   A Narrowing of the QRS complex during tachycardia
   B Widening of the QRS complex during tachycardia
   C Prolongation of the QT interval
   D Shortening of the QT interval

3 What is likely to happen when a Na channel is blocked?
   A Increase in intracellular Ca and increased contractility
   B Increase in EAD and DAD
   C Decrease in contractility
   D Increase in extracellular Na

4 Which one of the following is not associated with Brugada syndrome?
   A Mutation in SCN5A resulting in loss of function
   B Increase in I_{to} current
   C Inhibition of I_{Ca} during the plateau phase
   D Mutation in SCN5A, resulting in gain of function

5 What type of channel block, by lidocaine, results in effective suppression of arrhythmias during myocardial ischemia?
   A Inactivated state block
   B Resting state block
   C Open state block
   D Closed state block

6 Which one of the following agents is likely to be effective in treating Flecainide-induced VT?
   A IV magnesium
   B IV lidocaine
   C IV amiodarone
   D IV digoxin

7 Which one of the following metabolic abnormalities is likely to decrease lidocaine dissociation from the channel sites?
  A Acidosis
  B Ischemia
  C Hyperkalemia
  D Hyponatremia

8 What electrophysiologic manifestations can be expected when I_{Nab} (the slow component of the background Na current) is blocked?
  A Lengthening of the QT interval
  B Positive inotropy
  C Occurrence of EAD
  D Bradycardia

9 Which one of the following interventions is likely to promote occurrence of TDP in patients with LQT3?
  A Beta blocker induced bradycardia
  B Permanent pacemaker
  C Mexiletine
  D Exercise-induced sinus tachycardia

1.3 CALCIUM CHANNELS AND CURRENTS

1 In which one of the following is there no contribution from Calcium current I_{CaL}?
  A EAD
  B Electrical remodeling of the atrium during AF
  C DAD
  D Depolarization of the SA and AV nodes

2 Which of the following statements is incorrect?
  A β-Adrenergic agonists increase I_{CaL} channel activity
  B β Blockers act as Ca channel blockers
  C Parasympathetic stimulation decreases I_{CaL} activity
  D T-type Ca channel density is increased by growth hormone, endothelin, and pressure overload

3 Which of the following agents has no effect on T-type Ca channel?
  A Amiloride
  B Flunarizine
  C Mibefradil
  D Digoxin

4 Which of the following statements for the sarcoplasmic Ca release channel (SCRC) is incorrect?

A Caffeine releases Ca from SCRC

B Doxorubicin depletes sarcoplasmic reticulum Ca

C It is blocked by verapamil

D Ischemia decreases Ca release from the sarcoplasmic reticulum

5 Which of the following agents does not block Ca channel?

A Terfenadine

B Magnesium

C Diltiazem

D Sotalol

6 Which of the following statements is incorrect?

A I_{CaL} participates in the occurrence of DAD

B Phase-3 EAD shares the mechanisms of DAD

C EAD is associated with bradycardia and prolongation of APD

D DAD is associated with increased heart rate and Ca overload

1.1 POTASSIUM CHANNELS AND CURRENTS[1-4]

- There are more than eight types of potassium currents.
- The plateau phase of the action potential (AP) depends on the balance between inward (depolarizing) and outward (repolarizing) currents.
- Potassium currents (outward movement of the K through the potassium channels) are the main contributors to repolarization.

Classification of potassium currents

Voltage gated currents	Inwardly rectifying currents	Background currents
I_{to}	I_{K1}	I_{Kp}
I_{Kur}	I_{Kach}	
I_{Kr}	I_{Katp}	
I_{Ks}		

- AP duration (APD) determines the amount of calcium influx and tissue refractoriness. It is inversely related to heart rate. Prolongation of AP plateau increases the strength and duration of contraction. It also increases refractoriness.
- In congestive heart failure (CHF) and in left ventricular hypertrophy (LVH), repolarizing outward currents are reduced by 50%. This increases APD and results in early after depolarization (EAD) and arrhythmias. Use of class III drugs in patients with CHF needs reevaluation as the intended target (K channels) is down regulated or absent.
- In atrial fibrillation (AF) repolarizing outward currents (I_K, I_{to}) are reduced. Reduction of these currents may exacerbate the arrhythmic effect of hypokalemia and hypomagnesemia.
- Potassium channel expression is decreased in hypothyroid and hypoadrenal states.

Delayed and inwardly rectifying voltage sensitive potassium channels

- Rectification is a diode-like property of unidirectional current flow, which could be inwards or outwards. It limits the outward flow of potassium through I_{Kr} and I_{Ks} during a plateau. Delayed rectifier potassium channels have slow onset of action.
- Voltage gated potassium channels are activated during an upstroke of AP.
- Rapidly activating and inactivating voltage-sensitive transient outward current produces phase 1 of repolarization.
- Slowly activating delayed rectifier potassium current, and inward rectifier I_{K1}, which includes fast inactivating rapid component I_{Kr} and slow component I_{Ks}, contributes to plateau and phase 3 of AP.

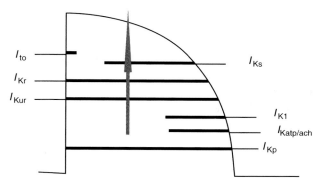

Fig 1.1 Outward currents.

- K channels carry a positive charge, which acts as a voltage sensor.
- Potassium channels are closed at resting potential and open after depolarization.
- Two types of voltage-gated channels play a major role in repolarization.
  i Transient outward current (I_{to}), which is characterized by rapid activation and inactivation.
  ii Delayed rectifier I_K, which has several components (Fig. 1.1):
   - I_{Kr} is a rapidly activating current with inward rectification.
   - I_{Ks} is a slowly activating current.
   - I_{Kp} is a time independent background plateau current.
   - I_{Kur} is an ultra rapid current.

Transient outward potassium current (I_{to})[5]

- There are two types of I_{to} currents: I_{to1} and I_{to2}.
- I_{to} is present in ventricular epicardium but not in endocardium. It is responsible for spike and dome morphology of AP in epicardium.
- In human atrium it recovers rapidly from inactivation, thus allowing rapid repolarization at a fast heart rate.
- Flecainide, Quinidine, and Ambasilide inhibit I_{to}. Flecainide binds to inactivated I_{to1}. It also demonstrates fast unbinding. Quinidine binds to open channel; its slow recovery from block causes a rate dependent effect.
- Inhibition of I_{to} prolongs repolarization in diseased human ventricle.
- I_{to2} is calcium activated.

I_{to} and J wave

- J wave (Osborn wave), elevated J point and T wave alternans may be due to a transmural gradient between epicardium and endocardium as a result of uneven distribution of I_{to}.
- Prominent J waves are often seen in the presence of hypothermia and hypercalcemia.

Rapidly activating delayed rectifier I_{Kr}

- It is blocked by methane sulfonamide, class III agents (D-Sotalol).
- Inward rectification of I_{Kr} results in a small outward current.
- It plays an important role in atrial pacemaker cells. It rapidly recovers from inactivation and it peaks at -40 mV.
- KCNH2 (HERG, Human Ether Related-a-go-go gene protein) encodes I_{Kr} channel.
- I_{Kr} is increased in the presence of elevated extracellular potassium. Normally, increased extracellular potassium will decrease the outward potassium current by decreasing the chemical gradient, but the activity of I_{Kr} is increased.
- Increase in serum potassium by 1.4 mEq/L decreases QTc by 24% and decreases QT dispersion.
- The efficacy of I_{Kr} blockers is limited by inverse rate dependency. The drug is more effective at a slower heart rate. A high heart rate increases the prevalence of I_{Ks}, which is insensitive to I_{Kr} blocker. This offsets the k blocking effects of the I_{Kr} blockers.
- The effect of I_{Ks} but not of I_{Kr} is enhanced by β-adrenergic stimulation. Thus, the effects of pure I_{Kr} blockers will be antagonized by sympathetic stimulation.
- Selective I_{Kr} blockers (D-Sotalol) lose efficiency at high rates and during sympathetic stimulation.
- I_{Kr} and I_{Ks} are present in the human atrium and ventricle.

Slowly activating delayed rectifier I_{Ks}

- I_{Ks} is controlled by the gene KvLQT1 (voltage-dependent potassium controlling protein) and MinK (minimal potassium current controlling protein). MinK combined with protein of KvLQT1 induces I_{Ks}. Expression of both these proteins is necessary for normal function of I_{Ks}^1.
- MinK, a protein, acts as a function altering β subunit of KvLQT1. MinK modifies KvLQT1 gating and pharmacology.
- Mutation in MinK and KvLQT1 causes congenital long QT syndrome (LQTS).
- MinK suppression leads to inner ear abnormalities and deafness, seen in the Jarvell Lange-Nielson syndrome.
- Reduced activity of I_{Ks} in M cells prolongs APD.
- Bradycardia and class III drugs, which reduce I_{Ks} in M cells, prolong APD and predispose to arrhythmias.
- Slow deactivation of I_{Ks} is important for rate dependent shortening of AP. As the heart rate increases, I_{Ks} has less time to deactivate during shortened diastole, it accumulates in an open state, and contributes to faster repolarization.
- Increase in intracellular magnesium decreases and increase in intracellular calcium increases I_{Ks}.

- Indapamide (Diuretic), Thiopental, Propafol (Anesthetics) Benzodiazepine, and chromanol block I_{Ks}.
- Increasing cAMP either by β-adrenergic stimulation or by phosphodiesterase inhibitors increases I_{Ks}.
- Activation of protein kinase C increases I_{Ks}.

I_{Kur} *current*

- It is responsible for atrial repolarization. It is a potassium selective outwardly rectifying current. Short APD of the atria is due to I_{Kur}.
- I_{Kur} is also found in intercalated disks.
- I_{Kur} is absent from the human ventricular myocardium.
- It is enhanced by β-adrenergic agonists and is inhibited by α-adrenergic agonists.
- Drugs inhibiting I_{Ks} (Amiodarone, Ambasilide) or I_{Kur} (Ambasilide) will be therapeutically superior.
- The presence of I_{Kur} in the human atrium makes atrial repolarization relatively insensitive to agents that fail to inhibit this current (D-Sotalol and Flecainide). Quinidine and Ambasilide block I_{Kur} in a rate independent fashion.
- I_{Kur} decreases with increasing heart rate.

Inwardly rectifying currents

Inward rectifier I_{K1}

- I_{K1} rectification allows it to carry substantial current at negative potentials which maintains the resting potential.
- Resting potassium conductance is produced by voltage independent inwardly rectifying potassium channels.
- These channels permit inward potassium flux on membrane hyperpolarization but resist outward potassium flux on depolarization. It prevents potassium ion leak during prolonged depolarization. In addition to I_{K1}, I_{Katp} and I_{Kach} are also inward rectifiers.
- Intracellular magnesium, calcium, and polyamines block I_{K1}. Increase in intracellular pH inactivates I_{K1}. Increase in extracellular potassium depolarizes the resting membrane.
- Inwardly rectifying potassium channels (K1) produce less outward currents than inward currents. They stabilize the resting membrane potential by high resting potassium conductance, but during depolarization produce little outward current.

ATP sensitive potassium channel (Katp)[6,7]

- K_{atp} channel opens when the intracellular ATP level falls and closes when the ATP levels rise. ATP produced by the glycolytic pathway is preferentially sensed by the K_{atp} channel.
- I_{Katp} is a weak inward rectifier but produces a large outward current during depolarization and its activation decreases APD.

- It is responsible for ischemia preconditioning where brief episodes of ischemia protect the myocardium from prolonged episodes of ischemia.
- During ischemia, intracellular magnesium and sodium levels increase, I_{Katp} current decreases, and extracellular potassium increases.
- Protons, lactates, oxygen free radicals, adenosine, and muscarinic receptor stimulation desensitize the K_{atp} channel to the effects of the ATP level.
- Sodium and potassium pump and other ATPases degrade ATP.
- Cromakalim, Bimakalim, Aprikalim, Nicorandil, Adenosine, and protein kinase C open the K_{atp} channel and mimic preconditioning. Sulfonylureas such as Glipizide and Tolbutamide block K_{atp} and abolish preconditioning.
- During ischemia there is loss of intracellular potassium and increase in extracellular potassium resulting in membrane depolarization, slow conduction, and altered refractoriness resulting in reentrant arrhythmias. K_{atp} counteracts these effects by shortening APD, decreasing workload, promoting inexcitability, and increasing potassium conductance during ischemia and hypoxia. Increased potassium conductance is a result of an increased level of intracellular sodium that occurs during ischemia.
- I_{Katp} decreases APD and calcium influx. It preserves high-energy phosphates.
- Diazoxide does not activate I_{Katp} in sarcolemma but mimics preconditioning. This suggests that there may be other pathways involved in preconditioning.
- I_{Katp} causes coronary vasodilatation.

I_{Kach} (Acetylcholine-dependent K current)
- Stimulation of muscarinic receptors activates this current. It is mediated by acetylcholine. I_{Kach} is inwardly rectifying potassium current.
- Parasympathetic stimulation slows heart rate by activating muscarinic receptors, which reduces I_f (hyperpolarizing cation current; f stands for funny) in pacemaker cells.
- The effect of potassium channel blockers on atrial repolarization depends on their ability to counteract cholinergic activation of I_{Kach}, either by direct blocking of the channel (Quinidine) or by muscarinic receptor antagonism (Ambasilide, Disopyramide).

Background K currents I_{Kp}

- These currents contribute to repolarization and resting membrane potential.
- These currents are inhibited by decreasing intracellular pH.
- Arachidonic acid and polyunsaturated fatty acids modulate these channels.

Characteristics of potassium channel block[5,8,9]
- Voltage gated potassium channels are activated during upstroke of AP.
- Rapidly activating and inactivating voltage sensitive transient outward current produces phase 1 of repolarization.

- Slowly activating delayed rectifier potassium current, and inward rectifier I_{K1}, which includes fast inactivating rapid component I_{Kr} and slow component I_{Ks}, contributes to plateau and phase 3 of AP.
- Potassium channel blockers prolong APD. This is characteristic of Class III action.
- Some potassium channel blockers produce less block at a fast heart rate and more blocks at a slower heart rate. This phenomenon is called reverse use dependence.
- Potassium channels contribute to repolarization; therefore, reverse use dependent block will manifest itself during repolarization at the channel level.
- Blocking of K channel may not consistently affect repolarization because of the following:
  - i Many potassium channels are involved in repolarization.
  - ii Blocking of potassium channels (outward currents) may be counterbalanced by inward currents I_{Ca}, I_{Na}, and $I_{Na/Ca}$. Thus no one current dominates repolarization.
  - iii Nonspecific effects of potassium channel blockers.
  - iv Extracellular potassium level may affect K currents.
  - v Potassium channel distribution may be variable. Potassium channel expression varies within different layers of myocardium. I_{Kur} is found in the atria but not in the ventricles.
  - vi I_{Kr} block could shift repolarization to I_{Ks} at rapid rates. Inability of I_{Ks} to deactivate rapidly and fully will produce less of an increase in APD.
  - vii Many antiarrhythmics are capable of causing potassium channel block and other ion channel blocks simultaneously.
  - viii Drugs that need a long plateau phase to work will be more effective in the ventricle than the atrium.
- Open channel block occurs when the drug is present during activated or open state.
- Trapping block occurs when the channel closes around the drug without need for the drug to unbind. Activation is required to remove the drug from the binding site.
- The drug may bind the channel during the inactive state, but cannot bind it during the resting state.

Effect of pharmacologic agents on action potential

- Acetylcholine in low concentration prolongs and in high concentration produces abbreviation of epicardial AP. These effects are as follows:
  - i Reversed by atropine.
  - ii Do not occur when I_{to} is blocked.
  - iii Accentuated by isoproterenol.
  - iv Persist in the presence of Propranolol.
  - v Caused by inhibition of I_{Ca} or activation of I_{Kach}.

- Isoproterenol causes epicardial AP abbreviation more than endocardial. It influences I_{to}, I_{Ca}, I_K, and I_{Cl}. These currents contribute to phase 1 and phase 3 of AP.
- Organic calcium channel blockers (Verapamil) and inorganic calcium channel blocker $MnCl_2$ decreases the I_{Ca} (inward current) and leaves the outward currents unopposed, resulting in decrease of APD and loss of dome in epicardium and not in endocardium.
- I_{to} block may establish electrical homogeneity and abolish arrhythmias due to dispersion of repolarization caused by drugs and ischemia.
- Quinidine inhibits I_{to}.
- Amiloride, a potassium sparing diuretic, prolongs APD and refractoriness.
- Antiarrhythmics, Antimicrobial, Antihistamine, Psychotropic, GI prokinetic, and a host of other pharmacologic agents may alter repolarization.

M cells, potassium currents, and APD

- M cells are found in the mid-myocardium of anterior, lateral wall, and outflow tract.
- Electrophysiologically they resemble Purkinje cells.
- M cells show disproportional AP prolongation in response to slow heart rate. This may be due to weaker I_{Ks} and stronger late I_{Na}.
- M cells may enforce pump efficiency at slow rates. Long depolarization permits longer efficient contraction.
- Epicardium and endocardium electrically stabilize and abbreviate APD of M cells.
- Loss of either layer by infarction will lead to prolongation of APD. This may be the mechanism of increase in QT interval and QT dispersion seen in non-Q wave myocardial infarction (MI). These differences could be aggravated by drugs that prolong QT interval or in patients with LQTS.
- M cells play an important role in the inscription of T waves by producing a gradient between epicardium, endocardium, and M cells.
- U waves are due to repolarization of His Purkinje cells.
- Amiodarone prolongs APD in epicardium and endocardium and to a lesser extent in M cells; this may prevent transmural dispersion of refractoriness.

1.2 SODIUM CHANNELS AND CURRENTS[10-13]

- Inward movement of the Na or Ca across the cell membrane through the specific channels produces inward current. Na current depolarizes the cell membrane and is voltage dependent (Fig. 1.2).
- The process of channel opening is called activation and the process of closing is called inactivation. During inactivation phase channel enters a nonconducting state while depolarization is maintained.
- The gating process measures current movement rather than ion movement.
- Channels flip between conducting and non-conducting states.

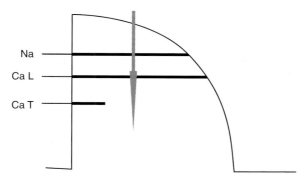

Fig 1.2 Inward currents.

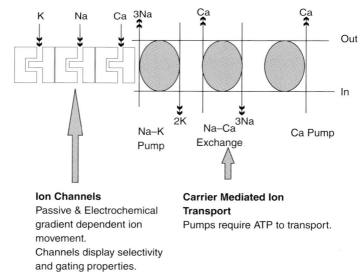

Ion Channels
Passive & Electrochemical
gradient dependent ion
movement.
Channels display selectivity
and gating properties.

**Carrier Mediated Ion
Transport**
Pumps require ATP to transport.

Fig 1.3 Ion pumps and channels.

- When all the gates (active or inactive) are open would a channel allow the passage of the ions.
- During the early part of repolarization Na channels become inactive. On completion of repolarization the Na channel returns from the inactive to the closed state. During resting potential the sodium channel is closed. Na ion conduction through the channel occurs when the channel is in the open state and not during the resting state.
- Movement of the sodium occurs through channels and pumps (Fig. 1.3).
- Repolarization occurs due to outward K currents. It will be delayed if the K currents are blocked as in LQT1 and LQT2 or when inward depolarizing currents

persist during repolarization as in LQT3. In LQT3 SCN5A, an Na channel remains open during repolarization resulting in continued inward current. This causes prolongation of the QT interval.

- Voltage-dependent opening of Na channel occurs as voltage decreases and conformational change in channel protein occurs (activation).
- There are no β_2 subunits of sodium channel in cardiac myocytes. Both β_1 and β_2 subunits are expressed in the Na channels of the brain neurons.
- Lidocaine inhibits the inactivated state of the sodium channel.
- Chronic exposure to Na channel blocking antiarrhythmic drugs increases the sodium channel messenger RNA which counteracts the effects of channel blockade.

Sodium channel block

- There are two types of Na channel block:
  i **Tonic** block results in a reduction of the peak current with the first pulse of the train of pulses. It is seen in drug-induced reduction of current during infrequent stimulation.
  ii **Phasic** block occurs when there is a sequential decline in the peak current from beat to beat. It is also called use dependent or frequency dependent block. It decreases AP upstroke and slows conduction velocity. This type of block increases with repetitive stimulation. If the interval between AP is less than four times the recovery constant of the channel, block accumulates.
- During phase 0 Na channels open (open state) for less than 1 millisecond and then become inactive.
- During phase 2 and phase 3 (plateau phase) less than 1% of sodium channels remain open (inactivated state).
- Most depressants of conduction such as elevated extracellular potassium (as may occur in ischemia) produce membrane depolarization and increase the fraction of inactivated Na channels. Lidocaine produces inactivated state block; thus, it is effective in ischemic zones. The fraction of channels available in the open state is reduced during ischemia.
- Quinidine, Disopyramide, and Propafenone produce open channel block.
- During the resting state dissipation of block occurs (drugs dissociate from the site).
- Drugs can produce Na channel block during the resting, open, or inactivated state. These are called state dependent blocks. The other type of channel block is voltage dependent.
- Two different sodium channel blocking drugs may act synergistically.
- Class 1A drugs increase APD, thus increasing the time sodium channels spend in the inactivated state. This will enhance the effectiveness of the drugs that bind to the inactivated state (Class 1B drug such as lidocaine).

- Drugs with different binding kinetics may interact. For example, drugs with fast kinetic may displace drugs with slower kinetic, thus reducing the overall block.
- Lidocaine may reverse the Quinidine, Propafenone Flecainide induced block.
- Ventricular tachycardia due to Flecainide, Yew needle toxin, dextropropoxylene can be treated with Lidocaine.
- Class 1B drugs have dissociation constant of less than one second. These drugs have no effect on the conduction of normal tissue but decrease the conduction following closely coupled premature ventricular contractions (PVCs) and in diseased (ischemic) cells.
- Class 1C drugs have the slowest dissociation of 12 seconds. This results in slowing of conduction and widening of QRS.
- Class 1A drugs have intermediate kinetics of more than 1 second but less than 12 seconds, this may result in slowing of conduction and widening of QRS at the normal heart rate, which increases during tachycardia.
- Lidocaine blocks I_{Na} by shifting voltage for inactivation to more negative. It binds to the activated and inactivated states of the sodium channel.
- Lidocaine, Quinidine, and Flecainide exert use dependent block with fast, intermediate, and slow kinetics, respectively.

Drug kinetics and channel state

- Membrane depressants such as increased extracellular potassium, hydrogen, and stretch reduce the resting membrane potential. This increases the fraction of inactivated channels and potentiates the effects of the drugs that act on the inactivated state. Fewer channels are available in the open state, thus decreasing the effectiveness of the drugs that are open state blockers.
- Decrease in extracellular pH slows the rate of dissociation of Lidocaine from the sodium channel. A combination of acidosis and membrane depolarization increases the block produced by Lidocaine.
- Class 1C drugs are slow to unbind from the channel site and cause slowing of conduction, which may produce incessant tachycardia.
- Marked sinus bradycardia may be proarrhythmic for drugs with fast half time of recovery from the block because the channels are left unprotected for the major part of APD.

Slow sodium currents (inward)

- Agents that increase the slow component of sodium current (Diphenylmethyl-Piperanzinyl-Indole derivatives) are likely to increase inotropy by increasing the entry of Na during the plateau phase. This leads to an increase in intracellular calcium through sodium/calcium exchange. Increase in intracellular Ca may lead to EAD and PVC.
- Methanesulfonalide Ibutilide prolongs APD by increasing the slow sodium channel current.

- Lidocaine and other class 1B agents block the slow component of sodium current and decrease QT in patients with LQT3[5].
- Negative inotropy by sodium channel blockers may be due to blockage of the slow sodium channel current.
- Slowing of heart rate produced by class 1B agents is due to blocking of background sodium current that contributes to the phase 4 of pacemaker AP.
- β-Adrenergic stimulation reverses the effects of class I drugs.
- Proarrhythmia from class IC drugs develops during increased heart rate when sympathetic activity is enhanced. Beta blockers may reverse this phenomenon[5].
- Angiotensin II increases the frequency of reopening of the sodium channel and increases the Na current.

1.3 CALCIUM CHANNELS AND CURRENTS[14–17]

- The process of channel opening and closing is called gating.
- Open channels are active. Closed channels are inactive. Calcium and sodium channels open in response to depolarization and enter the nonconducting state during repolarization, a gating process known as inactivation.
- Alpha 1 subunit of the Ca channel contains the binding site for calcium channel blocking drugs.
- Calcium channels are very selective and allow Ca permeability 1000-fold faster.
- There are four types of calcium channels:
  - i L-type expressed on surface membrane.
  - ii T-type expressed on surface membrane.
  - iii Sarcoplasmic reticulum (SR) Ca release channel.
  - iv Inositol triphosphate (IP3) receptor channels are present on internal membrane.

L-type calcium channel (L = Large and lasting)
- It is a major source of Ca entry into the cell. It opens when depolarization reaches positive to −40 mV.
- It is responsible for excitation in sino atrial node (SAN) and atrio-ventricular node (AVN). It produces inward current that contributes to depolarization in SAN and AVN.
- It produces inward current responsible for plateau of AP.
- Increased calcium current prolongs depolarization and increases the height of the AP plateau.
- Calcium channel dependent inward current is responsible for EAD.
- I_{CaL} is responsible for excitation, contraction, and coupling. Blockade of these channels results in negative inotropic effects.
- In AF decrease activity of the I_{CaL} channel shortens APD and perpetuates arrhythmia (electrical remodeling).

Regulation of pacemaker and Ca currents

β-Adrenergic receptor stimulation
- It increases L-type calcium channel activity.
- This results in increased contractility, heart rate, and conduction velocity.
- Stimulation of receptors activates guanosine triphosphate binding protein Gs, which in turn stimulates adenylyl cyclase activity, thus increasing the cAMP level.
- β-Blockers have no direct effect on calcium channel.
- Sympathetic stimulation may also activate alpha1 receptors.

Parasympathetic stimulation
- It decreases L-type calcium activity through muscarinic and cholinergic receptors.
- Acetylcholine, through G protein, activates inwardly rectifying I_{Kach}, which makes MDP more negative and decreases the slope of diastolic depolarization. This results in slowing of the heart rate.
- Magnesium acts as an L-type calcium channel blocker.

T-type calcium channel
- These are found in cardiac and vascular smooth muscles, including coronary arteries.
    - i It opens at more negative potential.
    - ii It rapidly inactivates (Transient T).
    - iii It demonstrates slow deactivation.
    - iv Has low conductance (tiny T).
- It is found in high density in SAN and AVN.
- It does not contribute to AP upstroke which is dominated by sodium channel.
- It is implicated in cell growth.
- T-type Ca channel density is increased in the presence of the growth hormone, endothelin-1, and pressure overload.
- Failing myocytes also demonstrate increase density of T-type Ca channels.
- Drugs and compounds that block T-type Ca channels include the following:
    - i Amiloride
    - ii 3,4-Dichrobenzamil
    - iii Verapamil
    - iv Diltiazem
    - v Flunarizine
    - vi Tetradrine
    - vii Nickel
    - viii Cadmium
    - ix Mibefradil
- T-type Ca channel is up regulated by norepinephrine, alpha agonist (phenylephrine), extracellular ATP, and LVH.

Sarcoplasmic calcium release channels (also called Ryanodine receptors)

- These are intracellular channels that are regulated by calcium.
- These channels mediate the influx of calcium from SR into cytosol.
- It provides calcium for cardiac contraction. SR controls the cytoplasmic Ca level by release or uptake during systole and diastole, respectively.
- Calcium release from SR is triggered by increase in intracellular calcium, produced by L-type Ca channel. It is called calcium-induced calcium release (CICR).
- When a cell is calcium overloaded SR releases calcium spontaneously and asynchronously causing DAD (delayed after depolarization) seen in digitalis toxicity.
- Caffeine releases calcium from SR.
- Doxorubicin decreases cardiac contractility by depleting SR calcium.
- Magnesium and ATP potentiates channel flux.
- In ischemia decreased intracellular ATP decreases calcium release and causes ischemic contractile failure.
- Verapamil has no effect on sarcoplasmic Ca release channel (SCRC).
- SR also has potassium, sodium, and hydrogen channels.

Inositol triphosphate receptors (IP3)
- These receptors are found in smooth muscles and in specialized conduction tissue.
- These are up regulated by angiotensin II and α-adrenergic stimulation.
- Stimulation of myocytes angiotensin II receptor by angiotensin increases intracellular IP3.
- The arrhythmogenic effect of angiotensin II in CHF may be due to elevated IP3.
- These receptors have been implicated in apoptosis.

Tetrodotoxin (TTX) sensitive calcium channel
- It produces inward current. It is blocked by TTX.
- The channel that carries this current is permeable to both sodium and calcium.
- Elevated intracellular Na may activate reverse Na/Ca exchange, thus increasing the levels of intracellular Ca which may trigger SR calcium release.
- It may contribute to cardiac arrhythmias.

Sodium and calcium exchange
- Opening of voltage operated calcium channel, during the plateau phase of APD, increases the flux of calcium into cytoplasm. This causes CICR from SR.
- During diastole calcium is removed from the cell by sodium/calcium exchange located in the cell membrane.
- Lowering of pH blocks sodium/calcium exchange.

- SR calcium ATPases, Sarcolemmal calcium ATPases and sodium/calcium exchange decrease cytoplasmic calcium from elevated systolic level to baseline diastolic level by pumping Ca back into SR or by extruding Ca out of the cell.
- During calcium removal inwardly directed current is observed, which may cause DAD.
- DAD occurs when there is pathologically high calcium load either due to digitalis toxicity or following reperfusion.
- Na/Ca exchange is able to transport calcium bi-directionally. Reverse mode will increase intracellular calcium, which may trigger SR calcium release.

Effect of antiarrhythmic drugs on calcium channel
- Most Na and K channel blocking drugs also affect Ca channels.
- Quinidine, Disopyramide, Lidocaine, Mexiletine, Diphenylhydantoin, Flecainide, Propafenone, Moricizine, and Azimilide suppress L-type calcium current.
- Amiodarone blocks both L and T-type Ca currents.
- Sotalol has no effect on Ca channel.
- Digoxin inhibits sodium/potassium ATPases. This inhibition results in an increase in intracellular Na, which in turn leads to an increase in intracellular Ca through Na/Ca exchange.
- Verapamil blocks Ca current and decreases calcium activated chloride current.

References

1 Delisle BP. Anson BD. Rajamani S. January CT. Biology of cardiac arrhythmias: ion channel protein trafficking. *Circ Res.* 94:1418–28, 2004.
2 Rosati B. McKinnon D. Regulation of ion channel expression. *Circ Res.* 94:874–83, 2004.
3 Priori SG. Inherited arrhythmogenic diseases: The complexity beyond monogenic disorders.*Circ Res.* 94:140–5, 2004.
4 Enkvetchakul D. Nichols CG. Gating mechanism of KATP channels: Function fits form. [Review] [100 refs] *J Gen Physiol.* 122:471–80, 2003.
5 Sah R. Ramirez RJ. Oudit GY. Gidrewicz D. Trivieri MG. Zobel C. Backx PH. Regulation of cardiac excitation–contraction coupling by action potential repolarization: Role of the transient outward potassium current (*I*to). *J Physiol.* 546(Pt1):5–18, 2003.
6 Kass RS. Moss AJ. Long QT syndrome: Novel insights into the mechanisms of cardiac arrhythmias. *J Clin Invest.* 112:810–5, 2003.
7 Gross GJ. Peart JN. KATP channels and myocardial preconditioning: An update. *Am J Physiol Heart Circ Physiol.* 285:H921–30, 2003.
8 Clancy CE. Kass RS. Defective cardiac ion channels: From mutations to clinical syndromes. *J Clin Invest.* 110:1075–7, 2002.
9 Hubner CA. Jentsch TJ. Ion channel diseases. *Hum Mol Genet.* 11: 2435–45, 2002.
10 Schram G. Pourrier M. Melnyk P. Nattel S. Differential distribution of cardiac ion channel expression as a basis for regional specialization in electrical function. *Circ Res.* 90:939–50, 2002.
11 Clancy CE. Kass RS. Defective cardiac ion channels: From mutations to clinical syndromes. *J Clin Invest.* 110:1075–7, 2002.

12 Towbin JA. Friedman RA. Provocation testing in inherited arrhythmia disorders: Can we be more specific? *Heart Rhythm.* 2:147–8, 2005.

13 Fish JM. Antzelevitch C. Role of sodium and calcium channel block in unmasking the Brugada syndrome. *Heart Rhythm.* 1:210–17, 2004.

14 Dolphin AC. G protein modulation of voltage-gated calcium channels. *Pharmacol Rev.* 55:607–27, 2003.

15 Yamakage M. Namiki A. Calcium channels – basic aspects of their structure, function and gene encoding; anesthetic action on the channels – a review. *Can J Anaesth.* 49:151–64, 2002.

16 Marks, AR. Cardiac intracellular calcium release channels: Role in heart failure. *Circ Res.* 87:8–11, 2000.

17 Grossman E. Calcium antagonists. *Prog Cardiovasc Dis.* 47:34–57, 2004.

2 Electrophysiologic Effects of Cardiac Autonomic Activity

Self-Assessment Questions

1 Which one of the following is the likely cardiac manifestation of β_3 receptor stimulation?
   A Increase in contractility
   B Decrease in contractility
   C Decrease in heart rate
   D Increase in heart rate

2 Which one of the following muscarinic receptors is predominantly found in the heart?
   A M_1
   B M_2
   C M_3
   D M_4

3 What is the likely cardiac effect of muscarinic receptor stimulation by acetylcholine?
   A Coronary vasoconstriction
   B Positive chronotropic response
   C Enhanced inotropic response
   D Negative dromotropic effect

4 Which one of the following is likely to occur with cardiac adenosine receptors stimulation?
   A Negative chronotropic effect
   B Positive dromotropic effect
   C Enhanced contractility
   D Coronary vasoconstriction

5 Which one of the following currents is activated by purinergic agonists?

   A $K_{Ach,Ado}$
   B I_{Na}
   C I_{CL}
   D $I_{Ca(T)}$

6 Which of the following effects is due to adenosine?

   A Increase in Ca current
   B Decrease in atrial APD and refractory period
   C Stimulation of P_2 receptors
   D Decrease in I_{Katp} current

7 Which of the following electrophysiologic effects is least likely to occur with vagal denervation of the atrium?

   A Increases atrial APD and ERP
   B Abolishes sinus arrhythmia
   C Decreases heart rate variability and baroreflex sensitivity
   D Decreases the ventricular effective refractory period

8 Which one of the following observations may suggest that in the treatment of CHF nonselective β blockers are likely to be superior to selective β blockers?

   A $\beta 1$ receptors are up regulated
   B $\beta 2$ and $\beta 3$ receptors are up regulated
   C Peripheral vascular resistance is increased
   D Glomerular filtration rate is decreased

2.1 ADRENERGIC RECEPTORS[1-4]

The human adrenergic receptor family consists of nine subtypes originating from different genes: α1A, α1B, α1D, α2A, α2B, α2C, β1, β2, and β3.

β-adrenergic receptors

- β_1 is a predominant adrenergic receptor in the myocardium. 75% of the total β receptor population is β_1.
- β_1 stimulation causes positive inotropic, chronotropic, and lusitropic (relaxation) response. cAMP-dependent activation of protein kinase A (PKA) phosphorylates and activates β-adrenergic receptor.
- Even in the presence of continuing β stimulation cAMP response wanes. This phenomenon is called receptor desensitization. Persistent agonist stimulation decreases the total number of receptors (receptor down regulation).
- In ageing heart, β_1 receptor is down regulated and β_2 becomes dominant.
- In congestive heart failure (CHF) sustained adrenergic stimulation leads to desensitization and down regulation of β_1 receptors. β_2 receptor expression is preserved. α1 receptor subtypes remain constant or may even be up-regulated. Under these conditions β_2 and α1 stimulation results in atrial and ventricular arrhythmias.
- This supports the notion that nonselective β blockers reduce cardiac mortality in post-myocardial infarction (MI) and CHF patients.
- In general, the type-2 adrenergic receptors (α2 and β2) are found at the pre-junctional site in the central and peripheral sympathetic nervous system, where activation of α2 receptors inhibits and activation of β2 receptors enhances norepinephrine release (Table 2.1).
- Presynaptically localized α2A-receptor and α2C-receptor subtypes are important in decreasing sympathetic activity in the central nervous system as well as in decreasing the norepinephrine release in cardiac sympathetic nerve terminals.
- β_2 receptor is up regulated in denervated, transplanted heart.
- Stimulation of the β_2 receptors of sino atrial node (SAN) results in sinus tachycardia.
- β_2 receptor stimulation elevates intracellular pH, which increases responsiveness to calcium.
- β-Adrenergic stimulation increases I_K.
- In cardiomyocytes, endothelial or smooth muscle cells, the type-2 adrenergic receptors are also present postsynaptically together with α1, β1, and β3 receptors.
- Acute changes in myocardial function are exclusively governed by the β receptors.
- α1-Receptor contribution is negligible in humans under normal conditions.

Table 2.1 Characteristics of the subtypes of adrenergic receptors

Receptor	Agonist	Antagonist	Tissue	Responses
α_1	Epi > NE ≫ Iso phenylephrine	Prazocin	Heart	↑Contractility, arrhythmias
		Intestinal SM	Relaxation	
			Urinary and vascular SM	Contraction
			Liver	Glycogenolysis Gluconeogenesis
α_2	Epi > NE ≫ Iso, clonidine	Yohimbine	Pancreatic β cells	↓Insulin Aggregation
			Platelets	↓NE
			Nerve terminal	Contraction
			Vascular SM	
β_1	Iso > Epi = NE, dobutamine	Metoprolol	Heart	↑Inotropy, chronotropy and AV conduction
			Juxtaglomerular	↑Renin
β_2	Iso > Epi ≫ NE terbutaline	Propranolol	Heart	↑Inotropy Automaticity Arrhythmias
			Vascular GI GU bronchial SM	Relaxation
			Skeletal muscle	Glycogenolysis K uptake
			Liver	Glycogenolysis
β_3	Iso = NE > Epi		Adipose tissue	Lipolysis
			Heart	↓Contractility

Epi, epinephrine; NE, norepinephrine; Iso, isoproterenol; SM, smooth muscle; GI, gastrointestinal; GU, genitourinary; ↑, increased release; ↓, decreased release.

- Although all three types of $\alpha1$ receptors are expressed in the heart, the $\alpha1A$ is the dominant subtype.
- No direct $\alpha2$-receptor mediated effects are discernible on the myocardium.
- $\alpha1$-Adrenergic receptor stimulation induces growth.

$\beta3$ receptors

- $\beta3$ receptor is an important regulator of adipose tissue and gastrointestinal tract. It is also present in human heart and is implicated as an inhibitor of cardiac contractile function. In normal heart $\beta3$-adrenoceptors protects myocardium from the deleterious effects of excess catecholamines that may occur in hyperadrenergic states including heart failure.

- The negative inotropic effects of $\beta 3$-adrenoceptors are mediated through activation of constitutively expressed endothelial nitric oxide synthase. This action opposes the positive inotropic effects of catecholamines on $\beta 1$- and $\beta 2$-receptors, which are mediated via cyclic adenosine monophosphate (cAMP).
- Whereas $\beta 3$ receptor activation may protect against cardiac myocyte damage due to catecholamine excess during the early stage of heart failure, $\beta 3$-adrenoceptor up-regulation may contribute to decrease contractility in the later phases of disease.
- $\beta 3$-adrenoceptors are desensitization-resistant and their action may exceed that of impaired, down-regulated or desensitized $\beta 1$- and $\beta 2$-adrenoceptors. This may result in depression of contractility and exacerbation of heart failure.
- This supports the observation that non selective beta blockers reduce cardiac mortality in post MI and CHF patients.

2.2 CHOLINERGIC RECEPTORS[5,6]

- Cholinergic receptors are nicotinic or muscarinic depending on their ability to interact with nicotine or muscarine.
- Cholinergic receptors are activated by acetylcholine (Ach) from parasympathetic nerve terminals.
- The effects of Ach that are mimicked by muscarine and blocked by atropine are called muscarinic effects. Other effects of Ach that are mimicked by nicotine and are not antagonized by atropine but are blocked by tubocurarine are labeled as nicotinic effects.
- Cardiac action of Ach is mediated by muscarinic cholinergic receptors.
- Five types of (M1–M5) muscarinic receptors have been identified.
- M1 and M3 receptors cause mobilization of intracellular Ca by activating phospholipase C. M2 and M4 receptors inhibit adenylyl cyclase and enhance K conductance through K channels.
- M1 receptor is found in autonomic ganglion and central nervous system.
- M2 is a dominant muscarinic receptor of cardiac myocytes.
- M3 is a predominant receptor in smooth muscle cells, where its stimulation causes contraction, and in secretory glands.
- Inhibitory effects of Ach on calcium current and contractility are due to M2 receptors and can be blocked by M2 antagonist.
- ACh is hydrolyzed by acetylcholinestrase. Cardiac effects of ACh are characterized by vasodilatation, negative chronotropic effect, negative dromotropic effect [decrease in conduction in SAN and atrio-ventricular node (AVN)], and negative inotropic effect.
- Commonly used synthetic choline derivatives are Methacholine, Carbachol, and Bethanechol.

- Muscarine, pilocarpine, and arecholine are naturally occurring alkaloids with pharmacological properties similar to Ach.
- Atropine and scopolamine are naturally occurring alkaloids that act as muscarinic receptor antagonist.

2.3 PURINERGIC RECEPTORS[1,7]

- Autonomic nonadrenergic and noncholinergic nerves were suggested to contain ATP.
- Nerves utilizing ATP as their principal transmitter were named "purinergic" based on the actions of purine nucleotides and nucleosides in a wide variety of tissues; P1- and P2-receptor classification was proposed.

Purinergic receptors

- There are two types of purinergic receptors, P1–P2.
- P1 is activated by adenosine.
- P2 is activated by extracellular ATP.
- Two types of P2 receptors have been identified. P2X are ion channels, while P2Y are G protein coupled receptor.
- P1 purinoceptors are much more sensitive to adenosine and AMP than to ADP and ATP. The reverse is true for P2 purinoceptors.
- P2 receptors are unaffected by Methylxanthines such as caffeine and theophylline that selectively and completely inhibits the P1 purinoceptors.
- Subclasses of P1 adenosine receptors were introduced when their stimulation was shown to inhibit (A1 subtype) or activate (A2 subtype) adenylyl cyclase activity.

Adenosine

- There are four subtypes of adenosine (P1 purinergic) receptors: A_1, A_2A, A_2B, and A_3. All four are expressed in the heart.
- A_1 and A_2 receptors are antagonized by xanthines.
- Electrophysiologic actions of adenosine on the heart are mediated by A_1 receptors. Blockade of this receptor abolishes negative chronotropic, dromotropic, inotropic and anti-β-adrenergic effects of adenosine.
- A_1 receptors inhibit adenylyl cyclase and activate K current and phospholipase C.
- A_2 receptors activate adenylyl cyclase.
- A_2A receptors are present in vascular endothelium and smooth muscles of coronary arteries and cause adenosine induced coronary vasodilatation.
- Effects of extracellular ATP, before its degradation to adenosine, are mediated by P_2 purinergic receptors.

- Stimulation of muscarinic and adenosine receptors causes activation of inhibitory guanine (G) proteins. This leads to production of cAMP mediated activation of I_{CaL}, I_K, and I_{CL}.
- Density of A_1 adenosine and M_2 muscarinic cholinergic receptor is greater in the atrium.

Acetylcholine and adenosine sensitive potassium currents

- Cholinergic and purinergic agonists activate inwardly rectifying potassium currents $I_{KAch,Ado}$.
- Inwardly rectifying means it is easier for the current to flow inwards than outwards through $I_{KAch,Ado}$ channels. Inward rectification is attributed to voltage dependent block of potassium channels by intracellular Mg and polyamines (Spermine and Spermidine).
- These currents are also activated by extracellular ATP, arachidonic acid (Prostacycline), somatostatin, and sphingosine 1 phosphate.
- Lipooxygenase potentiates and cyclooxygenase inhibits $I_{KAch,Ado}$.
- Hyperpolarizing current (I_f) is an inward current and is responsible for diastolic depolarization of SAN. This is a time-dependent, nonspecific cation current.
- Ach and adenosine inhibit I_f. This effect is due to inhibition of adenylate cyclase.
- Adenosine has no effect on ventricular AP of myocytes.
- In the SAN and AVN adenosine and Ach cause hyperpolarization and reduce the rate of diastolic depolarization. These actions result in slowing of the heart rate (negative chronotropy) and delay in AVN conduction (negative dromotropy).
- Adenosine's effects occur at the atrial-His and nodal region, it has no effect on the nodal-His bundle region (NH) of the AVN.
- Ach and adenosine decrease atrial action potential duration (APD) and contractile force (in the absence of β-adrenergic stimulation) due to activation of $I_{KAch,Ado}$ and inhibition of I_{CaL}.
- Adenosine and Ach attenuate β-adrenergic stimulated I_{CaL} in ventricular and atrial myocytes and inhibit transient inward current and delayed after depolarization (DAD). Adenosine may be effective in catecholamine sensitive ventricular tachycardia by abolishing cAMP-dependent triggered activity.
- Ach and adenosine decrease atrial action potential duration (APD) and effective refractory period (ERP) and facilitate induction of atrial fibrillation (AF).
- During AV nodal ischemia local production of adenosine may be responsible for bradycardia seen in patients with inferior wall MI.
- Extracellular ATP causes DAD, and early after depolarization by stimulating P_2 receptors and inducing I_{CaL} (Table 2.2).

Cardiac autonomic innervations[1]

- Vagal postganglionic neurons to sinus node are located in the left pulmonary vein left atrial junction, and neurons to AVN are found in the IVC-LA fat pad.

Table 2.2 Effect of Ach, adenosine, and extracellular
ATP on cardiac currents

	Ach	Adenosine	ATP
Receptor	M_2	A_1	P_2
$I_{KAch,Ado}$	↑	↑	↑
I_K	No effect	No effect	↑
I_{KATP}	↑	↑	↑
I_{CaL}	↓	↓	↑In atria ↓ in V
I_{Na}	No effect	No effect	Variable
I_f	↓	↓	No effect
I_{CL}	No effect	↓ I_f stimulated	↑

↑,increase; ↓, decrease; V, ventricle.

- SVC/aorta fat pad innervates both atria.
- Vagal denervation of atria prevents induction of acute AF, abolishes sinus arrhythmias, decreases heart rate variability, and eliminates baroreflex sensitivity without affecting vagal innervation to the ventricle.
- Efferent vagal fibers to ventricle do not travel through three epicardial fat pads.
- Changes in sinus node function may not reflect changes at the ventricular level.
- Sympathetic efferent fibers are epicardial along coronary arteries, and parasympathetic efferent fibers are subendocardial in the ventricle.
- Block of nitric oxide synthase attenuates cholinergic action and increases calcium current. L-Arginine reverses these effects.
- L-Arginine also reduces the effects of sympathetic stimulation such as shortening of ERP and induction of ventricular arrhythmias.
- Vagal stimulation facilitates AF.
- Decrease in refractory period may be due to activation of sodium/hydrogen exchanger induced by atrial ischemia during AF.
- After MI there is regional sympathetic denervation which results in post-denervation supersensitivity to circulating catecholamines and predisposes to ventricular arrhythmias.
- Beneficial effects of β blockers in reducing the incidence of sudden cardiac death in post-MI patients are due to reduction in the heart rate and other anti-sympathetic activities.
- Initial sympathetic stimulation and subsequent withdrawal resulting in hypotension and bradycardia may be responsible for neurocardiogenic syncope.
- Pure I_{Kr} blockers may not reduce sudden death (SWORD and DIAMOND) because sympathetic stimulation may activate I_{Ks} and I_K.
- I_{Ks} blockers prolong APD and refractoriness; however, this effect is lost with sympathetic stimulation.
- Alpha blocking agents have no antifibrillatory effects.

- In post-MI patients LCSD confers the same survival benefit as β blockers (3% mortality). This provides an alternative to patients who cannot take β blockers.
- Vagal stimulation decreases the heart rate and lethal arrhythmia during ischemia. These effects are reversed by atropine.
- Muscarinic agonists such as Morphine, Methacholine, and Oxotremorine reduce ischemic ventricular arrhythmias.
- Exercise training increases parasympathetic tone, increases heart rate variability (HRV), baroreflex sensitivity and decreases the density of β-adrenergic receptor. In HRV low frequency component reflects sympathetic and high frequency component reflects vagal activity.

References

1 Kirstein SL. Insel PA. Autonomic nervous system pharmacogenomics: A progress report. *Pharmacol Rev.* 56 (1): 31–52, 2004.
2 Taylor MR. Bristow MR. The emerging pharmacogenomics of the beta-adrenergic receptors. *Congest Heart Fail.* 10 (6): 281–8, 2004.
3 Reiter MJ. Cardiovascular drug class specificity: Beta-blockers. *Prog Cardiovasc Dis.* 47 (1): 11–33, 2004.
4 Metra M. Nodari S. Dei Cas L. Beta-blockade in heart failure: Selective versus nonselective agents. *Am J Cardiovasc Drugs.* 1: 3–14, 2001.
5 Harvey RD. Belevych AE. <http://ezproxy.ttuhsc.edu:2524/entrez/query.fcgi?cmd=Retrieve&db=pubmed&dopt=Abstract&list_uids=12871825> Muscarinic regulation of cardiac ion channels. *Br J Pharmacol.* 139: 1074–84, 2003.
6 Brodde OE. Bruck H. Leineweber K. Seyfarth T. <http://ezproxy.ttuhsc.edu:2524/entrez/query.fcgi?cmd=Retrieve&db=pubmed&dopt=Abstract&list_uids=11770070> Presence, distribution and physiological function of adrenergic and muscarinic receptor subtypes in the human heart. *Basic Res Cardiol.* 96: 528–38, 2001.
7 Vassort G. Adenosine 5-Triphosphate: A P2-purinergic agonist in the myocardium. *Physiological reviews.* 2: 81, 2001.

3 Mechanisms of Arrhythmias

Self-Assessment Questions

1 Which one of the following statements about the Osborn wave is incorrect?
   A It is due to transmural voltage gradient
   B It may occur in hypothermia
   C It may be seen in hypercalcemia
   D It is a manifestation of intracranial bleed

2 Which of the following statements about DAD is incorrect?
   A It is caused by inward currents produced by Ca overload
   B Most common cause of DAD is Digoxin
   C Occurs during phase 2 of APD
   D Lidocaine may decrease the tendency for DAD

3 Which of the following statements about EAD is correct?
   A Occurs after the completion of the AP
   B Occurs during tachycardia
   C It is caused by reactivation of the I_{CaL} during the plateau phase
   D It is caused by Na channel blockers

4 Which of the following statements about reentry is correct?
   A It occurs when there is prolongation of phase 2 of AP
   B It is caused by spontaneous depolarization during phase 4
   C It is a result of sarcoplasmic reticulum Ca overload
   D It requires an area of slow conduction and unidirectional block

Conduction and block

Electrophysiology of action potential (AP)

- Normal APD is 180 milliseconds.
- Maximum negative membrane potential is defined as a resting potential.
- I_k repolarizes the membrane to the resting potential.
- When the membrane potential reaches the threshold level it results in the onset of AP. When the threshold stimulus excites the cell, I_{Na} depolarizes the membrane at 382 V/s. This produces phase 0 of AP. Phase 1 of AP is a result of early repolarization produced by I_{to}. Plateau phase is phase 2 of AP.
- I_{CaL} (inward current) supports AP plateau against repolarizing (outward current) I_k. I_{CaL} triggers calcium release from sarcoplasmic reticulum (SR) through calcium induced calcium release (CICR).
- $I_{Na/Ca}$ pump, during repolarization, extrudes calcium. It takes in three sodium ions for each calcium ion that is removed. This causes significant inward current, which slows repolarization and prolongs APD.
- I_{Kr} increases during the early phase of AP. Its level of activity is low due to instantaneous inward rectification. I_{Kr} is potassium selective.
- I_{Ks} attains a large magnitude during a plateau. It is a major repolarizing current.
- The end of the plateau phase heralds the beginning of phase 3 of AP. During this phase depolarizing Ca and Na currents decline and K currents enhance repolarization. The end of phase 3 occurs when the resting potential is reached.
- Cells capable of producing spontaneous depolarization initiate phase 4 of AP.

Depolarizing and repolarizing currents

- Inward movement of positive ions depolarizes the cell by increasing the positive charge on the inner surface of the cell membrane as compared with the outer surface of the membrane. Outward movement of positive ions repolarizes the cell membrane by making the inner surface more negative than the outer surface.
- Potassium currents are outward currents.
- During the plateau phase of AP current flow activity is reduced. It separates phase 2 from phase 3 of AP.
- The length of the plateau phase of the AP determines the strength and duration of cardiac contraction and produces a cardioprotective window during which reexcitation by sodium and calcium channel cannot occur.
- A small net current is needed to maintain the plateau and a small change in the current markedly influences the time course of the plateau.
- Repolarization begins when the net current flow becomes outward either by an increase in outward or by a decrease in inward currents.

Supernormal conduction

- During a recovery phase of APD supernormal conduction may exist when a subthreshold stimulus may evoke a response. The same stimulus may fail to produce a response before or after the supernormal conduction period.

- An Impulse arriving during supernormal excitability conducts better than expected or conducts when the block was expected. It is not faster than normal.
- Supernormal conduction depends on supernormal excitability and exists only in Purkinje fibers, not in His bundle or myocardium. It may be noted in the presence of a complete AV block.
- Supernormal conduction is recorded in diseased cardiac tissue.
- Improved AV conduction (not supernormal conduction) may be due to gap phenomenon, peeling of refractory period and dual AV nodal physiology.
- The period of supernormal excitability correlates with the end of the T wave and the beginning of diastole.
- Supernormal conduction may manifest as unexpected normalization of bundle branch block at a shorter RR interval.
- The PR interval remains unchanged or is shorter, thereby excluding equal delay in both bundles as a cause of normalization of the QRS.
- In the presence of acceleration dependent aberration during atrial fibrillation (AF) or sinus rhythm with premature atrial contractions (PACs), supernormal conduction may manifest as normalization of QRS.
- Atrial impulse may propagate during a supernormal period and result in displacement of the subsidiary pacemaker due to concealed conduction.
- The duration of the preceding cycle length (CL) determines the location of supernormal conduction. Longer CL shifts the supernormal period to the right.
- During AV block a sinus impulse may conduct or an electronic pacemaker may capture during the period of supernormal excitability.

Concealed conduction

- It is characterized by unexpected behavior of a subsequent impulse in response to incomplete conduction of a preceding electrical impulse. Its diagnosis is made by deductive analysis and exclusion of the other conduction abnormalities such as block of conduction.
- A concealed impulse may become intermittently manifest in other parts of the same tracing.
- ECG reflects conduction and electrophysiologic properties of the myocardium.
- Propagation of an impulse through specialized conduction tissue is not recorded on a surface electrocardiogram but can be inferred.
- Concealment is commonly encountered at the level of AVN or bundle branches.

Exit block

- It is commonly seen in sino atrial, junctional, and ventricular pacemaker.
- A repetitive pattern or group beating of type I or II periodicity is suggestive of exit block.
- **Type I** exit block presents with gradual shortening of PP or RR interval and failure to record P or R resulting in a pause that is less than the sum of two basic CLs. This is typical of Wenckebach periodicity.
- Atypical Wenckebach delay may resemble sinus arrhythmia.

- **Type II** exit block is characterized by a pause that is a multiple of basic CL.
- In a parasystole, failure of the impulse to manifest may be due to an exit block or physiologic refractoriness.
- If a tachycardia presents with two different CLs in which short CL is longer than basic CL and long CL is less than the sum of two basic CL and the sum of short and long CL equals three basic CL then 3 : 2 type I exit block is present.

Gap junction

- Gap junctions are for intercellular transfer of current. Connexion 43 (CX43) is a major gap junction protein. It is found in human atrium and ventricles.
- A 50% reduction in CX43 produces a marked slowing of conduction velocity.
- These are located at or near the ends of working atrial and ventricular myocytes where intercalated discs connect adjacent cells.
- Longitudinal conduction velocity in myocardium is 0.7 m/s and transverse velocity of 0.2 m/s. This produces the substrate for anisotropic conduction.
- In crista terminalis the ratio of longitudinal to transverse conduction is 10 : 1.
- Slow conduction in the SA and AV nodes is due to small and sparsely distributed gap junctions.
- Gap junctions in Purkinje tissue facilitate rapid conduction.
- CX40 is a major conductor of intercellular currents in atrium. CX43 is a major conductor of intercellular currents in ventricle.

Continuous and discontinuous conduction

- The difference between the electrical potential of excited and nonexcited tissue produces a flow of current.
- As the current flows through the cell membrane it shifts membrane potential to threshold potential by activating sodium and calcium currents.
- During normal propagation, sodium (inward) current provides the charge for membrane depolarization except in atrio-ventricular node (AVN) and sino atrial node (SAN).
- Delay in propagation may occur in the gap junction. Calcium inward current is essential for allowing the current to pass through the cell junction.
- Atrial trabeculation may contribute to conduction discontinuities.
- In ventricle connective tissue, hypertrophy, a scar from myocardial infarction (MI) may add to discontinuities.
- Impedance of a scar is lower than that of normal myocardium.
- Capillaries may contribute to anisotropic conduction.

Electrical heterogeneity

- AP of ventricular epicardium and M cells shows a prominent notch due to I_{to} mediated phase 1.
- Absence of a notch in endocardium correlates with weaker I_{to}.
- Spike and dome morphology of AP is absent in the neonate. Its gradual appearance correlates with the appearance of I_{to}.
- I_{to2} is a calcium activated chloride current.

- The magnitude of I_{to} and spike and dome in right ventricular epicardium is more prominent than left ventricular epicardium.

I_{to} and J wave

- Transmural voltage gradient between epicardium and endocardium due to I_{to} results in J wave (Osborn wave).
- Prominent J waves may occur in the presence of hypothermia and hypercalcemia.
- Occurrence of elevated J point may be due to transmural gradient and dispersion of early repolarization.

Automaticity

- Automaticity occurs due to spontaneous diastolic depolarization as a result of inward Na currents or due to decay of outward K currents during phase 4 of AP.
- Normal automaticity occurs during physiologic conditions utilizing the currents that are normally involved in impulse generation. It is present in SA node, some atrial tissue such as crista terminalis and Bachmann's bundle, AV node and His Purkinje fibers.
- Ionic currents which are normally not involved in pacemaker current may produce these currents in the presence of disease state and cause abnormal automaticity and induce arrhythmias.
- The rate of impulse formation in the pacemaker cell depends on resting potential, slope of diastolic depolarization and threshold (take-off) potential.
- Norepinephrine accelerates spontaneous depolarization of SAN by stimulating β_1 receptors. Acetylcholine (Ach) slows spontaneous depolarization via muscarinic receptors.
- Increase in adenylyl cyclase and cyclic adenosine monophosphate (cAMP) and I_f current activity accelerates and decrease in the activity slows the sinus rate.
- Ach slows the sinus rate by opening I_{KAch}. This results in more negative maximum diastolic potential (MDP).
- Ventricular myocytes also have pacemaker current (I_f). β Stimulation increases pacemaker current in Purkinje fiber. Ach reverses the effects of β stimulation by reducing cAMP generated by β stimulation; it has no direct effect on pacemaker current.
- Pacemaker cell depolarization is inhibited when it is driven faster than its intrinsic rate (overdrive suppression). This is mediated by sodium/potassium exchange pump and possible inactivation of I_{CaL} current.
- Atrial and ventricular myocytes do not have spontaneous diastolic depolarization.
- When membrane potential is depolarized to less than $-60\,\text{mV}$ spontaneous depolarization may occur (abnormal automaticity). This is mediated by slow inward calcium current.
- Decrease in membrane potential may be due to ischemia.
- Extracellular Na and Ca may affect abnormal automaticity.
- Overdrive suppression is less likely to affect abnormal automaticity.

Pacemaker channels

- Pacemaker channels are dominant in SAN and subsidiary pacemakers.
- Subsidiary pacemakers are located in AVN and His purkinje system (HPS).
- Cells from SAN demonstrate steeper diastolic depolarization and therefore reach the threshold earlier than subsidiary pacemakers. This may cause overdrive suppression of subsidiary cells.
- Diastolic depolarization is caused by activating inward currents or by deactivating outward currents. At least one of these currents is time dependent.
- Delayed rectifier (I_K I_{Kr} I_{Ks}) and I_f are present in SAN.
- I_f is a hyperpolarizing current. Its conductance is increased by extracellular hyperkalemia.
- L- and T-type calcium currents are also present in pacemaker cells.
- Inward rectifying I_{K1} is present in purkinje cells but not in SAN. This current increases with elevated extracellular potassium. This may contribute to suppression of pacemaker activity in HPS during hyperkalemia.
- Decay of I_K appears to facilitate pacemaker current.

Autonomic regulation of pacemaker currents

- β Agonist stimulates G protein through the β receptors located on the cell membrane. This increases the level of cAMP and promotes phosphorylation of I_{CaL}, I_f, I_K, and $I_{Na/K}$ pump through protein kinase A. These actions promote increase in heart rate as a result of increase in MDP and increase in the slope of diastolic depolarization.
- Parasympathetic agonist Ach activates muscarinic receptors.
- Ach, through G protein, activates inwardly rectifying I_{KAch}, which makes MDP more negative and decreases the slope of diastolic depolarization. This results in slowing of the heart rate.

Triggered activity[1,2]

- Triggered activity is initiated by after-depolarization. There are two types of after-depolarizations, early and delayed.
- Early after-depolarization (EAD) occurs before and delayed after depolarization (DAD) occurs after the completion of AP repolarization.

Delayed after-depolarization

- DAD occurs after repolarization of AP. It is caused by inward currents produced by an increase in the intracellular Ca load.
- DADs are associated with fast heart rate and Ca overload.
- Increase in the level of catecholamines and cAMP enhances Ca uptake and causes DAD in atrial and ventricular myocytes.
- Catecholamines increase sarcolemmal calcium by stimulating sodium/calcium exchange.

- The most common cause of DAD is Digoxin. It inhibits the sodium/potassium pump and leads to an increase in intracellular calcium.
- Increase in the extracellular ATP levels potentiates the DAD effect of catecholamines.
- Withdrawal of cholinergic stimulation increases calcium in atrial myocytes and may cause DAD.
- Longer APD favors DAD. Longer CL allows for more calcium entry into cells. The amplitude of the DAD depends on CL.
- Quinidine may increase DAD by prolonging APD. Lidocaine shortens APD and thus decreases DAD.

Sodium and calcium exchange and DAD
- Opening of voltage-operated calcium channels, during the plateau phase of APD, increases the flux of calcium into cytoplasm. This causes CICR from SR.
- During diastole calcium is removed from the cell by the sodium/calcium exchange pump, located in the cell membrane.
- Lowering of pH blocks sodium/calcium exchange.
- SR calcium ATPase, Sarcolemmal calcium ATPase, and sodium/calcium exchange decrease cytoplasmic calcium from the elevated systolic level to the baseline diastolic level by pumping Ca back into SR or by extruding Ca out of the cell.
- During calcium removal, inwardly directed current $I_{Na/Ca}$ is observed, which may cause DAD.
- DAD occurs when there is a pathologically high calcium load either due to digitalis toxicity or fallowing reperfusion.
- Na/Ca exchange is able to transport calcium bi-directionally. Reverse mode will increase intracellular calcium, which may trigger SR calcium release.
- DAD is induced by a spontaneous release of calcium from the overloaded SR, which in turn activates the Na/Ca exchanger to extrude Ca from the cell. This generates, because of the $3:1$ ratio of Na/Ca exchange, a large inward current that causes depolarization and DAD. I_{CaL} does not participate in DAD.

Early after-depolarizations

Phase 2 EAD
- EAD occurs when a large inward current during the plateau phase occurs, resulting in prolongation of plateau. This provides time for reactivation of I_{CaL}. It is this second phase of reactivation of inward I_{CaL} that produces EAD by depolarizing the membrane.
- EAD does not require a spontaneous release of calcium from SR and does not require inward activation of $I_{Na/Ca}$.
- I_{CaL} is a primary depolarizing factor responsible for EAD.
- The delicate balance between depolarizing and repolarizing currents controls the plateau phase of the AP. An increase in the inward current and/or a decrease in

the outward current may induce EADs. Examples include persistent inward I_{Na} in LQT3 and reduced I_{Kr} and I_{Ks} in LQT2 and LQT1, respectively.
- Once the plateau is prolonged, reactivation of I_{CaL} induces EAD. This mechanism applies to phase 2 (plateau) EAD.
- EAD occurs in Purkinje fibers and M cells of the myocardium.
- Other conditions that can cause EAD are bradycardia, which reduces the outward current caused by delayed rectifier I_K, hypokalemia, and increase in calcium current induced by sympathetic stimulation in the presence of ischemia or injury.
- Pharmacological agents such as potassium channel blockers (Quinidine, Sotalol), in the presence of hypokalemia and bradycardia prolong repolarization and induce EAD.
- I_{Kr} blockers such as Erythromycin, Piperidine derivatives that block histamine H_1 receptors such as Astemizole and Terfenadine, and Cisapride increase APD and cause EAD.
- Magnesium, Flunarizine, and Ryanodine can abolish EAD by decreasing the intracellular calcium load.
- EAD caused by inward sodium current are abolished by sodium channel blocker Mexiletine.

Phase 3 EAD
- These occur during fast repolarization and share the mechanism of DAD (spontaneous Ca release from SR and activation of the $I_{Na/Ca}$). They are called EAD because they occur before the completion of AP repolarization (Fig. 3.1).
- EAD may occur during the plateau phase and are caused by L-type Ca current. EAD that occur during phase 3 of APD are due to the Na/Ca exchange current.

Torsades De Pointes (TDP)
- TDP is a polymorphic ventricular tachycardia (VT) associated with long QT syndrome (LQTS).
- Quinidine and hypokalemia produce EAD and triggered activity resulting in TDP. Initial event in TDP is EAD-induced triggered activity.
- TDP often follows short long short CL.

Excitability and conduction
- Excitability is dependent on the availability of sodium channels; thus reduced Na channel activity will reduce excitability and conduction velocity.
- Reduced membrane excitability and reduced gap junction coupling slows conduction, which may predispose to reentrant arrhythmias.
- Reduced gap junction coupling also slows conduction velocity, which may allow I_{CaL} to induce inward depolarizing currents.
- I_{CaL} plays a dominant role in maintaining conduction in the setting of reduced coupling. While I_{Na} controls excitability, I_{CaL} influences conduction during reduced coupling.

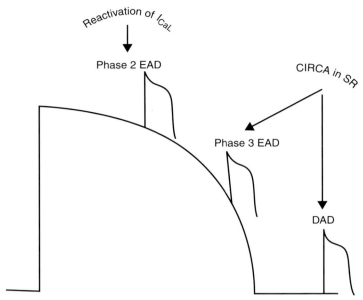

Fig 3.1 Mechanisms of EAD and DAD.

Summary

- DADs occur during calcium overload due to Ca release from SR. This activates $I_{Na/Ca}$.
- EAD is generated by recovery and reactivation of I_{CaL}.
- Phase 3 EAD shares the mechanism of DAD.
- Slow conduction could be due to decreased membrane excitability or reduced gap junction coupling.
- I_{Na} causes slow conduction, due to decreased excitability.
- Slow conduction due to decreased gap junction coupling requires contribution of I_{CaL}.

Reentry

- The size of reentry circuit depends on tissue excitability.
- It overdrive suppresses normal pacemaker cells.
- Decrease in conduction velocity, increase in the refractory period and/or decrease in the circuit length will make reentry less likely.
- Decreasing wavelength will increase the tendency to cause reentry arrhythmias.
- Restitution is described as the recovery of excitability after the refractory period.
- Multiple reentries may result in fibrillation.
- The reentry wave dies when it reaches the border of the tissue.
- The spiral of reentry wave may drift or it could be fixed (pin) around the obstacle.

- Reentry can be classic (anatomical) or functional.
- If a stimulus enters a vulnerable window of an anatomical reentry, it terminates it.
- Functional reentry is not terminated by entry of the stimulus inside the vulnerable window.
- Pacing induces a drift in the reentry circuit.
- Decrease in tissue excitability, by slowing conduction, eliminates reentry.
- When an electrical shock is applied to the heart, the tissue near the cathode (negative electrode) is depolarized (positive charge on the membrane) and the tissue near the anode (positive electrode) is hyperpolarized (negative charge on the membrane). This terminates the arrhythmia.
- For initiation and maintenance of reentry, whether anatomic or functional, unidirectional conduction block and the presence of excitable tissue ahead of propagating wave front (excitable gap) are essential. Slowing of conduction or shortening of the refractory period or both facilitate the excitable gap.
- Half of all cell-to-cell connections are side to side and the other half are end to end. The gap junction membrane provides resistance to current flow that results in slower conduction transversely than longitudinally. This results in anisotropic conduction through the myocardium. Reduction in myocardial CX43 results in slowing of conduction velocity.
- During myocardial ischemia slowing of the conduction occurs due to changes in ion channel function and increased resistance at gap junctions. After 60 minutes of ischemia irreversible damage occurs to the gap junction membrane and CX43. This results in slowing and non-uniform conduction.
- Crista terminalis and pectinate muscle produce anisotropic conduction and act as facilitators of reentry. Conduction along the longitudinal axis of the crista and pectinate muscle is faster than along the horizontal axis.
- Crista and Eustachian ridge act as anatomic barrier (isthmus) during reentrant activation.
- Discordant activation of atrial epicardium and endocardium at a faster rate promotes reentry.
- Crista, pectinate muscles, and Backman bundle propagate sinus impulses rapidly.
- Ectopic beat may alter normal conduction and produce changes in refractoriness which promotes reentry.

Phase 2 reentries[2]
- Prominent outward current due to I_{to} results in shortening of the APD.
- This may occur during ischemia and may result in a decrease of the plateau phase of AP. These changes may occur nonuniformly throughout the myocardium and cause dispersion of repolarization and phase 2 reentries.
- When I_{to}, an outward current, is dominant it results in APD shortening and loss of plateau of AP in some epicardial sites producing dispersion of repolarization. This results in local reexcitation and premature beats. This mechanism is termed as phase 2 reentry.

- Phase 2 reentry may occur in the presence of potassium channel opener Pinacidil, sodium channel blockers Flecainide, increase in extracellular calcium, and ischemia.
- I_{to} blockers restore homogeneity and abolish reentrant activity.
- I_{to} is present in ventricular epicardium but not in endocardium. It is responsible for spike and dome morphology of AP in epicardium.
- Reduced activity of I_{Ks} in M cells prolongs APD. Bradycardia and class III drugs prolong APD in M cells and predispose to arrhythmias.
- Repolarization is sensitive to changes in the heart rate.

Pharmacological differences in epicardium and endocardium
- Ach may alter the epicardial repolarization pattern by blocking I_{Ca} or activating I_{KAch}. It has no effect on I_{to}.
- Isoproterenol causes epicardial AP abbreviation more than it does in the endocardium.
- Organic calcium channel blockers (Verapamil) and inorganic calcium channel blocker $MnCl_2$ can cause loss of AP plateau phase in epicardium but only a slight abbreviation of AP in endocardium.
- Sodium current block decreases APD in epicardium.
- Block or decrease in calcium current leaves outward currents unopposed, which may result in shortening of APD.
- I_{to} block may establish electrical homogeneity and abolish arrhythmias due to dispersion of repolarization caused by drugs and ischemia. Quinidine inhibits I_{to}.
- Amiloride, a potassium sparing diuretic, prolongs APD and refractoriness.
- M cells, found in mid-myocardium of anterior, lateral wall, and outflow tract exhibit marked AP prolongation in response to bradycardia and on exposure to class III agents.
- This may be due to weaker I_{Ks} activity and stronger late I_{Na} activity.
- At slower rates M cells may contribute to pump efficiency because prolonged depolarization permits longer and more efficient contraction.
- Epicardium and endocardium electrically stabilize and abbreviate APD of M cells.
- Loss of either layer by infarction will lead to prolongation of APD. This may be the mechanism by which QT prolongation and dispersion occurs in non-Q wave MI. These differences could be aggravated by drugs that prolong the QT interval or in patients with LQTS.
- M cells play an important role in the inscription of T waves by producing a gradient between epicardium, endocardium, and M cells.
- U waves are due to repolarization of His Purkinje cells.

Post myocardial infarction arrhythmias
- Post MI hypertrophy of non-infracted myocytes occurs by three weeks due to volume overload.

- β Blockers and ace inhibitors may decrease post MI left ventricular hypertrophy (LVH).
- APD increases in LVH.
- In LVH, the following changes in ionic current occur that favor prolongation of APD and generation of EAD:
  - i Decreased I_{to}.
  - ii Decreased I_K.
  - iii Delayed inactivation of I_{Ca}.
- DAD is easily induced in hypertrophied myocytes in the presence of increased calcium load and β-adrenergic agonist.
- Increase in intracellular Ca load is through the Na/Ca exchange mechanism.
- Hyperpolarization activated current (I_f) and T-type calcium currents also become active in hypertrophied myocytes.
- Non-homogeneous prolongation of the APD in LVH results in dispersion of refractoriness and reentrant arrhythmias.
- **Acute** arrhythmias occur within a few minutes of the onset of ischemia.
- **Delayed** arrhythmias occur 5–48 hours after the onset of MI. These arrhythmias may be due to abnormal automaticity of Purkinje fibers and may result in accelerated idioventricular rhythm.
- **Late** arrhythmias occur within a few days to a few weeks after MI. Surviving cells within the MI zone demonstrate shortening of APD, diminished AP upstroke. Reentrant tachycardia can be easily induced.
- Post-MI VT originates in the subendocardial region.
- Infarct size, surviving cells in the MI zone, nonhomogeneous sympathetic denervation of myocardium distal to infarct are arrhythmogenic.
- After successful reperfusion the incidence of spontaneous VT appears to be less than 1%; however inducible arrhythmias occur more frequently. This suggests that the substrate for VT is present but triggers such as premature ventricular contractions (PVCs), ischemia, and increase in sympathetic activity may be absent.
- VT often occurs at the border of an infarcted and normal myocardium close to endocardium.
- Occurrence of the arrhythmias is facilitated by the presence of the **substrate** for arrhythmia such as scar or other conduction slowing abnormalities, electrical **triggers** such as PVCs, **electrical modulating factors** such as altered conduction, transmural dispersion of refractoriness and **physiologic modulating factors** such as ischemia, electrolyte abnormalities, hypoxia, and proarrhythmic drugs.
- Ventricular fibrillation (VF) is due to multiple random reentries. Electrical shock results in elimination of these reentries and renders a large portion of myocardium unexcitable, resulting in a successful defibrillation. When 65% or more of myocardium is depolarized VF terminates.
- There is a correlation between the shock strength that does not induce VF when applied on a T wave during sinus rhythm and the shock energy that successfully defibrillates during VF.

Ionic basis for prolongation of APD in LVH

- Increased activity or slow inactivation of I_{CaL} does not contribute to prolongation of APD.
- In hypertrophied myocytes there is a decrease in density without a change in the kinetics of I_{to}. Loss of I_{to} contributes to prolongation of APD.
- Na/Ca exchange generates inward current. This current is increased in LVH and may contribute to prolongation of APD.
- Hyperpolarization activated (I_f) current normally activates at $-120\,mV$; however, in hypertrophied myocytes it may activate at less negative potential and cause spontaneous diastolic depolarization.
- In post-MI hypertrophy there is a decrease in CX43 more so in endocardium than in epicardium. This may result in inhomogeneous conduction.
- In the presence of LQT1 sympathetic stimulation prolongs the QT interval and causes Torsade. Sympathetic stimulation abbreviates APD in epicardium and endocardium but not in M cells resulting in transmural dispersion.
- Differences in the response of the three cell types to adrenergic stimulation is related to the level of augmentation of I_{Ks}, which is strong in epicardium and endocardium and weak in M cells.
- Augmented I_{Ks} in epicardium and endocardium but not in M cells abbreviates APD and causes dispersion of repolarization and broad base T waves.
- D-Sotalol, an I_{Kr} blocker, prolongs the QT interval and mimics LQT2. It causes greater prolongation of APD in M cells and slows phase 3 repolarization in all cell layers of the myocardium, resulting in prolongation of the QT interval and low-amplitude T waves.
- Hypokalemia in the presence of I_{Kr} block results in a marked slowing of repolarization and low-amplitude notched T waves.
- The onset of the T wave corresponds to the onset of epicardial AP plateau. Final repolarization of epicardium causes the peak of the second component of the T wave. Final repolarization of M cells defines the end of the T wave.
- ATX II augments late I_{Na} by slowing inactivation of I_{Na} and mimics LQT3. This delays the onset of the T wave and causes marked prolongation of APD in M cells. M cells have large late sodium current.

References

1 Huffaker R. Lamp ST. Weiss JN. Kogan B. Intracellular calcium cycling, early after-depolarizations, and reentry in simulated long QT syndrome. *Heart Rhythm.* 1:441–8, 2004.
2 Gilmour RF. Early afterdepolarization-induced triggered activity: Initiation and reinitiation of reentrant arrhythmias. *Heart Rhythm.* 1:449–50, 2004.

4 Sinus Node Dysfunction and AV Blocks

Self-Assessment Questions

1 Which of the following currents contribute to the AP of SAN?
   A I_{CaL}
   B I_{Na}
   C I_f
   D I_{to}

2 What are the characteristics of type I SA exit block?
   A There is progressive lengthening of the PP interval preceding the pause
   B The duration of the pause is less than the sum of the two preceding sinus beats
   C It is caused by non-conducted PACs
   D It may progress to complete AV block

3 A 65-year-old man presents with an AV block where the PR interval of all captured complexes are constant in spite of varying RP interval. These characteristics are suggestive of which type of AV block?
   A Type I second degree AV block
   B Fascicular block
   C Type II second degree AV block
   D Functional block

4 Which one of the following statements is incorrect regarding paroxysmal AV block?
   A It occurs below the His
   B It is initiated by concealed conduction of the P waves
   C Resumption of normal conduction is due to peeling of the refractory period
   D Permanent pacing is not indicated

5 A 65-year-old female presents with acute anterior MI, RBBB, left anterior fascicular block and intermittent complete AV block. What are the likely characteristics of this AV block?
   A Permanent pacemaker is indicated
   B Mortality is less than 5%
   C Complete AV block is preceded by progressive changes in AV conduction
   D The site of the AV block is in the AV node

6 A 25-year-old male was admitted to a hospital following an episode of syncope. He was diagnosed to have myotonic dystrophy 5 years ago. Echocardiogram revealed left ventricular hypertrophy. The most likely cause of his syncope is:
   A Ventricular tachycardia
   B Preexcitation
   C Seizure disorder
   D Complete AV block

7 A 72-year-old male had an episode of syncope. Perfusion studies and the echo-cardiogram are normal. ECG rhythm strip, recorded during event monitor, is shown below.

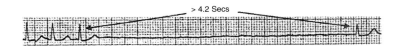

Which of the following is the most appropriate choice of therapy?
   A Dual chamber permanent pacemaker implant
   B Biventricular pacemaker implant
   C VVI pacemaker implant
   D Oral theophylline administration

8 ECG, shown below, was recorded in an 81-year-old patient who presented with episodes of dizziness.

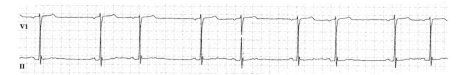

What is the likely diagnosis?
   A Type 1 sino atrial exit block
   B Type 1 second degree AVN block
   C Type II sino atrial exit block
   D Nonconducted PACs

Sino atrial node[1]

- Upstroke velocity of action potential (AP) in sino atrial node (SAN) cells is 4–9 V/s. Maximum diastolic potential (MDP) is −40 to −70 mV. AP amplitude is 70–80 mV. Action potential duration (APD) is 100–120 ms.
- I_f current is activated at less than −50 to −60 mV. It is an inward current, carried by Na and K ions (decay of I_K).
- I_f current is found in spider cells. It is a safety current.
- I_{CaL} is responsible for the upstroke of AP. It is activated in the last third of diastolic depolarization. Block of I_{CaL} stops spontaneous depolarization.
- I_{CaT} is present in SAN cells and has a more negative threshold and more rapid rate of inactivation.
- I_{Na} does not contribute to AP in SAN, a more positive MDP of the pacemaker cells inactivates this current; however, in the presence of hyperpolarizing agents such as acetylcholine (Ach) it may contribute to increased upstroke.
- I_{Nab} is a background inward current selective for sodium and potassium. Like I_f current it contributes to spontaneous depolarization.
- I_K is also present in pacemaker cells and influences APD by the rate of its inactivation. Blockade of this current may cause loss of spontaneous activity in pacemaker cells.
- I_{Kach} is present in pacemaker cells. It is a strong outward current and is responsible for hyperpolarization of the membrane.
- I_{to} and I_{K1} are not present in pacemaker cells. Absence of I_{K1} in pacemaker cells is responsible for diastolic depolarization.
- $I_{Na/K}$, a sodium/potassium pump current, produces significant outward current during diastolic depolarization. It can be blocked by Ouabain.
- Sodium calcium, exchanger $I_{Na/Ca}$, contributes to diastolic depolarization and produces increased inward current in the later third of diastolic depolarization. Elimination of these currents stops spontaneous activity.
- Adrenergic stimulation increases I_{CaL} and I_f.
- Cholinergic stimulation decreases I_{CaL} and I_f by shifting activation to more negative potential.
- I_{CaL} block slows the rate of propagation velocity in pacemaker cells but not in the atrium.
- Cholinergic stimulation activates I_{Kach} and hyperpolarizes SA cells by producing outward current. This outward current can result in sinus arrest and make cells unexcitable to normal levels of the currents.
- Adrenergic and cholinergic activity is modulated by β_1 and M_1 receptors, respectively. These receptors activate and increase the level of the cAMP.
- SAN has a large number of β_1 receptors, which play a role in chronotropic response.
- Increase in atrial pressure increases the heart rate by stimulating mechanically sensitive ion channels. This phenomenon is called the *Bainbridge effect*.

- When pacemaker cells are stimulated by adjacent cells during the first half of diastole there is a decrease in the rate, when the cells are stimulated in the latter half of diastole, the rate increases.

Sinus tachycardia and SA reentry tachycardia[2,3]

- The sinus node is located in the epicardial groove of the sulcus terminalis and its activity may extend along the crista terminalis. The sinus node artery runs through the center of the node.
- With an increasing heart rate the site of impulse formation moves superiorly and with a decreasing rate it shifts inferiorly.
- The resting potential of sinus pacemaker cells is −55mV.
- Parasympathetic stimulation decreases the sinus rate while sympathetic stimulation increases it.
- Common causes of sinus tachycardia include fever, anemia, hypotension, hyperthyroidism, and drugs such as atropine, catecholamines, caffeine, nicotine, aminophylline, and amphetamines.
- Persistent sinus tachycardia in the absence of any identifiable cause is called inappropriate sinus tachycardia (IST). Possible mechanisms include:
  - i Autonomic dysfunction. Increased sympathetic and/or decreased parasympathetic tone.
  - ii Abnormal sinus node automaticity.
  - iii Atrial tachycardia arising in close proximity to the sinus node.
- Unpredictable sudden onset suggests the presence of atrial tachycardia.
- Diagnostic features of IST include the following:
  - i The resting heart rate is more than 100 beasts per minute (bpm).
  - ii P wave morphology is similar to sinus P wave.
  - iii Persistent tachycardia in the absence of any physiologic cause.
- Symptoms include palpitation, near syncope, and exercise intolerance.
- It is common in females. It is not associated with mitral valve prolapse.
- Diagnostic evaluation includes EKG, 24-hour Holter monitor, stress test, and assessment of the intrinsic heart rate using autonomic blockade by intravenous administration of 0.2 mg/kg of propranolol and 0.4 mg/kg of atropine.
- Intrinsic heart rate = 118.1−(0.57 × age).
- Electrophysiologic study may be helpful in excluding atrial tachycardia or sinus node reentry tachycardia.
- Reentrant tachycardias are induced by extra stimulus.
- Most right atrial tachycardias arise from crista terminalis. With adrenergic stimulation the rate of atrial tachycardia increases without any shift of the focus. Onset is often abrupt.
- In IST, the rate and focus shift gradually with adrenergic stimulation.

Treatment of IST

- Treatment includes β-blockers and/or calcium channel blockers.
- Amiodarone, propafenone, and flecainide decrease SN automaticity and may be useful in severe cases.

- Successful radiofrequency (RF) ablation of IST or sinus node modification remains difficult. Although short-term success rates may be favorable (range 76–100%), long-term outcomes are disappointing.
- The endpoint of successful sinus node ablation remains unclear. Heart rate below 80–90 bpm, with or without isoproterenol infusion (usually 1–2 μg/min), at the conclusion of the procedure is considered a reasonable end point.
- Most of the cardiac and extra-cardiac symptoms persist despite documented slower heart rates, suggesting that sinus tachycardia and symptoms of palpitations are likely secondary manifestations of autonomic dysregulation.
- In the absence of atrial or other supraventricular tachycardia and autonomic and other multisystem symptoms RF ablation can be considered.
- Three-dimensional mapping or intracardiac echocardiography in localizing the crista may improve the outcome of the ablation.
- Surgical or RF ablation of the SAN and insertion of a permanent pacemaker may be considered. Fatigue, awareness of the paced rhythm and other symptoms may persist in spite of rate reduction.
- To avoid diaphragmatic paralysis high output pacing should be performed with an ablation catheter along the crista terminalis before delivering RF current.
- The clinical features of IST significantly overlap with postural orthostatic tachycardia syndrome (POTS).
- A multidisciplinary approach involving neurologist, cardiovascular rehabilitation, and psychiatrist may be necessary in managing patients with IST.

Sinus node dysfunction (SND)

Causes of sinus node dysfunction
Intrinsic (primary) SND may result from fibrosis and ageing-related loss of pacemaker cells.

Extrinsic (secondary) causes of SND are listed in Box 4.1.

Pathophysiology
- The sinus node is located near the superior anterolateral portion of RA near the SVC junction and the superior end of the crista terminalis.
- Cells in the SAN demonstrate diastolic depolarization and its AP is calcium channel dependent. Phase 0 demonstrates slow upstroke velocity.
- SAN cells do not have connexion 43 ($\times$43) gap junctions.
- Impulses may originate along the crista. With sympathetic stimulation the source of impulse formation shifts more superiorly and with vagal stimulation it shifts more inferiorly.
- The primary pacemaker area is located in the center of the node. Sympathetic and parasympathetic nerves innervate it.
- The AP of the pacemaker cells is characterized by phase 4 depolarization, relatively positive MDP and slow upstroke velocity.

Box 4.1 Extrinsic causes of SND

Hypothyroidism
SAN or atrial ischemia
Post-atrial surgery
Medications: Antiarrhythmics: Class I agents, Amiodarone
                 Beta blockers: Ca channel blockers
                 H2 receptor blockers: Ranitidine, Cimetidine
                 Psychotropic drugs: Lithium, Tricyclic antidepressants, Phenothiazines
Neurologic diseases: Myotonic dystrophy, Emery–Dreifuss syndrome, Tuberous sclerosis
Infiltrative disorders: Amyloidosis, Hemochromatosis, Systemic Lupus, Sarcoidosis,
Lymphoma
Myocarditis
Familial
Carotid sinus hypersensitivity
Increased vagal tone
Jaundice
Hypothermia
Elevated intracranial pressure

- Phase 4 depolarization is the result of four different ionic currents:
  - i I_K delayed rectifier.
  - ii Increase I_f inward current.
  - iii Inward calcium current.
  - iv Background current.
- Sympathetic stimulation enhances phase 4 depolarization by increasing I_f and I_{Ca}. Parasympathetic stimulation decreases phase 4 depolarization.
- Two potassium currents I_{to} and I_K and Na/Ca exchanger are responsible for sinus node repolarization.
- Drugs causing negative chronotropic response aggravate SND.
- Sensitivity to parasympathetic transmitters increases with age.
- Increase in APD of atrial myocardium may cause bradycardia. This may be the mechanism of bradycardia in LQTS.
- Bradycardia-related dispersion of refractoriness might cause tachyarrhythmia.

Clinical manifestations

- The SAN intrinsic rate decreases as the number of cells declines with increasing age.
- Long pauses may occur due to exit block from SAN after premature atrial contractions (PAC) or termination of the tachycardia. This may result in syncope or near syncope. Bradycardia may cause fatigue and/or dyspnea.
- Atrial asystole may predispose to thromboembolic complications.
- SND may present as abnormality of impulse formation such as bradycardia or sinus arrest or as abnormality of impulse conduction such as exit block or loss of physiologic responsiveness such as chronotropic incompetence.

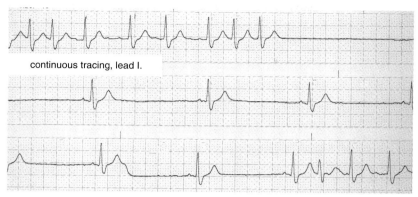

Fig 4.1 Sinus pause (sino atrial exit block) following rapid paroxysmal AF, followed by extreme sinus bradycardia. Typical of Brady Tachy syndrome.

- SND could be intrinsic due to structural disease of the sinus node or it could be due to extrinsic influences.
- Bradycardia, SA exit block, sinus arrest, chronotropic incompetence, atrial fibrillation (AF), or arrhythmias are the common manifestations of SND.
- SND may appear intermittently.
- Extrinsic factors causing SND include carotid sinus syndrome, vasovagal syncope, and increased vagal tone.
- Bradycardia may cause fatigue and dyspnea. Palpitation and embolism may occur due to AF.
- Carotid sinus pressure or tilt test may uncover the abnormalities.
- Carotid sinus hypersensitivity, sternocleidomastoid denervation syndrome and neurocardiogenic syncope may coexist with SND.

Electrocardiographic characteristics of SND
- Persistent sinus bradycardia, in the absence of drugs, is common.
- A sinus pause of 3 seconds or more may occur (Fig. 4.1). The duration of the pause is not a multiple of the basic heart rate. Following the pause the heart rate may accelerate (not seen in exit block). Non-conducted PAC may mimic sinus pauses. (Fig. 4.1).
- SA exit block is a common manifestation of SND. In type 1 SA exit block there is progressive shortening of the PP interval preceding the pause. The pause is less than the sum of two preceding sinus cycle lengths (CLs).
- In type 2 SA block the pause is equal to a multiple of sinus CL. (Fig. 4.2).
- In SND there may be concomitant suppression of subsidiary pacemaker.

Diagnosis
- Exercise test may uncover chronotropic incompetence.
- Administration of adenosine bolus, if results in slowing of sinus CL, by more than 2 standard deviations, is indicative of SND.

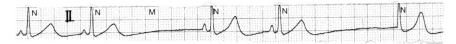

Fig 4.2 SA exit block.

- Sinus node recovery time (SNRT) is an interval from the last paced beat to the first sinus impulse. It is considered abnormal if it exceeds 1400 milliseconds.
- Corrected SNRT is derived by subtracting base line sinus CL from SNRT. A CSNRT of greater than 530 milliseconds is considered abnormal.
- CSNRT, if divided by 2, yields sino atrial conduction time (SACT). Normal SACT ranges from 70 to 120 milliseconds.
- Atropine by decreasing the vagal tone and enhancing retrograde conduction into SN may worsen SNRT.
- Low intrinsic heart rate after autonomic blockade is suggestive of SND.
- After complete autonomic blockade the intrinsic heart rate can be calculated by $118.1 - [0.57 \times age]$.
- During electrophysiologic study a normal corrected SNRT does not exclude the possibility of SND.

Prognosis and treatment
- Prognosis is good; however, occurrence of a stroke in the presence of AF, congestive heart failure (CHF) and AV block may alter the outcome.
- Atrial based pacing for symptomatic bradycardia lowers the incidence of AF and thromboembolic events and CHF.
- Atrial based pacing should be considered for symptomatic patients. The incidence of AV block is 1% per year.
- Drugs responsible for bradycardia should be discontinued.
- DDD pacing should be considered for patients with His Purkinje disease and neurocardiogenic syncope.
- Pacing may allow the use of antiarrhythmic drugs.
- Anticoagulation should be considered in the presence of atrial flutter/fibrillation.
- Anticholinergics, sympathomimetic, or methylated xanthines can be used for patients with mildly symptomatic bradycardia.
- Discontinuation of the offending agents, treatment of hypothyroidism, use of vagolytic agents or theophylline may be helpful in the short term.
- VVI pacemaker implant is the treatment of choice for patients who present with a pause related syncope but otherwise have normal atrio-ventricular node (AVN) conduction.

AVN anatomy and electrophysiology[1]
- The AVN is located in the triangle of Koch, bound by the tendon of Todaro, orifice of the coronary sinus (CS) and the septal leaflet of the tricuspid valve.

- There are anterior and posterior inputs to the AVN from the atrium.
- There are two types of cells in the AVN: rod-and ovoid-shaped cells.
- Spontaneous activity correlates with I_f current, which is far greater in the ovoid cells.
- I_{Na} and I_{to} are present in the rod cells.
- AVN conduction delay is inversely related to the prematurity of the impulse that it receives from the atrium.
- The occurrence of longer S2H2 interval with shorter S1S2 is due to the slow recovery of excitability of N cells.
- Slow AVN pathway (posterior input) is located posteriorly and inferiorly between the orifice of the CS and the septal leaflet of the tricuspid valve.
- Fast pathway is located anteriorly and superiorly in the interatrial septum. It has a shorter distance to travel to the AVN but demonstrates longer effective refractory period (ERP).
- A sudden change in the AH interval with a minimal change in the input interval may be due to shift of conduction from anterior (fast) to posterior (slow) pathway.
- After the successful elimination of the AVNRT, discontinuous conduction may still be present.
- In AF slow pathway elimination may not alter the heart rate if impulses can reach the AVN via another route.
- Subthreshold stimuli delivered in the triangle of Koch cause postganglionic release of Ach, resulting in hyperpolarization of N cells and slowing AVN conduction.

AV block AV dissociation
- AV dissociation can be due to AV block or due to physiologic refractoriness, resulting in the failure of transmission of the atrial impulse to the ventricle.
- AV block is due to failure of conduction of the atrial impulse to ventricle in the absence of physiologic refractoriness. It is generally due to interruption of the normal conduction pathway or due to pathologic refractoriness.
- AV block can be proximal (above the His bundle) indicating block in the AVN or it can be intra-Hisian or it can be distal to His bundle (infra-Hisian).
- The prognosis depends on the site of the AV block. Block distal to His bundle implies poor prognosis.

Prolonged PR interval (first-degree AV block)
It is defined as PR interval of more than 200 milliseconds.
- This may represent conduction delay in the atrium, AVN or His Purkinje system (HPS).
- All P waves are conducted to the ventricle with prolonged but constant interval. The causes of variable PR interval are enumerated in Box 4.2.
- If the QRS duration is normal the delay is invariably in the AVN. Ninety percent of these cases will demonstrate prolonged AH interval.

Box 4.2 Causes of variable PR interval

Intermittent conduction over slow pathway
Intermittent conduction over accessory pathway
Type I (Wenckebach) AV block
Concealed conduction from premature beats into AV junction
Intermittent junction rhythm and AV dissociation
High adrenergic tone

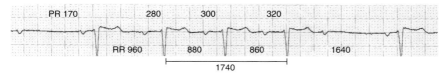

Fig 4.3 Type I AV block (intervals are in msecs).

- If the QRS duration is prolonged then the delay could be in the AVN (60%) or in HPS.
- Very long PR intervals favor delay in the AVN.
- Prognosis of the patients with prolonged PR interval is good and no therapy is indicated.
- In patients with prolonged PR interval and bifascicular block, the rate of progression to CHB is low and in asymptomatic patients pacing is not indicated even if the patient requires general anesthesia.
- If the HV interval exceeds 100 milliseconds, prophylactic pacing is indicated.

Second-degree AV blocks

These are of two types.

- Type I AV block (Mobitz I or Wenckebach) is characterized by the following (see Fig. 4.3):
    i Progressive prolongation of the PR interval at decreasing increments.
    ii Progressive shortening of the RR interval.
    iii A pause encompassing the blocked P wave. The duration of the pause is less than the sum of two PP intervals.
- Typical type I AV block is seen in 50% of cases, others are atypical and characterized by a varying sequence of PR and RR intervals. For example, PR and RR interval that terminates the cycle may be longest and PR interval may be constant or decrease.
- Long Wenckebach cycles tend to be atypical.
- Concealed conduction may be the mechanism for prolongation of PR RR in atypical sequence.
- Type I AV block, in asymptomatic subjects with normal heart, has excellent prognosis and requires no treatment.

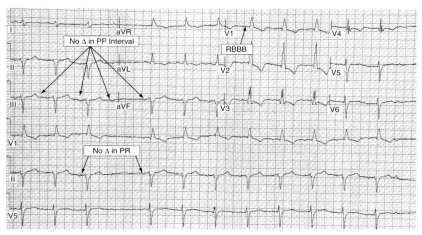

Fig 4.4 Type II AV block.

- Type I AV block with normal QRS complex is likely to be AV nodal; however, if the QRS duration is prolonged the block may be in the AVN, His bundle or infra-Hisian.
- Symptomatic patients with syncope, near syncope, worsening of CHF, or angina due to bradycardia produced by type I AV block may require pacing.
- Type II AV block is characterized by the following:
  - i Constant PP and RR intervals.
  - ii Constant PR interval before the blocked P wave.
  - iii The pause encompassing the P wave is twice as long as the preceding PP interval (Fig. 4.4).
- It often accompanies bundle branch block.
- Site of block is invariably in the His or infra-Hisian (Fig. 4.5).
- Second-degree AV block with narrow QRS complex is likely to be type I AV block with minimal increments in the PR interval and may be mistaken for type II block.
- 2 : 1 AV block with very long PR interval and narrow QRS suggests AV nodal block.
- Constant PR interval of all captured complexes, in spite of varying RP interval, suggests type II AV block. If the PR interval varies inversely with RP interval it is likely to be due to type I AV block.
- Functional infra-Hisian block may occur in the presence of long short HH CLs preceding the block. Rapid atrial pacing will not reproduce this type of block. Pacing is not indicated for functional infra-Hisian AV block.
- Type II AV block often progresses to complete AV block and requires pacing even in an asymptomatic patient.
- Type II AV block accompanied by alternating BBB would require a permanent pacemaker.

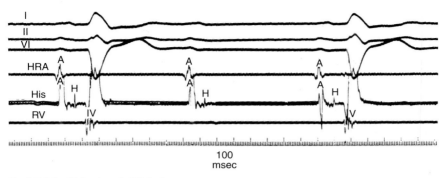

100
msec

Fig 4.5 Infra-Hisian type II AV block.

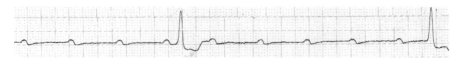

Fig 4.6 Complete AV block.

Third-degree AV block or complete AV block

- It could be congenital or acquired.
- The Site of the block could be AVN or below the His.
- It is characterized by the failure of all the P waves to conduct to the ventricle.
- Escape rhythm can be junctional with a rate of 40–60 bpm and narrow QRS complex or 20–40 bpm with wide QRS if it arises from the ventricle (Fig. 4.6).
- Drug-induced AV block may persist after discontinuing the offending agent.[5]
- Pacing is recommended for congenital AV block if
  - i The patient is symptomatic.
  - ii The QRS is wide.
  - iii The rate is less than 50 bpm.
  - iv The block is infra-Hisian.

  Other causes of the AV block are listed in Box 4.3.

Paroxysmal AV block[8]

- It presents as an abrupt and persistent AV block in the presence of normal AV conduction.
- It is produced by blocked or conducted PAC or PVC.
- It occurs below the His.

  Mechanisms include the following:
  - i Concealed conduction of non-conducted P waves into the AV junction.
  - ii Deceleration dependent depolarization of the lower AV junction.

Box 4.3 Causes of complete AV block

Drugs[5]	Beta blockers, Ca Ch blockers, Quinidine, Procainamide Amiodarone
Degenerative diseases	Lenegre disease, Lev disease, Sclerosis of conduction system
CAD	MI, Ischemia
Infection	Rheumatic fever, Myocarditis, Lyme disease, Chagas disease
Connective tissue diseases[6,7]	Ankylosing spondylitis, Reiter disease, Polychondritis, Scleroderma, Rheumatoid arthritis
Infiltrative disorders	Amyloidosis, Sarcoidosis, Tumors, Hodgkin disease, Myeloma
Neurologic disorders	Becker Muscular dystrophy, Myotonic dystrophy
Congenital	Fibroelastosis, Transposition of vessels, Septal defects, Collagen diseases in mother
Metabolic	Hypoxia, Electrolyte disorders
Traumatic	Surgical trauma, Cardiac contusion, Alcohol/surgical septal ablation

---

Resumption of normal AV conduction following paroxysmal block has been attributed to the following:

i Wedensky facilitation, where properly timed retrograde impulse allows sub-threshold antegrade impulse to conduct.

ii Peeling of refractory period (shortening of the refractory period with increasing frequency of stimulation).

- These patients require permanent pacing.

AV block in patients with acute myocardial infarction (MI)[4,9]

- It is common with inferior MI.
- It is probably due to increased vagal tone that accompanies early after an acute inferior MI. It presents as prolonged PR or type I AV block or advanced AV block.
- It responds to atropine.
- AV block occurring late after an acute MI is secondary to ischemia of the AVN, resulting in increased levels of adenosine in the AVN area. These effects can be blocked by theophylline.

Characteristics of AV block in the setting of inferior and anterior MI differ and are listed in Table 4.1.

AV dissociation

- During AV dissociation atrial and ventricular activity is independent.
- The mechanisms of AV dissociation could be physiologic or pathologic:
  i Physiologic refractoriness with interference. (Impulse may conduct if occurs during non-refractory window of CL).
    - The Rate of the primary pacemaker (sinus) is slower than the subsidiary (junctional) pacemaker, resulting in non-conduction of some of the impulses due to physiologic refractoriness.
    - Inappropriate acceleration of the subsidiary pacemaker. Accelerated junctional rhythm or ventricular tachycardia.

Table 4.1 Characteristics of AV block in the setting of acute MI

	Inferior MI	Anterior MI
Characteristic	Preceded by type I AV block	Preceded by type II AV block
Onset	Occurs in the first 2–3 days	Occurs in the first week
Duration	May last for 3–14 days	Could be permanent
Site	Nodal	Infra nodal
Pathology	AV nodal ischemia	Necrosis of conduction tissue
QRS duration	Narrow	Wide. Bundle branch block
Treatment	Temporary pacing	Permanent pacing
Mortality (%)	10–20	60–80

- Due to physiologic refractoriness and physiologic AV conduction delay when the primary pacemaker accelerates (Sinus or atrial tachycardia).

ii Pathologic failure of conduction of sinus impulses resulting in more P waves than QRS complexes as in complete AV block. (Impulse does not conduct even if it occurs during non-refractory period of the CL.)

References

1 James TN. Structure and function of the sinus node, AV node and His bundle of the human heart: Part I-structure. *Prog Cardiovasc Dis.* 45:235–6, 2002.

2 Shen WK. Modification and ablation for inappropriate sinus tachycardia: Current status. *Card Electrophysiol Rev.* 6:349–55, 2002.

3 Shen WK. How to manage patients with inappropriate sinus tachycardia. *Heart Rhythm.* 2:1015–19, 2005.

4 Brady WJ. Diagnosis and management of bradycardia and atrioventricular block associated with acute coronary ischemia. *Emerg Med Clin North Am.* 19:371–84, 2001.

5 Zeltser D. Justo D. Halkin A. Drug-induced atrioventricular block: prognosis after discontinuation of the culprit drug. *J Am Coll Cardiol.* 44:105–8, 2004.

6 Clancy RM. Buyon JP. Autoimmune-associated congenital heart block: dissecting the cascade from immunologic insult to relentless fibrosis. *Anat Rec A Discov Mol Cell Evol Biol.* 280:1027–35, 2004.

7 Qu Y. Xiao GQ. Chen L. Autoantibodies from mothers of children with congenital heart block down regulate cardiac L-type Ca channels. *J Mol Cell Cardiol.* 33:1153–63, 2001.

8 Silvetti MS. Grutter G. Di Ciommo V. Paroxysmal atrioventricular block in young patients. *Pediatr Cardiol.* 25:506–12, 2004.

9 Abidov A. Kaluski E. Hod H. Leor J. Vered Z. Gottlieb S. Behar S. Cotter G. Israel Working Group on Intensive Cardiac Care: Influence of conduction disturbances on clinical outcome in patients with acute myocardial infarction receiving thrombolysis (results from the ARGAMI-2 study). *Am J Cardiol.* 93:76–80, 2004.

5 Supraventricular Tachycardia

Self-Assessment Questions

5.1 ATRIAL FLUTTER

1 A 54-year-old male presents with progressively increasing dyspnea. ECG is shown below. Serum potassium was 3.2 mEq. Perfusion studies are normal. Echocardiogram revealed biatrial enlargement, enlarged and diffusely hypokinetic left ventricle, and ejection fraction of 26%. Eight months ago on a routine examination blood pressure of 120/70 and a heart rate of 70 b.p.m. were recorded. Six months ago a spot check in a drug store revealed a blood pressure of 110/70 and a heart rate of 150 b.p.m. The patient was asymptomatic.

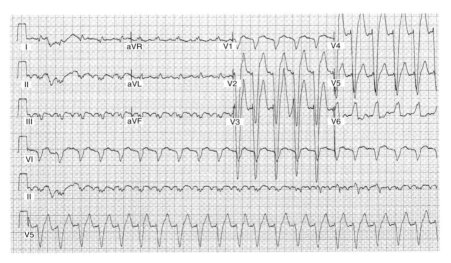

What will you recommend?
   A IV lidocaine
   B Bi V defibrillator implant
   C Radiofrequency ablation
   D Ca channel blockers

2 A 36-year-old sales representative was found to have an atrial flutter. Physical examination and echocardiogram were normal. Serum potassium was 3.9 mEq. The next day he reported to hospital outpatient area for chemical cardioversion. He received 1 mg of Ibutilide intravenously and converted to sinus rhythm within 10 minutes. Two hours later he insisted on leaving the hospital. While in a meeting he had an episode of syncope. He was in sinus rhythm and blood pressure was normal.

What is the most likely cause of his syncope?

A Recurrence of atrial flutter with rapid ventricular response

B Neurocardiogenic syncope

C Polymorphic ventricular tachycardia

D Embolic stroke from left atrial clot

3 A 45-year-old male who has persistent atrial flutter, undergoes radiofrequency ablation. During the second application of the energy flutter is terminated. What will you consider as a satisfactory end point for this procedure?

A Termination of atrial flutter is a satisfactory end point

B Bidirectional block across isthmus should be demonstrated

C Rapid atrial pacing should be performed in an attempt to induce flutter

D Additional RF lesions should be delivered near CS ostium

4 A 77-year-old female had paroxysmal atrial fibrillation. Echocardiogram and perfusion studies were normal. She was treated with propafenone 150 mg TID. Five weeks later she came to the clinic complaining of palpitations. ECG revealed persistent atrial flutter.

What will be your recommendation?

A Continue propafenone and consider ablation for atrial flutter

B Discontinue propafenone

C Consider ablation for atrial fibrillation

D Consider rate control using Ca channel blockers and β blockers

5.2 ATRIAL TACHYCARDIAS

1 A 56-year-old nurse presents with recurrent episodes of tachycardia. ECG is shown.

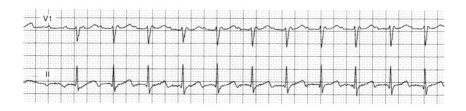

What is the most likely diagnosis?

A Sinus tachycardia

B Atrial tachycardia

C AVRT

D Atypical AVNRT

2 Ablation at which of the following sites is likely to cure the tachycardia?

A Accessory pathway

B AV nodal slow pathway

C Atrial tachycardia focus

D AV junction

3 A 25-year-old man is referred to you because of sustained tachycardia. During electrophysiologic study, following tracing was obtained.

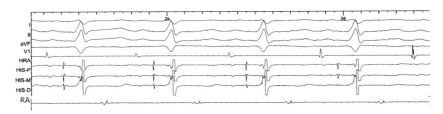

Which of the following is the most likely diagnosis?

A Atrial tachycardia

B Atypical AV reentrant tachycardia using a slowly conducting pathway as the retrograde limb

C Atypical (fast-slow) AV nodal reentrant tachycardia

D Sinus node reentrant tachycardia

5.3 ATRIAL FIBRILLATION

1 A 35-years-old female with mitral valve disease presents with history of several episodes of atrial fibrillation that lasted for 2–4 hours and spontaneously terminates. This could be classified as:

A Persistent AF

B Chronic AF

C Paroxysmal AF

B Lone AF

2 Most common symptom of the AF is:

A TIA/Stroke

B Fatigue and tiredness

C Syncope

D Chest pain

3 Which of the following is not a risk factor for thromboembolic complication in a patient with AF and therefore not an indication for anticoagulation with warfarin?

 A The patient is 57 year old
 B Hypertension
 C LVF
 D Diabetes

4 A 48-year-old patient presents with AF that has lasted for more than 48 hours. TEE is negative for intracardiac clots. What will be your recommendation following a successful cardioversion?

 A Begin Warfarin and continue indefinitely
 B Begin Aspirin
 C Begin Warfarin for 3 weeks
 D Patient does not need anticoagulation or antiplatelate therapy

5 Attempted cardioversion for AF is unsuccessful in a 60-year-old patient. His EF is 25%. Should he undergo repeat cardioversion after administration of IV ibutilide?

 A True
 B False

6 A 50-year-old female patient presents with paroxysmal AF. She was recently diagnosed to have chronic active hepatitis and abnormal liver function test. To maintain sinus rhythm which of the following drugs could be safely prescribed?

 A Sotalol
 B Mexiletine
 C Amiodarone
 D Procainamide

7 A 76-year-old woman has had persistent atrial fibrillation for three years. She also has hypertension and asthma. Current medications are warfarin; digoxin, 0.25 mg daily; atenolol, 25 mg twice daily; diltiazem, 30 mg every 8 hours; and inhaled bronchodilators. During 24-hour ambulatory ECG monitoring, the average ventricular response was 130 beats per minute (b.p.m.) with occasional episodes of 150 b.p.m. Echocardiogram shows a 6 cm left atrium and a dilated left ventricle. Estimated left ventricular ejection fraction is 35%.
Which of the following is the best treatment plan?

 A Increase the dose of atenolol
 B Increase the dose of diltiazem
 C Initiate amiodarone and consider elective cardioversion 4 weeks later
 D Radiofrequency catheter ablation of the AV junction, and insertion of rate-responsive ventricular pacemaker

5.4 AUTOMATIC JUNCTIONAL TACHYCARDIA

1 To differentiate AJT from AVNRT which of the following maneuvers could be helpful?

A PAC delivered near slow pathway when septal A has occurred

B Adenosine infusion

C Parahisian pacing

D Assessment of prematurity index

2 Which of the following therapeutic options is least likely to help in the treatment of AJT?

A AV node ablation and insertion of permanent pacemaker

B Amiodarone

C Digoxin

D Propafenone

5.5 AV NODE REENTRY TACHYCARDIAS

1 Dual AV node physiology is defined as:

A 50 milliseconds increase in H_1H_2 for 10 milliseconds decrease in A_1A_2 interval

B 50 milliseconds increase in A_2H_2 for 10 milliseconds decrease in A_1A_2 interval

C 50 milliseconds increase in H_2V_2 for 10 milliseconds decrease in A_1A_2 interval

D Occurrence of atrial echo beats in response to any A_1A_2

2 Which of the following properties is the result of distal insertion of fast pathway into AV junction?

A Increased decremental conduction

B Increased response to AV node blocking agents

C Greater response to Na channel blocking agents

D Preexcitation on surface electrocardiogram

3 After slow pathway ablation, the presence of A_2H_2 jump without induction of tachycardia is indicative of unsuccessful ablation.

A True

B False

4 In which of the following conditions is the HA interval during tachycardia likely to be shorter than the HA interval during RV pacing?

A AVNRT

B AVRT

C RVOT VT

D Atrial tachycardia

5 Which of the following conditions are likely to present with variable HA interval? (Choose more than one).
  A AVNRT
  B AVRT with dual AV node physiology
  C Atrial tachycardia
  D Multiple concealed accessory pathways

6 A 25-year-old female had recurrent episodes of palpitation. During electrophysiologic study wide complex tachycardia was induced. Tachycardia could be entrained by right atrial pacing; however, on repeated occasions, on termination of atrial pacing tachycardia resumed as shown in the following tracing.

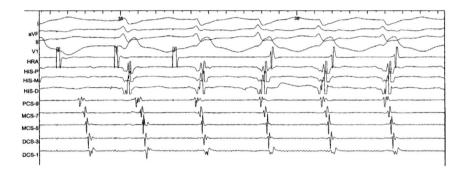

What is the most likely mechanism of this tachycardia?
  A AVNRT
  B AVRT
  C Atrial tachycardia
  D LVVT (fascicular tachycardia)

7 A 50-year-old female had recurrent episodes of tachycardia. During electrophysiologic study the following observations were made.

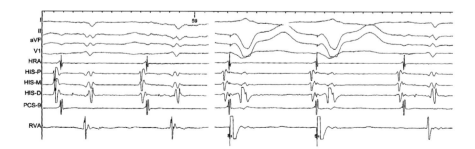

Ablation at which of the following sites is mostly likely to cure the tachycardia?

A Subeustachian isthmus

B Accessory pathway

C AV nodal slow pathway

D Atrial tachycardia focus

8 A 26-year-old woman, who is in the last trimester of pregnancy, complains of palpitations. Episodes last several minutes and terminate spontaneously; they are not associated with dizziness, chest pain, or syncope. One such episode was recorded while in primary care physician's office.

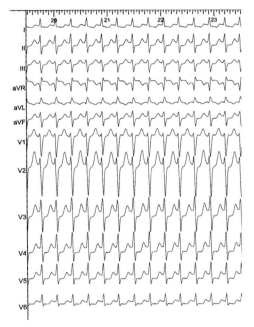

Tachycardia terminates spontaneously. Baseline ECG and echocardiogram are normal.

Which of the following is most appropriate at this time?

A Deliver the fetus as soon as possible

B Begin flecainide

C Begin metoprolol

D Reassure the patient

9 A 67-year-old man has had palpitations for the last 10 years. Recently the episodes have become more frequent and severe. Medical history includes hypertension, diabetes, and hypercholesterolemia. ECG recorded in the office was found to be normal.

Two days ago he came to hospital complaining of dyspnea, chest pressure, and palpitations. He was diaphoretic; the heart rate was 140 per minute, the blood pressure was 100/60 mm Hg. Electrocardiogram is shown.

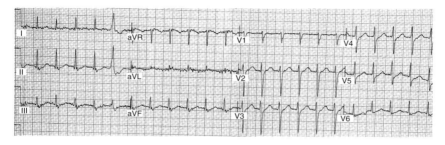

Today during electrophysiologic study anterograde dual AV nodal pathway is demonstrated; however, sustained supraventricular tachycardia (SVT) cannot be induced.

Which one of the following should be done next?

A Repeat electrophysiologic study in 4 weeks

B Prescribe Metoprolol

C Ablate the AV nodal slow pathway

D Prescribe amiodarone

10 A 32-year-old woman undergoes electrophysiologic study for recurrent palpitations. The following recording is obtained.

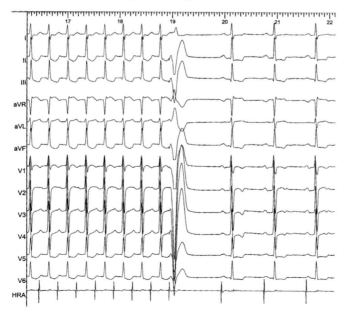

Which of the following is the most likely diagnosis?

A AV reentrant tachycardia using an accessory pathway

B Atypical (fast-slow) AV nodal reentrant tachycardia

C Intraatrial reentrant tachycardia

D Typical (slow-fast) AV nodal reentrant tachycardia

5.6 AV REENTRANT TACHYCARDIAS

1 A 27-year-old female patient presents with AVRT utilizing left lateral AP. There is a variation in the cycle length although the VA interval remains unchanged. The most likely explanation of this observation is:

A Slowing of conduction in AP

B Change in conduction through the AV node due to dual AV node physiology

C Multiple accessory pathways

D Accelerated conduction through His Purkinje system

2 Which one of the following is least likely to present with short RP tachycardia?

A AVNRT

B Ventricular tachycardia

C AVRT

D Sinoatrial reentrant tachycardia

3 On termination of the SVT the last complex recorded is a QRS. Which one of the following is the most likely mechanism?

A AVNRT

B AVRT

C Atrial tachycardia

D None of the above

4 His synchronous PVC terminates the SVT without depolarizing the atrium. In which of the following conditions is this phenomenon likely to be noticed?

A Atrial tachycardia

B AVNRT

C Automatic junctional tachycardia

D AVRT

5 In which of the following conditions is the VA interval likely to be shorter during RV apex pacing than RV base pacing?

A AV node

B Septal AP

C Left posterior AP

D Atrioventricular connection (Mahaim fibers)

6 Which one of the following is likely to present with a constant VA interval with or without His capture during parahisian pacing?
   A Dual AV nodal physiology
   B Septal AP
   C Nodo-fascicular pathway
   D Atriofascicular pathway

7 Which one of the following is unlikely to cause variable VA interval during AVRT?
   A Intermittent bundle branch block
   B Multiple retrogradely conducting accessory pathways
   C Decremental retrograde conduction through the AP
   D Dual AVN physiology

8 SVT is entrained by RV pacing. On termination of V pacing the response is AAV. This observation suggests the diagnosis of:
   A Atrial tachycardia
   B AVNRT
   C AVRT
   D Atrio fascicular tachycardia

9 SVT is entrained by RV pacing. On termination of V pacing the stimulus to A-VA interval is >85 msec and PPI-TCL interval is >115 msec. These observations suggests the diagnosis of:
   A Atrial tachycardia
   B Atypical AVNRT
   C Atriofascicular pathway
   D AVRT

10 Which of the following observations is least likely to suggest the presence of antidromic tachycardia as opposed to antegrade bystander utilization of AP during atrial tachycardia?
   A Earliest retrograde atrial activation is through AV junction
   B Late PAC advances the whole tachycardia circuit (V and following A)
   C PVC delivered at the ventricular insertion site of the AP abolishes the preexcitation but tachycardia continues
   D Ventricles are the integral part of the tachycardia circuit

11 During a wide complex tachycardia it is noted that the atrium and ventricle are an obligatory part of the circuit and retrograde atrial activation is eccentric. These observations suggest presence of:
   A Atrial tachycardia utilizing bystander AP
   B VT utilizing bystander AP
   C Antidromic tachycardia
   D Bypass to bypass tachycardia

12 PAC delivered during wide complex tachycardia advances the ventricular electrogram and the next atrial electrogram without any change in the atrial activation sequence. These findings are suggestive of:

A AVNRT utilizing bystander AP

B Atrial tachycardia utilizing bystander AP

C Antidromic tachycardia

D Ventricular tachycardia

13 During wide complex tachycardia, a short HV interval is recorded. This finding suggests the presence of:

A Ventricular preexcitation due to bystander AP

B Antidromic tachycardia

C Atrio fascicular pathway mediated tachycardia

D BBRVT

14 A 30-year-old male, who is known to have preexcitation, presents to ER with atrial fibrillation of 1 hour duration. The ventricular rate is 130–170 b.p.m. The patient is hemodynamically stable. Which of the following can be safely used to treat AF?

A IV Digoxin

B IV Verapamil

C IV procainamide

D IV metoprolol

15 A 19-year-old man who has paroxysmal supraventricular is referred to you for evaluation and recommendation. The patient has had tachycardia since age 10. Electrocardiogram obtained during sinus rhythm is shown. Echocardiogram is normal.

At which site, will delivery of radiofrequency result in resolution of the problem?

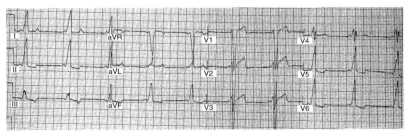

A Right anterior

B Posteroseptal

C Left lateral

D Anteroseptal

16 Surface and intracardiac electrograms recorded during tachycardia are shown in the following tracing.

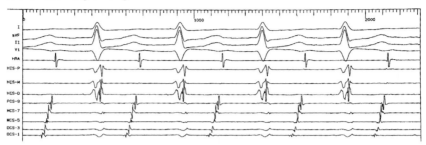

Which maneuver will help identify the correct mechanism of the tachycardia?

A Atrial pacing

B Ventricular pacing

C Isoproterenol infusion

D Mapping in the left superior pulmonary vein

17 A 20-year-old male presented with recurrent episodes of palpitations. During electrophysiologic study following arrhythmia was induced. Ablation at which one of the following sites is likely to terminate the tachycardia?

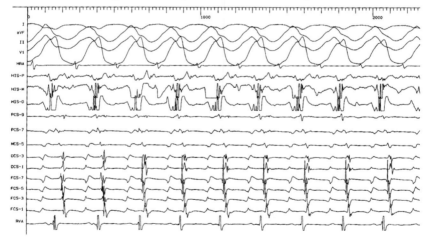

FCS = closely spaced (2 mm) electrograms recorded from CS using femoral approach. DCS, MCS and PCS are recorded from subclavian approach. (electrode spacing 10-2 mm)

A Left lateral mitral annulus

B LVOT

C Right lateral tricuspid annulus

D Right bundle

18 A 50-year-old woman has a long history of paroxysmal tachycardia despite treatment with digoxin, atenolol, and flecainide. She underwent electrophysiologic study and radiofrequency ablation (tracing A). Two months later she had a recurrence of the tachycardia. Electrophysiologic study was repeated (tracing B).

Tracing A

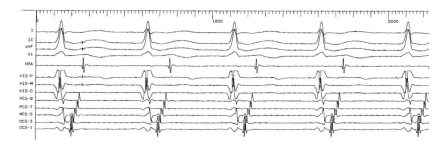

Tracing B

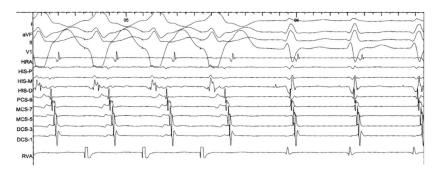

Which of the following best describes the mechanism(s) of the tachycardias?
A The patient had atypical AVNRT and now has typical AV nodal reentrant tachycardia
B The patient had AVRT utilizing the anteroseptal accessory pathway and now has atrial tachycardia
C The patient had AVRT utilizing the LLAP and now has typical AVNRT
D The patient had permanent junctional reciprocating tachycardia and now has atypical AV nodal reentrant tachycardia

19 A 15-year-old female fainted in a physician's office while the blood was being drawn. There is no previous history of syncope, chest pain, or palpitations. ECG rhythm strip recorded in the physician's office is shown below.

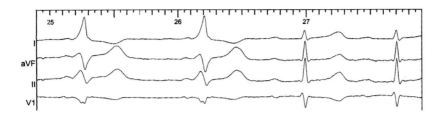

What will be your recommendation?

A Consider electrophysiologic study and RF ablation
B Begin procainamide
C Begin Metoprolol
D Reassure the patient

20 A 44-year-old man is referred to you because he has had three episodes of palpitations in the past year. Each episode began suddenly, lasted up to 30 minutes, and was associated with severe lightheadedness. The patient has not had syncope, dyspnea, or chest pain, and he has no family history of heart disease.

The findings of the physical examination are normal. Electrocardiograms recorded a few minutes apart are shown in tracings A and B.

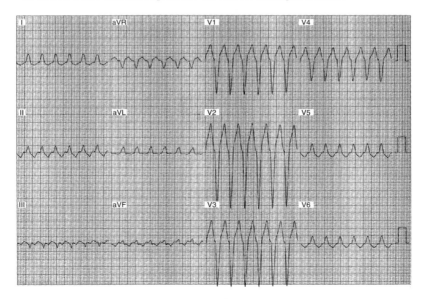

Tracing A

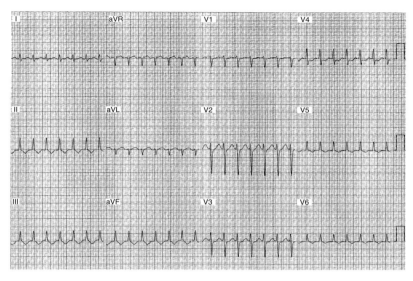

Tracing B

What is the most likely diagnosis?

A AVNRT

B Atrial tachycardia

C AVRT

D RVOT-VT and atrial tachycardia

5.1 ATRIAL FLUTTER

- Atrial Flutter is due to reentry.

Classification of atrial flutter

1 Typical atrial flutter
2 Reverse typical atrial flutter
3 Incisional scar related atrial flutter
4 Left atrial flutter

- Classical atrial flutter is confined to the right atrium where the impulse travels up the atrial septum and then travels inferiorly down the right atrial free wall to re-enter the atrial septum through the isthmus (Fig. 5.1).
- Atrial flutter produced by this mechanism is called typical atrial flutter. It has also has been called common or counterclockwise atrial flutter. A 12-lead ECG during typical atrial flutter produces negative "sawtooth" flutter waves[1] in leads II, III, and aVF (Fig. 5.2).

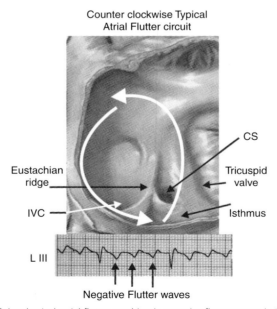

Counter clockwise Typical
Atrial Flutter circuit

CS

Eustachian
ridge

Tricuspid
valve

IVC

Isthmus

L III

Negative Flutter waves

Fig 5.1 Circuit of the classical atrial flutter resulting in negative flutter waves in LII, LIII, and aVF. CS, Coronary sinus ostium; IVC, inferior vena cava.

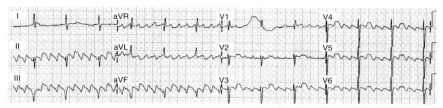

Fig 5.2 Typical atrial flutter.

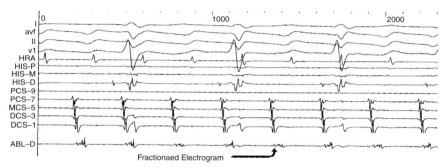

Fig 5.3 Fractionated electrograms recorded from the distal electrode of an ablation catheter located between the tricuspid annulus and the anterior wall of the CS.

- If the impulse travels in the opposite direction down the atrial septum and through the isthmus to travel up the right atrial free wall it is called *reverse typical atrial flutter* or clockwise atrial flutter. A 12-lead ECG during reverse typical atrial flutter produces positive flutter waves in leads II, III, and aVF.
- The isthmus is an area of slow conduction between the tricuspid valve annulus and the inferior vena cava (IVC). The eustachian ridge (ER), which extends to the posterior wall of the coronary sinus (CS) ostium (os), is an integral part of this isthmus and contributes to the slow conduction. Fractionated electrograms could be recorded from the area of slow conduction (Fig. 5.3).
- Entrainment occurs when pacing at shorter cycle length results in acceleration of the flutter. On termination of pacing flutter resumes without a change in its cycle length.
- Entrainment can be manifest when fusion occurs or it can be concealed when paced complexes are identical to spontaneously occurring flutter complexes (Fig. 5.4).
- Concealed entrainment of typical flutter occurs when pacing from the isthmus. If the post-pacing interval is the same as the flutter cycle length, this confirms that the flutter is isthmus-dependent.
- Incisional atrial re-entry is seen in patients with right atrial free wall incisions following cardiac surgery. The reentrant circuit travels around the line of block caused by the incision.

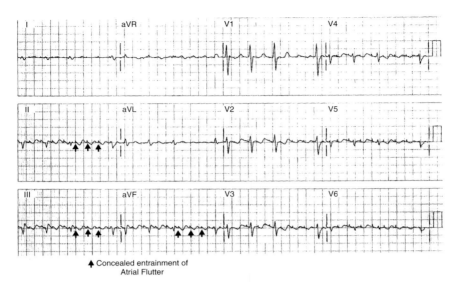

▲ Concealed entrainment of
Atrial Flutter

Fig 5.4 Pacing from the medial segment of the flutter isthmus results in concealed entrainment. Paced atrial complexes are identical to spontaneously occurring typical counterclockwise flutter waves. Short stimulus to F interval suggests that the capture is located at the exit site of the flutter isthmus.

- In left atrial flutter the area of slow conduction is between one or more of the pulmonary veins or the mitral valve annulus. It may occur spontaneously or following ablation for atrial fibrillation (AF) where an attempt to isolate pulmonary veins may result in a corridor of slowly conducting tissue between the mitral annulus and pulmonary veins.
- Left atrial flutter may also result from the gaps in ablation lines in the left atrium.
- Atrial flutter often presents with the same symptoms as AF. The atrial rate is typically between 250 and 350 beats per minute (bpm), with resultant 2 : 1 or 4 : 1 atrioventricular conduction block. Diagnosis is made on 12-lead ECG. The blocked flutter waves may not be readily apparent on 12-lead ECG because they may be masked by the QRS complex. The presence of a regular, narrow complex tachycardia at 150 bpm should raise suspicion of atrial flutter.
- Persistent atrial flutter with rapid ventricular response may result in tachycardia mediated cardiomyopathy.
- During atrial flutter atrio-ventricular node (AVN) conduction is often 2 : 1.
- Increase in AV block by vagal maneuvers or pharmacologic agents such as adenosine may clarify the diagnosis if the flutter waves are not clearly visible.
- Use of class IC drugs may slow the atrial rate and allow most of the atrial impulses to pass through the AV node, thus increasing the ventricular rate.

Treatment[2-6]

- The risk of thromboembolic events from atrial flutter is the same as with AF. Therefore, the recommendations for anticoagulation with atrial flutter are the same as with AF.
- New onset of flutter of short duration can be treated by the following:
  1 Intravenous Ibutilide if serum potassium is >4.0 mEq, QT_c is less than 440 milliseconds and left ventricle (LV) function is normal.
  2 Single oral dose of Flecainide (300 mg) or Propafenone (600 mg).
  3 Cardioversion 25–50 J can achieve cardioversion to sinus rhythm.
  4 Overdrive atrial pacing using high outputs.
- IV Ibutilide may prolong the QT interval and may induce Torsade. The patient should be monitored for the half life of the drug (4 h) following administration of the drug.
- Cardioversion should be considered if the patient is hemodynamically unstable.
- β-Blockers or calcium channel blockers can achieve rate control.
- For paroxysmal or chronic atrial flutter radiofrequency (RF) ablation of the isthmus is the treatment of choice. These patients should be anticoagulated for 4 weeks prior to cardioversion or ablation. Alternatively if the transesophageal echocardiogram is negative for intracardiac blood clots immediate cardioversion can be performed after starting anticoagulation.
- AV node ablation and insertion of a permanent pacemaker can be considered for rate control.
- Oral antiarrhythmic drug therapy to maintain sinus rhythm is not very effective.

Atrial flutter ablation[7-11]

- In a typical flutter the activation in the right atrium occurs in a counter-clockwise direction. This produces a negative sawtooth pattern in L2, L3, and aVF. It produces positive flutter waves in V1 and negative flutter waves in V6 (Fig. 5.1).
- In a clockwise flutter the pattern is reversed.
- The flutter wave travels along the broad area of the anterolateral wall of the right atrium. It then enters the narrow and slowly conducting isthmus area. The anterior boundary of the isthmus is the tricuspid annulus (TA) and the posterior boundary includes the IVC, ER and the CS os. In some patients the wave front after emerging from the isthmus may divide into two exits traveling anterior and posterior to the CS os. In other patients continuation of the ER into the posterior lip of the CS os prevents posterior exit. Thus the wave front only travels between the TA and the ER.
- The wave front then emerges in the low right atrium and ascends along the interatrial septum. Block along the crista terminalis prevents the impulse from entering the anterior trabeculated segment of the atrium. This prevents collision with the reentrant wave.

- The principle of ablation for reentrant tachycardia with the area of slow conduction bounded by two anatomical barriers is transaction of the circuit with lesion extending from one fixed barrier to the next.
- In typical atrial flutter that area is the narrow isthmus between the TA and the IVC and/or the ER and the CS os.
- Entrainment mapping should be used to confirm that the isthmus is an integral part of the flutter circuit. Sometimes a typical electrocardiographic pattern may be present in non-isthmus dependent atrial reentrant tachycardias.
- Flutter is entrained by pacing at the isthmus (6:00 or 7:00 clock position of the TA in the left anterior oblique view) at a cycle length 20 milliseconds shorter than flutter cycle length.
- The following features are suggestive of entrainment with concealed fusion and indicate that the flutter is isthmus dependent:
  1 A long interval from the pacing stimulus to the onset of the flutter wave.
  2 No change in flutter wave morphology on surface ECG.
  3 No change in endocardial activation pattern along the TA.
  4 Post pacing interval equals tachycardia cycle length.
- The width of the isthmus may vary from 2 to 4 cm. It may contain fibrous thebesian valve and pectinate muscles. In some patients the narrowest portion of the isthmus is towards the septum between the anterior lip of the CS os and the TA.
- During ablation special sheaths may be needed to maintain proper orientation and tissue contact.
- The goal should be to achieve adequate tissue temperatures (50–60°F) for 30 seconds before moving the catheter by a few millimeters till the ablation line is completed between the TA and IVC.
- Larger lesions can be achieved by using a large tip or irrigated tip ablation catheter.
- Transient isthmus block during RF application may terminate atrial flutter, but a complete and permanent block across the isthmus is essential for cure. Bidirectional block across the isthmus should be demonstrated by pacing from the low lateral right atrium and from the CS.
- RF energy can be applied during atrial flutter or during CS pacing. Block across the isthmus will change the activation sequence along the lateral aspect of the right atrium when pacing from the CS.
- Pacing from the lateral aspect of the isthmus, before isthmus block, results in negative P waves in inferior leads as activation proceeds through the isthmus to the CS os and the atrial septum. After the successful ablation the P wave morphology in inferior leads becomes positive and bifid, as activation along the septum is no longer possible.
- Split potential on the ablation line where the interval between the two potentials exceeds 100 milliseconds during CS pacing is also suggestive of block across the isthmus.

- When assessing block across the isthmus long pacing cycle lengths should be used. Shorter cycle lengths may result in slowing of conduction and appearance of a block (Pseudo block).
- Incomplete block across the isthmus may result in a "leak" across the isthmus on pacing from the lateral or medial aspect. The site of such a leak is generally located:
  1 Adjacent to TA.
  2 On the lip of the ER.
  3 At the anterior wall or base of the deep subeustachian sinus.
  4 On the large pectinate muscle in the isthmus.
- Gaps can be identified during CS pacing or during flutter by identifying narrowly split or single electrograms along the ablation line interposed by widely separated double potentials.
- Electroanatomical 3-dimensional mapping may help in identifying the "leaks" of conduction across the isthmus.
- Intracardiac echocardiography may help identify right atrial landmarks such as crista, CS.
- The acute success rate of flutter ablation is 90% and reoccurrence rate of 5–10%.
- In patients who present with paroxysmal atrial flutter/AF, ablation of the atrial flutter may make treatment of AF more manageable.
- If antiarrhythmic drug therapy organizes AF into atrial flutter, a hybrid approach of flutter ablation and continued antiarrhythmic drug therapy may be effective in maintaining sinus rhythm.

5.2 ATRIAL TACHYCARDIAS

Atrial tachycardia

- Five percent of all supraventricular tachycardias (SVTs), in adults, could be attributed to atrial tachycardia (AT). Electrocardiographically it is characterized by an atrial rate of less than 240 bpm and the presence of an isoelectric interval between P waves.
  Atrial tach can be classified into focal or macroreentrant (Fig.5.5).

Focal atrial tachycardia[13]

- AT could originate from any one of the following sites:

Along the crista terminalis
Pulmonary veins superior more common than inferior
Coronary sinus ostium
Mitral and tricuspid annulus
AV node fast pathway region
Superior vena cava
Left atrial appendage

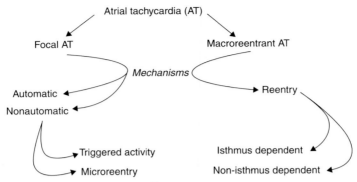

Fig 5.5 Classification of atrial tachycardia.[12]

Table 5.1 Characteristics of the different mechanisms of focal AT

	Automatic AT	Triggered activity	Microreentrant AT
PES	No response	CL dependent	Reproducibly initiates and terminates AT
Isoproterenol for induction	Yes	No	No
Entrainment	No	No	Yes
Warm up cool down	Yes	No	No
Response to adenosine	No*	Yes	Yes
Response to propranolol, verapamil	Propranolol	Propranolol, verapamil	Verapamil
Vagal maneuvers	No response	Terminates AT	No response

PES, programmed electrical stimulation. *Yes if AT is induced by Isoproterenol. Major drawback of the above observations is the overlap of responses.

- Electrophysiologic mechanism of the atrial tachycardia can be reentry, abnormal automaticity or triggered activity (Table 5.1).
- Focal tachycardias are characterized by centrifugal spread of electrical impulse from a single focus.
- Activation covers less than 20% of the tachycardia cycle length (CL).
- Localization of the focal AT can be achieved by multielectrode catheters or point-to-point exploration of the atrium after regionalizing the focus.
- Some focal AT origin sites may produce misleading activation results. These sites include the following:
  1 Right superior pulmonary vein (RSPV) focus could be mistaken for superior right atrium (RA).
  2 Superior vena cava (SVC) focus may be mistaken for right AT.
  3 Focal AT arising from the left-hand side of the interatrial septum.
  4 Epicardial focus and Marshall's ligament. Tachycardia arising from these sites may be difficult to ablate due to epicardial origin and can be mistaken for tachycardia arising from the left pulmonary vein or atrial appendage.

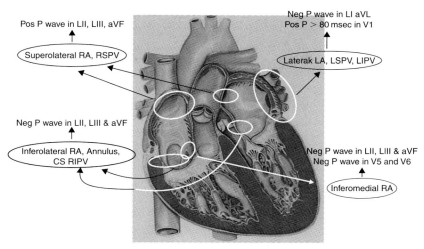

Pos P wave in LII, LIII, aVF
↑
Superolateral RA, RSPV

Neg P wave in LI aVL
Pos P > 80 msec in V1
↑
Laterak LA, LSPV, LIPV

Neg P wave in LII, LIII & aVF
↑
Inferolateral RA, Annulus, CS RIPV

Neg P wave in LII, LIII & aVF
Neg P wave in V5 and V6
↑
Inferomedial RA

Fig 5.6 Site of origin of focal AT and respective P wave morphology.

Clinical presentation[14]

- Patients present with palpitation, dyspnea, dizziness, or chest pain.
- Rapid firing of the focal AT may induce atrial fibrillation (AF), thus the patient may present with AF.

Electrocardiographic characteristics of the focal atrial tachycardia[15,16]

- In focal AT P waves are separated by an isoelectric line.
- P wave morphology may help identify the approximate origin of the AT (Fig. 5.6).
- The commonest location of right AT in patients with structurally normal heart is crista terminalis. P wave morphology is positive in LII, LIII, and aVF.
- The presence of anisotropy and automaticity in the cells of crista terminalis may facilitate the occurrence of the tachycardia in this location.
- Tachycardias arising from the atrio-ventricular (AV) annulus or coronary sinus (CS) os account for approximately 20% of all AT.

Ablation for atrial tachycardia[17–25]

- AT arising from the atrial septum (right or left) or triangle of Koch may require electrophysiologic study and multielectrode or three-dimensional (3D) mapping for precise localization prior to ablation.
- Dense mapping in the area of interest, using a 3D sequential mapping system, may help in precise localization of the focal AT. Incomplete mapping may result in erroneous results and failed ablation.
- If earliest activation appears to be on the right side of the interatrial septum but activation time from the onset of the P wave is less than 15 milliseconds, earliest site appears to be near Bachmann bundle, or a narrow monophasic P wave

is present in V1, consider further mapping on the left side of the interatrial septum.

- Tachycardia arising from the RSPV may be mistaken for right AT. When multiple sites in posterior superior RA register the same activation time, it is likely that the tachycardia is arising from RSPV.
- The presence of a diffuse area of activation near LSPV, LIPV, and the posterolateral mitral annulus may suggest an epicardial focus.
- Focal ablation site can be further confirmed by the presence of fractionated electrograms, negative unipolar atrial electrogram, or transient termination of the tachycardia during mechanical pressure from the ablation catheter.
- AT should be differentiated from AVRT and atypical AVNRT (Table 5.1 in Section 5.6).
- The target for ablation is the earliest activation preceding P wave by more than 30 milliseconds. Energy 30–50 W is delivered for 30–60 seconds.
- Acceleration of the tachycardia and termination within 10 seconds of radiofrequency (RF) application is a sign of a successful outcome.
- Ablation in the lateral wall of the RA, crista terminalis, may result in phrenic nerve damage.
- Ablation from the atrial septum, Koch's triangle carries the risk of AV block. Titrating energy delivery from 5 to 40 W and closely monitoring AV conduction may avoid occurrence of AV block.
- Ablation of the AT arising from the annulus requires documentation of the small A and larger V electrogram at the site of ablation.
- If ablating in venous structures, CS veins, SVC, lower power and temperature not exceeding 50°C may help avoid thrombus formation or stenosis.
- The success rate from RF ablation of the focal AT is 90% and the recurrence rate is 10%.
- Predictors of lower success rate or recurrences include:
  1 Left AT.
  2 Multiple focal origin.
  3 Older patients.

Macroreentrant atrial tachycardia[16–25]

- Macroreentrant tachycardia can be classified into isthmus or non-isthmus dependent type of AT (Fig. 5.7).

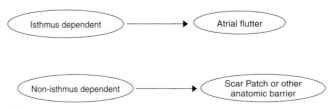

Fig 5.7 Classification macroreentrant AT

- Activation and recording of the fractionated electrograms identifies the area of slow conduction. (Please refer to Section 5.1.)
- Pacing for concealed entrainment from the isthmus at CL 30 milliseconds shorter than flutter CL results in acceleration of the tachycardia to pacing CL without any change in the morphology of the P waves, recorded on surface ECG. On termination of pacing, the post-pacing interval is the same as the tachycardia CL. The sensitivity and specificity of this maneuver for the diagnosis of reentrant isthmus dependent tachycardia is approximately 90%.

Entrainment mapping[18,23,25]

- Entrainment mapping can be used to determine if the tachycardia is originating from the RA or the left atrium (LA).
- If the PPI-TCL = <50 milliseconds in HRA and PCS then it is suggestive of right atrial flutter.
- If the PPI-TCL = <50 milliseconds in HRA but >50 milliseconds in PCS then it is suggestive of lateral RA tachycardia.
- If the PPI-TCL = >50 milliseconds in HRA and PCS then it is suggestive of left PV tachycardia.
- If the PPI-TCL = >50 milliseconds in HRA and <50 milliseconds in PCS and DCS consider left atrial flutter utilizing mitral annular isthmus.
- If the PPI-TCL = >50 milliseconds in HRA and <50 milliseconds in PCS and >50 milliseconds in DCS consider right PV or septal tachycardia.
- Computerized 3D mapping allows recording of the isochronal maps of the tachycardia circuit.
- Scar-related macroreentrant right ATs have been characterized as atypical atrial flutter.
- Scar-related AT may require higher energy and temperatures for successful ablation. This could be accomplished by a large/irrigated tip catheter.
- Combination of the electroanatomical and electrophysiologic mapping improves ablation outcome.
- As opposed to focal AT, atrial activation during macroreentrant tachycardia occupies 90% or more of the tachycardia CL. Earliest and latest activation tend to be adjacent.
- Left atrial macroreentrant tachycardia is characterized by the following:[16]
  1 Negative P waves in LI and aVL.
  2 Area of slow conduction between mitral annulus and anatomic barrier which could be pulmonary vein, scar, or atrial appendage.
  3 Post-pacing interval in the RA is >40 milliseconds longer than the tachycardia CL at three or more sites including cavotricuspid isthmus, thus excluding right atrial flutter or macroreentrant tachycardia.
  4 CL variation in the LA precedes the RA.
  5 Right atrial activation accounts for less than 50% of the tachycardia CL during sequential catheter mapping.

- Macroreentrant tachycardias are common after surgical repair procedures such as Mustard and Senning, Fontan or repair of tetralogy of Fallot.
- Identification and elimination of areas of slow conduction between the scars or scars and anatomical barriers is the preferred approach during RF ablation.
- Incisional (scar-related) reentry may occur following:
  1 Surgery for congenital heart disease.
  2 Partially successful Maze procedure.
  3 Catheter based ablation for AF.
- Following a patch repair of the ASD the isthmus for reentrant tachycardia may be between the patch and the CS.
- Atriotomy scar-related macroreentrant tachycardia may occur from the scar that extends from the atrial appendage to the inferoposterior right atrial free wall. Incision typically does not extend to IVC or TA producing a narrow isthmus.
- Entrainment with concealed fusion can be demonstrated from the entry, mid portion, or the exit site of this isthmus.
- Following observations are likely to identify the optimum site for successful ablation:
  1 PPI is the same as TCL.
  2 Earliest electrogram precedes the onset of surface P wave by more than 50 msec.
  3 On pacing from the site of the earliest electrogram, at cycle length 20 to 30 msec shorter, results in concealed entrainment.
  4 Interval from the electrogram to the onset of P wave is same as the interval from the stimulus to the onset of P wave. (Figs. 5.8 and 5.9.)
- Electroanatomical mapping can identify activation pattern, scar by using voltage map, and sites for ablation.

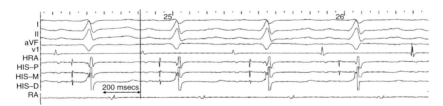

Fig 5.8 Electrogram to onset of P wave 200 milliseconds.

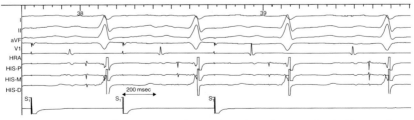

Fig 5.9 Stimulus to onset of P wave 200 milliseconds. Tachycardia is entrained without a change in activation or P wave morphology.

5.3 ATRIAL FIBRILLATION

Mechanism, pathophysiology, and classification of atrial fibrillation[26-28]

- Atrial fibrillation (AF) is the most common chronic rhythm disorder1, affecting 5% of adults over age 65. AF occurs in 40% of the patients suffering from congestive heart failure (CHF).
- Mortality in patients with AF is twice as high when compared with patients in sinus rhythm.
- AF could be due to persistent rapid firing from the single focus termed as focal driver or it could be maintained by multiple wavelets after being initiated by premature atrial beats called focal triggers.
- These episodes of paroxysmal focal AF tend to occur in young patients without structural heart disease and are often preceded by frequent premature atrial contractions (PACs) of short coupling interval.
- Factors affecting the conduction and refractoriness in the atrium such as inflammation, fibrosis, and ischemia are conducive to initiation and maintenance of AF.

AF can be classified into the following categories:
1 Paroxysmal AF: starts and stops spontaneously.
2 Persistent AF: requires electrical or pharmacologic cardioversion to terminate an episode.
3 Chronic AF: persists in spite of therapeutic intervention or based on a decision not to restore sinus rhythm.
- Lone AF can either be paroxysmal, persistent, or chronic. It is defined as AF occurring in patients less than 60 years of age who have no associated cardiovascular diseases.
- Paroxysmal AF often progresses to chronic AF. Conversion and maintenance of sinus rhythm becomes increasingly difficult with chronic AF.
- Chemical and electrical cardioversion for maintenance of sinus rhythm is easier in AF of short duration.

During chronic AF the following structural and electrical changes may occur:
1 Atrial dilatation.
2 Apoptosis, resulting in loss of myofibrils.
3 Fibrosis, which alters conduction velocity.
4 There may be reduction in Connexion 43.

Shortening of the atrial refractory period occurs for the following reasons:
- A rapid atrial rate induces atrial ischemia, which results in shortening of the atrial refractory period. Inhibitors of Na/H exchanger abolish ischemia-induced shortening of the refractory period.
- There is a decrease in sodium channel density and current.
- Increase in the intracellular calcium load shortens the refractory period.

- Rate adaptation of the refractory period is lost.
- In AF I_{CaL} is reduced. This results in shortening of action potential duration (APD) and refractory period.
- Shortening of the refractory period may persist after recovery from AF and predispose one to reoccurrences.
- Atrial dilatation and stretch may result in a decrease in the refractory period.
- Shortening of the effective refractory period (ERP) and APD and an increase in dispersion of refractoriness perpetuates AF.
- Human atrial repolarization uses I_{KUR}. I_{to} and I_{KUR} are decreased in AF, resulting in shortening of the refractory period.

Neurohumoral changes during AF:
- Atrial natriuretic factor increases due to atrial stretch and dilation.
- Elevated ANF decreases after cardioversion.
- ANF may shorten the atrial refractory period.

Clinical presentation

- Most common symptoms are fatigue, reduced exercise tolerance, dyspnea, and palpitation, although most episodes of AF remain asymptomatic.
- Tachycardia from AF can exacerbate angina or CHF.
- Irregular rhythm is consistent with but not diagnostic of AF. Other conditions, such as sinus rhythm with frequent supraventricular or ventricular ectopic beats, sinus arrhythmia, or multifocal atrial tachycardia, can cause irregular pulse. An ECG is necessary to confirm the diagnosis. The absence of P waves is characteristic of AF. Extremely rapid ventricular response may appear regular.
- AF with rapid ventricular response and aberrant ventricular conduction can result in a wide complex tachycardia which may be mistaken for ventricular tachycardia.[6]

Treatment[29–34]

- If the patient is hemodynamically unstable immediate cardioversion should be considered.
- Rate control can be achieved by AV node (AVN) blocking drugs.
- Digoxin is least effective in controlling the rate especially in physically active patients.
- β-Blockers and/or calcium channel blockers are effective AVN blocking agents.
- Calcium channel blockers are preferred in patients with bronchial asthma. The aim should be to achieve a ventricular response between 80 and 100 bpm.
- AVN blocking agents should be avoided in the presence of ventricular preexcitation. Amiodarone could be used in this setting because it prolongs the refractory period of accessory pathway.
- The duration of AF and risk factors for thromboembolic complication determine the need for anticoagulation. AF increases the risk of stroke by 8-fold.

Risk factors for thromboembolic events in the presence of AF include:
1 Age >65 years.
2 Hypertension.
3 LVF.
4 Enlarged left atrium (LA).
5 Diabetes mellitus.
6 History of TIA.
7 Valvular heart disease.

Evidence that anticoagulation with warfarin prevents thromboembolic complication is supported by the following studies.

1. Benefit of anticoagulation versus placebo: SPAF trial
• It was concluded that aspirin or warfarin significantly reduces events when compared with a placebo. SPAF is not a comparison of aspirin with warfarin.
• Retrospective analysis suggested a lack of benefit of anticoagulation for patients younger than 60 years.

2. Benefit of warfarin over aspirin: Atrial Fibrillation, Aspirin, Anticoagulation (AFASAK) trial
• There was a substantial reduction of thromboembolic events with warfarin versus aspirin or placebo (2% per year versus 5.5% per year).
• There was no significant difference in mortality. The bleeding rates were 6% per year with warfarin and 1% per year with aspirin or placebo.
• This study supported the conclusion that warfarin is superior to aspirin and placebo in preventing thromboembolic events among a largely elderly population.

3. The Boston Area Anticoagulation Trial for Atrial Fibrillation (BAATAF)
• There was a significant reduction in events in the warfarin-treated group (0.4% per year versus 2.98% per year in the control group, an overall 86% reduction).
• Increased mortality was noted in the control group.
• There was no significant difference in bleeding events.
• It was concluded that warfarin is superior to placebo in reducing thromboembolic events and mortality.

4. SPAF-II trial
• SPAF-II demonstrated higher event rates in high-risk patients over 75 years old. This is reduced with warfarin anticoagulation.
• Increased risk for bleeding was noted.

5. Aspirin in low-risk patients: SPAF-III trial
• SPAF III supports the use of aspirin for thromboembolic prophylaxis in low risk patients and suggests that patients with prior hypertension may be at sufficient risk to justify anticoagulation with warfarin.

Rate control versus rhythm control[35–37]

- The issue of treating patients with AF with rate control agents versus using anti-arrhythmic drugs to maintain sinus rhythm has been addressed by two clinical trials.

AFFIRM

- The Atrial Fibrillation Follow-up Investigation of Rhythm Management (AFFIRM) trial: Patients were randomized between a strategy of rate control with β blockers and calcium channel blockers targeted to a resting heart rate of 80 bpm versus rhythm control using anti-arrhythmic drugs.
- There was a non-significant trend toward higher total mortality in the rhythm control group, the study's primary endpoint.
- Pre-specified subgroup analysis demonstrated a statistically significant mortality benefit with rate control for patients above the age of 65. There was no significant difference in the incidence of stroke (roughly 1% per year); the majority (73%) of ischemic strokes occurred in patients who had discontinued warfarin or had an INR < 2.0.
- These findings support the recommendation that anticoagulation be continued in patients even if AF is successfully suppressed.
- AFFIRM demonstrated no advantage to a rhythm control strategy for recurrent AF, and suggests a rate control strategy may be superior in patients above the age of 65.
- Patients enrolled in this study were minimally symptomatic.
- These results do not apply to patients with symptomatic AF.
- Higher mortality in rhythm control group may be due to proarrhythmic effects of antiarrhythmic drugs rather than due to maintenance of sinus rhythm.

RACE

- The RACE (Rate Control versus Electrical Cardioversion for Persistent Atrial Fibrillation).
- No significant difference in cardiovascular death or thromboembolic events was noted, but 83% of all thromboembolic events occurred in patients who had discontinued warfarin or had an INR <2.0.
- The study demonstrated no significant advantage to a rhythm control strategy for the management of persistent AF. Any benefits derived by rhythm control may have been neutralized by the proarrhythmic effects of the antiarrhythmic drugs.
  1 A rate control strategy is an acceptable approach to management of patients with AF, particularly if they are asymptomatic and elderly.
  2 Rhythm control should be reserved for patients with symptomatic AF. This strategy should also be considered in minimally symptomatic young patients with AF.

Anticoagulation for conversion to sinus rhythm
- If AF is of less than 48 hours' duration, cardioversion can be attempted.
- The presence of AF for more than 48 hours necessitates three to four weeks of therapeutic anticoagulation prior to conversion, unless transesophageal echocardiography (TEE) demonstrates absence of clot in the LA and its appendage.
- Regardless of whether a TEE is performed, systemic anticoagulation is required for three weeks following cardioversion in all patients with AF of greater than 48 hours' duration.

The ACUTE trial[38]
- Patients were assigned to TEE followed by DC cardioversion (if no intracardiac clot was found) versus conventional therapy consisting of three weeks of anticoagulation before DC cardioversion.
- All subjects (TEE group and conventional therapy group) received therapeutic anticoagulation for four weeks after cardioversion.
- At eight weeks (from the time of enrollment), there was no significant difference in primary endpoint of cerebrovascular accident, TIA, and peripheral embolus.
- Fewer bleeding events were noted in the TEE group.
- The risk of thromboembolic events is higher in the first three to four weeks immediately following conversion to sinus rhythm.
- This may be due to atrial stunning, a term describing the observation of reduced atrial systolic function following conversion to sinus rhythm.
- Atrial stunning can allow relative stasis of blood within the atrium, potentially resulting in thrombus formation.
- Patients should receive anticoagulation with warfarin for three weeks following conversion to sinus rhythm even if they are in a low risk category for thromboembolic events.
- Patients with the indications for chronic anticoagulation with warfarin mentioned above (valvular heart disease, age above 65, prior thromboembolic event, hypertension, heart failure, coronary artery disease, or diabetes) should receive long-term anticoagulation following cardioversion.

DC cardioversion[39,40]
- Emergent electrical cardioversion is indicated if the patient is hemodynamically unstable as a result of tachycardia.
- Cardioversion can either be performed with a standard monophasic or biphasic defibrillator. If a standard defibrillator fails, cardioversion should be repeated using a biphasic defibrillator.

Rectilinear biphasic defibrillation
- During biphasic defibrillation there is a change in the polarity of the waveform during delivery of energy.

- Biphasic defibrillation allows for similar current delivery (which is the most important variable for achieving cardioversion) with lower energy.
- The number of shocks required to achieve cardioversion is also reduced.
- Biphasic defibrillation is superior to monophasic defibrillation.

Chemical cardioversion[3]

- Ibutilide: Class III anti-arrhythmic can be used for cardioversion alone or as an adjuvant to facilitate DC cardioversion, particularly when initial DC cardioversion is unsuccessful.
- Ibutilide is administered intravenously 1 mg over 10 minutes.
- Ten to fifteen percent of the patients with new onset AF may convert to sinus rhythm with ibutilide alone.
- When cardioversion is performed after the administration of ibutilide, the success rate may approach 100% and the amount of energy required may also be less.
- Patients should be monitored for 4 hours after administration of ibutilide.
- Risk factors for ibutilide induced ventricular arrhythmias include prolonged QT, depressed left ventricular function (ejection fraction <0.30), hypokalemia, or hypomagnesemia.

Maintenance of sinus rhythm[41–44]

- Anti-arrhythmic therapy is indicated for patients with symptomatic AF.
- Rate control alone can be used for elderly minimally symptomatic patients.
- For moderate to severe left ventricular systolic dysfunction the agent of choice is amiodarone. Dofetilide can be used.
- All other antiarrhythmics are relatively contraindicated in patients with LV dysfunction because of the potential for proarrhythmias.
- For patients with ischemic heart disease and preserved left ventricular systolic function, sotalol may be useful because of its β-blocker effects.
- Disopyramide can be used in patients suspected of having AF due to increased vagal tone.
- Class IC agents such as flecainide and propafenone can be used in patients without ischemic heart disease and normal LV wall thickness and function.
- These agents can be administered daily for maintenance of sinus rhythm.
- They can also be used on an as needed basis for acute conversion of symptomatic paroxysmal AF.
- 300 mg of Flecainide or 600 mg of propafenone can be administered orally.
- β-Blocker or calcium channel blocker should be administered 30–60 minutes prior to administration of the anti-arrhythmic agent to prevent accelerated AV conduction.
- The first trial of this approach should be performed while the patient is being monitored.
- Treatment of lone AF with Class IC agents can result in conversion to atrial flutter because of prolongation of the atrial refractory period and slowing of conduction velocity.

- This "Class IC atrial flutter" can be treated with ablation of the right atrial cavotricuspid isthmus followed by continuation of the AAD.[45]
- Class III agents include amiodarone, sotalol, and dofetilide.

Amiodarone

- Evidence supporting the efficacy of amiodarone comes from the Canadian Trial of Atrial Fibrillation (CTAF) trial.
- At 1 year follow-up, 69% of patients treated with amiodarone were in sinus rhythm compared with 39% of individuals treated with sotalol or propafenone.
- Amiodarone was associated with a higher discontinuation rate due to side effects that was not statistically significant.
- There was no significant difference in total mortality between the groups.
- Amiodarone has multiple adverse reactions; patients receiving amiodarone need monitoring of pulmonary function tests (carbon monoxide diffusion test), thyroid function, liver function, and ocular examination for corneal deposits.
- Although there is no FDA indication for amiodarone in AF this is a most commonly prescribed anti-arrhythmic agent for treatment of AF.
- Amiodarone can be initiated as an outpatient, usually at 400 mg per day for a period of two to four weeks, then decreasing the dose to 200 mg per day.

Dofetilide

- It requires in-hospital initiation and monitoring for arrhythmias.
- Safety of dofetilide in patients with heart failure is supported by the Danish Investigations of Arrhythmia and Mortality on Dofetilide in Congestive Heart Failure (DIAMOND-CHF) Study. Patients with left ventricular ejection fractions <35% were enrolled. The dofetilide dose was 500 μg BID. It was adjusted to 250 μg BID for creatinine clearances between 40–60 ml/min and 250 μg QD for patients with creatinine clearance of <40 ml/min. Patients with creatinine clearance of less than 20 ml/min were excluded.
- There was no significant difference in total mortality. Retrospective analysis of the results demonstrated that 12% of patients with AF in the treatment arm converted to sinus rhythm, compared with 1% in the placebo arm, with a significant reduction in the subsequent development of AF.

Sotalol

- It should not be given to patients with renal dysfunction, left ventricular hypertrophy, prolonged QT intervals, bradycardia, or electrolyte abnormalities (hypokalemia).
- Nodally active agents should be stopped or decreased before initiation of sotalol because of the risk of bradycardia from β-blocking properties seen at 40 mg bid. The Class III anti-arrhythmic effect (action potential prolongation) appears at 120–160 mg bid.
- Sotalol should be initiated in hospital while monitoring for proarrhythmias and prolongation of the QT interval.

- Sotalol can be administered as follows:
  1 80 mg tid for 1 day.
  2 Then 120 mg bid on the second day.
  3 Then 160 mg bid on the third day.
  4 Discharge on 120 mg bid, with increase to 160 mg bid if needed.

Nonpharmacologic options in the management of AF

Radiofrequency (RF) ablation[46–51]

- Arrhythmias are produced by abnormality of impulse generation or impulse propagation. RF ablation seeks to eliminate these abnormalities.
- When RF current passes through the tissue it produces heat, which is proportional to the power density within tissue. It is an alternating current.
- Maximum heating occurs at the tip of the electrode and it diminishes as the distance from the tip increases. Increase in the radius (distance) from the tip will decrease the heat by 4-fold. For this reason the depth and the volume of the tissue that is affected by heat is small (2 mm). Deeper tissue heating is due to heat conduction.
- Commonly used RF is 300–1000 kHz. Lower frequency may produce muscle stimulation. At higher frequency mode of heating changes from resistive to dielectric.
- RF energy is delivered in a unipolar fashion from the catheter tip to the dispersive patch electrode placed on the skin.
- The surface area of catheter electrode is 12 mm^2 and the surface area of the patch electrode is 100–250 cm.^{2} This results in an increase in power density and heating at the catheter tip.
- Catheter tip electrodes with a large surface area or when the catheter tip is cooled by irrigation allows lower system impedance and delivery of higher power. This results in deeper and larger lesion. Since the temperature is measured at the catheter tip it does not reflect actual tissue temperature, which may be very high.
- Very high tissue temperature results in heat expansion of the tissue, crater formation and may produce tissue pop.
- RF energy delivery should be at least for 60 seconds.
- Rise in temperature at deeper tissue level may continue if high power or temperature settings are used, producing thermal latency even after termination of energy delivery.
- RF generated heat produces coagulation necrosis of the myocytes. Healing by fibrosis is complete by eight weeks.

Radiofrequency ablation for AF

- This procedure is typically reserved for patients with lone or paroxysmal AF who have failed one or more trials of anti-arrhythmic therapy.
- AF can be cured with catheter ablation techniques.

- The best results of this procedure (up to 85% success) have been achieved in patients with lone AF. Lower success rates (50–70%) have been reported in other subsets of AF patients.
- Potential complications of this procedure include pulmonary vein stenosis, stroke, LA esophageal fistula, and pericardial tamponade.
- The approach to AF ablation could be classified as elimination of the triggers, substrate, or autonomic facilitators (parasympathetic ganglion).

Elimination of the triggers
- It was noted that the AF is initiated by rapidly firing triggers located in pulmonary veins.
- This may manifest as frequent PACs or clearly discernible atrial activity in the form of atrial tachycardia at the onset of AF or during AF.
- These foci arise from the myocardial muscular sleeve that extends few centimeters into the pulmonary veins.
- Initial approaches included identification of PACs with earliest activation and elimination of these foci within the pulmonary vein. A possible risk of pulmonary vein stenois shifted the focus to ablation outside the orifice of the pulmonary vein in a quadrantic fashion.

Pulmonary vein isolation using RF ablation in LA
- In this approach an attempt is made to isolate all the four pulmonary vein orifices from the LA. It reduces the probability of the pulmonary vein stenosis.
- The rationale is that PACs (triggers) could arise from any of the four pulmonary veins.
- It may also produce compartmentalization and "debulking" of the LA.
- The drawback of this approach includes reoccurrences, creation of the isthmus that may predispose to atrial tachycardia.
- Esophageal perforation following posteromedial left atrial or right superior pulmonary vein ablation may occur. This is a serious and often fatal complication.

Elimination of the substrate
- Identification and elimination of the fractionated electrograms may result in termination of the AF during the procedure. A success rate of 80% has been reported.
- Fractionated electrograms may be recorded from the LA around the pulmonary veins, left atrial appendage or interatrial septum. In the right atrium (RA) the fractionated electrograms could be recorded from the crista terminalis, the orifices of the vena cava, the orifice of the coronary sinus (CS), or up to 2–3 cm within the CS.
- Like pulmonary veins, muscular extension into proximal CS may produce rapidly firing automatic foci responsible for initiating AF.

Modification of the autonomic substrate

- The posterior wall of the LA is richly innervated by vagal (parasympathetic) fibers.
- Parasympathetic stimulation produces bradycardia and shortening of the atrial refractory period. These electrophysiologic changes are conducive to initiation and maintenance of AF, termed as vagally induced AF.
- Vagally induced AF occurs during sleep and may be responsible for the atrial arrhythmias that occur during sleep apnea.
- During ablation of the vagal neural terminals, located in the posterior wall of the LA, bradycardia, or junctional rhythm may occur.
- It may be necessary to tailor these three approaches when using ablation as the therapeutic modality in the management of AF. For example, a paroxysmal AF in a young patient with a structurally normal heart where focal tachycardia or premature beats are identified as the initiator of the AF may benefit from elimination of that focus.

Atrioventricular node ablation with permanent pacemaker implantation[52]

- Patients with left ventricular dysfunction or chronic pulmonary disease or those who cannot tolerate the doses of AVN blocking agents necessary to achieve rate control or the agents for rhythm control may be candidates for this approach.
- AVN blocking agents may produce negative inotropic effects or bronchospasm in these patients.
- The overall survival of patients undergoing AVN ablation and pacemaker insertion is the same as a matched group of patients treated with antiarrhythmic drugs.
- The drawback of AVN ablation and the pacemaker approach include persistence of AF, need for anticoagulation, pacemaker dependence and ventricular dys-synchrony from RV pacing.
- AVN ablation should rarely be performed in young patients with AF.

Electrical therapies for AF

- In patients who have or need pacemaker for other indications, programming to eliminate PACs or abolish post-PAC pauses may decrease the burden of AF.
- Defibrillators with atrial arrhythmia therapy options such as high frequency pacing at 50 Hz and cardioversion may decrease the frequency and duration of the AF. These features can be set to automatically cardiovert the patient upon detection of AF using specified criteria or it can be triggered by the patient or the physician.[67]
- Defibrillator with atrial therapy features is implanted in patients who are undergoing ICD implant and also have paroxysmal AF.

Surgical Maze procedure

- Incisions are made in the LA around the pulmonary veins, posterior wall and extended to the mitral annulus.
- This procedure can be performed in conjunction with other cardiac surgery such as mitral valve replacement. Success rates are approximately 80–90%.
- The epicardial approach, using minimally invasive thoracotomy and microwave, attempts to isolate the pulmonary veins.

5.4 AUTOMATIC JUNCTIONAL TACHYCARDIA

Junctional tachycardia[53,54]

- Automatic junctional tachycardia (AJT) is common in infants. It carries high mortality.
- In older patients it has a more benign course and is not associated with structural heart disease.
- AJT arises from transitional cells of atrio-ventricular (AV) junction and is due to abnormal automaticity. Tachycardia is sensitive to catecholamines.
- Electrocardiogram shows narrow QRS (wide if bundle branch block present) tachycardia. Ventriculo atrial (VA) block may be present. Sinus capture beats may occur.
- AJT is often irregular and may be mistaken for atrial fibrillation or multifocal atrial tachycardia.
- If the QRS is wide it may be mistaken for ventricular tachycardia.
- Intra-cardiac electrograms show that each QRS is preceded by His and a normal HV interval.
- Initiation termination is spontaneous without critical AH delay.
- AV dissociation is common. The tachycardia is unaffected by atrial or ventricular pacing.
- AJT should be differentiated from non-paroxysmal junctional tachycardia (NPJT), which tends to be slower and regular. It occurs in the setting of digitalis toxicity, COPD, myocardial ischemia, carditis, and post cardiac surgery.
- NPJT is believed to be due to triggered activity.
- To differentiate AJT from AV node re-entry tachycardia (AVNRT), premature atrial beats are delivered in the region of slow pathway when septal A is committed. This will advance His in AVNRT but not in AJT.
- AVNRT is initiated by premature atrial contraction (PAC), needs critical AH interval and demonstrates dual AV nodal physiology.
- Orthodromic nodofescicular tachycardia is often initiated by PACs or premature ventricular contractions (PVCs), demonstrates preexcitation during atrial pacing, occurrence of bundle branch block results in a change in CL and advancement of next His or termination of tachycardia with PVC delivered when His is refractory.

Treatment

- In young patients AVN blocking drugs are ineffective. Amiodarone may be more effective.
- Abrupt onset of AV block may occur. Insertion of permanent pacemaker is recommended.
- If drug therapy fails ablation at the site of earliest activation along the septum or AVN ablation and insertion of permanent pacemaker could be considered.
- In adult patients β-blockers may be effective.
- AJT may occur following surgery for congenital heart disease. It may last for 1–4 days after surgery.
- The use of inotropic agents, such as catecholamines and digoxin, may induce AJT.
- It responds well to IV propafenone, procainamide, or amiodarone.

5.5 AV NODE REENTRY TACHYCARDIAS

AV node reentry tachycardia[55–59]

- Dual atrio-ventricular (AV) nodal physiology is defined as 50 milliseconds increase in A2H2 for a 10 milliseconds decrease in A1A2.
- Fast and slow pathways represent different atrionodal connection as suggested by different sites of earliest retrograde activation during tachycardia or retrograde conduction during ventricular pacing.
- Resetting of the tachycardia by late premature atrial contraction (PAC) delivered outside the AV node (AVN) near the posterior right atrial septum or coronary sinus (CS) also suggests the presence of reentrant loop.

Fast pathway

- Retrograde earliest atrial activation during atrio-ventricular reentry tachycardia (AVNRT) suggesting a fast pathway insertion site is located 5 mm posterior and 8 mm superior to His bundle electrogram recording. Atrial electrogram at this site may precede atrial activation on His electrogram by 10–20 milliseconds. This site is located superior to tendon of Todaro outside the triangle of Koch.
- Retrograde fast pathway activation at the posterior superior right atrial septum may demonstrate two components. Initial low frequency component reflects far field atrial potential from the left-hand side of the septum.
- Application of radiofrequency (RF) current superior to tendon of Todaro will eliminate antegrade fast pathway conduction.
- The right side component of the fast pathway begins in the anterior limbus of the fossa ovalis, as atrial cell then becomes a transitional cell on crossing the tendon of Todaro and inserts into the common AV bundle distal to the compact AVN.

- This distal insertion may explain why the fast pathway has less decremental properties, is less responsive to AVN blocking agents and has greater response to sodium channel blocking agents.
- During decremental atrial pacing block in the fast pathway occurs proximally, closer to the anterior limbus of the fossa ovalis.

Slow pathway
- It is located in the posterior septum between the tricuspid annulus and the CS ostium.
- The SP connects to the posterior extension of the AVN.
- Retrograde slow pathway activation proceeds from the proximal CS to the left atrium (LA) and across the septum to the right atrium (RA). From here it proceeds anteriorly towards the His bundle and posteriorly behind the CS ostium and the Eustachian ridge.
- CS musculature electrically connects the RA and the LA.
- The Eustachian valve and ridge form a line of block that confines SP potential/impulse to within the triangle of Koch. This may allow dissociation of slow pathway potential from the right atrial electrograms.
- This line of block may explain the late occurrence of SP potential during sinus rhythm when compared with atrial electrogram at His location.
- In sinus rhythm slow pathway activation proceeds from posterior to anterior in the area of the triangle of Koch.
- During SP ablation accelerated junctional rhythm occurs with retrograde conduction over the fast pathway.
- There may be multiple slow pathways with multiple jumps in the AH interval.
- Linear ablation from the tricuspid annulus to the CS ostium is likely to eliminate most of the SP conduction.
- After slow pathway ablation the presence of A2H2 jump and echo beat may indicate the presence of additional SP, which may enter the triangle of Koch anterior to the CS ostium. These slow pathways may not be capable of causing arrhythmias.
- 84% of patients without a history of AVNRT demonstrated dual AV nodal physiology.
- This may be due to sedation with midazolam and fentanyl, which depresses antegrade and retrograde conduction over the fast pathway, thus allowing SP conduction to become manifest.
- Isoproterenol speeds up conduction in the fast pathway.
- Equal delay in conduction over the slow and the fast pathways may mask dual AV nodal physiology.
- A2H2 greater than 200 milliseconds may suggest conduction over SP.
- A shift in retrograde conduction from fast to slow will change the atrial activation sequence.

Common or typical AVNRT

- During tachycardia antegrade conduction is over the slow pathway and retrograde conduction over the fast pathway.
- It is induced by PAC and rarely by premature ventricular contraction (PVC).
- An abrupt increase in AH by 50 milliseconds with PAC before induction is common.
- Lack of increase in the AH interval may be due to equal delay in conduction in both pathways.
- AH during tachycardia usually exceeds 200 milliseconds.
- The HA interval is short, <50 milliseconds.
- Earliest retrograde atrial activation is superior to tendon of Todaro, suggestive of retrograde fast pathway activation.
- A short HA interval results in the superimposition of P waves on the QRS, thus obscuring P waves on the surface electrocardiogram. This may result in a pseudo R wave in V1 or pseudo S in inferior leads (Fig. 5.10a and 5.10b).
- During tachycardia, if there is simultaneous activation of the atrium and ventricles, late PVC may separate atrial and the ventricular potentials and help identify the atrial activation sequence.
- The reentry circuit between the atrial ends of the fast and the slow pathways includes a large atrial component. This may explain extremely rare VA block to the atrium during AVNRT.
- Late PAC delivered to the atrium that is incorporated in the tachycardia circuit may advance next His and reset tachycardia. PACs should be late and reach after retrograde earliest activation by the fast pathway.
- Post-pacing interval (stimulus to next A) may be longer than the tachycardia CL due to delay in AVN.
- Resetting with the shortest post pacing interval occurs from the posteroseptal RA and the proximal CS.
- Retrograde activation of the atrial septum occurs through the fast pathway, the impulse then propagates along the left-hand side of the interatrial septum to the proximal CS, the CS ostium, and the posterior end of the slow pathway.
- During decremental RV pacing there is little decremental conduction in the lower common pathway.
- The HA interval during tachycardia reflects retrograde conduction over the fast pathway minus simultaneous antegrade conduction over the lower common pathway. The HA interval during V pacing reflects retrograde conduction time over the lower common pathway and the fast pathway.
- HA during tachycardia tends to be shorter than during RV pacing.
- To record retrograde His, RV pacing should be performed near the anterobasal RV septum close to right bundle.
- In the left-sided variant of S/F AVNRT the slow pathway is located in the posterior mitral annulus. These patients tend to have a short HA interval of less than 15 milliseconds. This may be due to the longer lower common pathway.

(a)

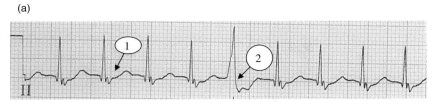

(b)

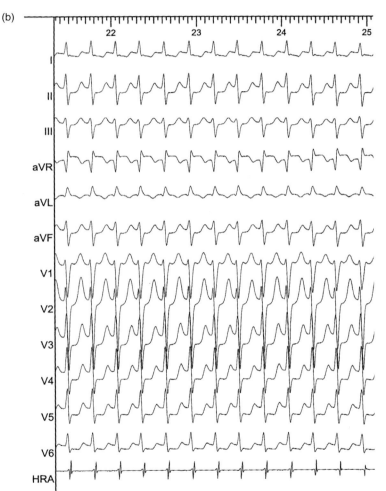

Fig 5.10 (a) AVNRT: spontaneously occurring PVC (2) does not reset the tachycardia. P waves (1) are noted in the terminal portion of the QRS. (b) Simultaneous activation of the atrium and the ventricles results in superimposition of P and QRS. P wave location is evident by simultaneous recording of atrial electrograms.

- During the onset of AVNRT, block below the AVN may occur, resulting in 2 : 1 conduction.
- Two for 1 phenomenon may occur during programmed atrial stimulation, when there is antegrade conduction of the atrial impulse once through the fast pathway and the same impulse conducts through the slow pathway, resulting in two ventricular electrograms for each atrial electrogram. This may indicate absence of retrograde penetration of the slow pathway by the antegrade fast pathway (Fig. 5.11).

Slow/slow (S/S) AVNRT

- During this tachycardia antegrade conduction is through the slow pathway as manifested by a long AH interval (240 milliseconds or more). Retrograde conduction is through slow pathway with earliest atrial activation at posteroseptal RA between the tricuspid annulus and the CS ostium or within the CS. This atrial activation may precede atrial activation in His electrogram by 30–60 milliseconds.
- The VA interval is long and may exceed 70 milliseconds.
- There may be multiple jumps in A2H2 during programmed atrial stimulation indicative of multiple slow pathways. There may be multiple HA intervals during tachycardia.
- Half of these patients may have S/F AVNRT.
- During ventricular pacing retrograde atrial activation may shift from the anterior to the posterior atrial septum, indicating the shift in conduction from the fast to the slow pathway.
- Tachycardia may be induced by programmed ventricular stimulation, resulting in a block in the retrograde fast pathway and retrograde conduction over the slow pathway.

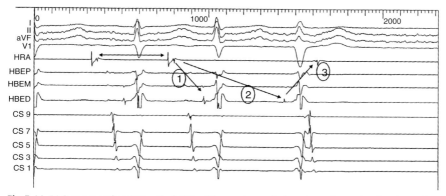

Fig 5.11 PAC at a coupling interval of 440 milliseconds results in antegrade conduction through the fast pathway (1) followed by antegrade conduction through the slow pathway (2) thus producing two QRS complexes for a single PAC. The same impulse then conducts retrogradely through the fast pathway (3).

- S/S AVNRT has a longer lower common pathway, which is located posteriorly.
- HA during ventricular pacing tends to be longer than HA during tachycardia in patients with S/S AVNRT.
- The HA interval represents retrograde conduction over the slow pathway minus antegrade conduction over the lower common pathway. Because of the longer lower common pathway the HA interval may be short or negative during S/S AVNRT.
- Fast pathway ablation will not eliminate S/S AVNRT.
- The reoccurrence rate is higher after ablation in patients with S/S AVNRT and may require more extensive ablation in the posteroseptal RA and the CS ostium.

Fast/slow or uncommon type of AVNRT

- It is characterized by a short AH (30–180 milliseconds) and a long HA interval (260 milliseconds).
- Antegrade conduction is over the fast pathway and retrograde conduction over the slow pathway.
- Earliest retrograde atrial activation is in the posteroseptal RA or the CS ostium.
- On the surface electrocardiogram the RP interval is longer than the PR interval. P waves are inverted in the inferior leads.
- On termination of the V pacing, where V pacing has successfully entrained AVNRT, post-pacing interval minus tachycardia cycle length (PPI–TCL) of >120 milliseconds and Stim to A minus VA interval of >85 milliseconds suggests the diagnosis of atypical AVNRT and excludes the diagnosis of AVRT utilizing septal accessory pathway (Fig. 5.12).

Differential diagnosis of AVNRT (Table 5.1)

- Single late PVC is delivered 50 milliseconds after the onset of His electrogram and advanced by 10 milliseconds without retrogradely activating His. Advancing of atrial activation without first retrogradely activating the His will suggest the presence of accessory pathway.

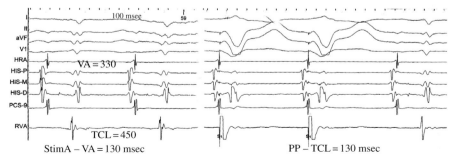

Fig 5.12 Atypical AVNRT response to ventricular pacing.

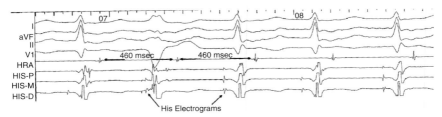

Fig 5.13 His synchronous PVC does not reset atrial electrogram.

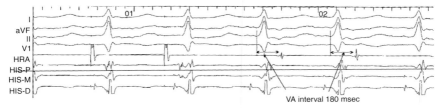

Fig 5.14 Termination of A pacing first VA is similar to subsequent VA intervals.

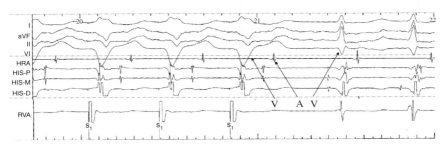

Fig 5.15 Termination of V pacing response is VAV.

- Atrial activation sequence remains unchanged and may advance next His electrogram. In AVNRT His synchronous PVC fails to advance atrial electrogram (Fig. 5.13).
- PVCs during supraventricular tachycardia (SVT) should be delivered at the base of right ventricular septum for posteroseptal accessory pathway (AP) and in parahisian location for anteroseptal AP.
- On termination of atrial pacing the first VA is identical to subsequent VA (Fig. 5.14) and on termination of V pacing the response is VAV (Fig. 5.15). These observations make the diagnosis of atrial tachycardia (AT) unlikely.
- Parahisian pacing is performed during sinus rhythm from the anterobasal right ventricle, anterior and apical to His recording, where high output captures the His, resulting in a narrow QRS and timing of His is advanced. At lower output His RB capture is lost, resulting in a wide QRS and delay in the timing of atrial

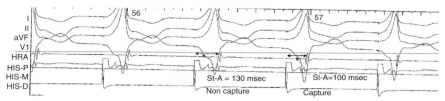

Fig 5.16 Parahisian pacing: stimulus to A is shorter during His capture.

activation (equal to the delay in His activation) without a change in activation sequence. This suggests conduction over the AVN (Fig. 5.16).
- With loss of HB RB capture, absence of change in the timing and sequence of atrial activation suggests conduction over AP.

Treatment
- For immediate termination of the tachycardia, vegal maneuvers, IV adenosine; calcium channel blockers or β-blockers can be used.
- Ablation of the slow pathway is the treatment of choice.

Ablation for AVNRT
- The preferred site of ablation for AVNRT is the slow pathway, which is located in the triangle of Koch.
- The boundaries of the triangle of Koch are delineated by CS ostium, tendon of Tedaro posteriorly, and septal leaflet of the tricuspid valve anteriorly and bundle of His at the apex of the triangle.
- Mean distance from His bundle to the mid-portion of the anterior lip of the CS ostium is 15–20 mm.
- The fast pathway is located anteriorly in close proximity to His bundle. The slow pathway is located posteriorly near the CS ostium.
- Discrete potentials noted in the posteroseptal RA may be due to anisotropic conduction and not due to activation of the slow pathway.
- Ablation of the slow pathway can be achieved by anatomic or electrogram approach or a combination of both.
- Area of interest is identified on fluoroscopic examination between His bundle electrogram and the CS ostium along the posteromedial aspect of TA. Multipolar electrograms are recorded at this site. The AV electrogram ratio should be less than 0.5.
- Electrogram and anatomic approaches should be combined to achieve successful ablation.
- The majority of successful ablation sites are located between TA and CS ostium. Other sites include within the CS ostium or inferior or the superior lip of the CS ostium.
- Unsuccessful ablation is the result of imprecise mapping or inadequate tissue contact and heating.

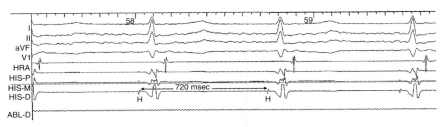

Fig 5.17 Junctional rhythm during RF application to the slow pathway.

- Target temperature should be 45–50°C. Slow junctional rhythm that may last for 15–20 seconds may occur (Fig. 5.17).
- If junctional rhythm does not occur within 20 seconds of achieving target temperature RF application should be terminated.
- Complete AV block may occur in 1% of patients, undergoing slow pathway ablation.
- Monitoring VA conduction during junctional rhythm or prolongation of the PR interval should be performed.
- Complete AV block is unlikely to occur in the presence of intact VA conduction during junctional rhythm. Application of RF energy should be discontinued with the first sign of VA block, slowing of VA conduction, or prolongation of the PR interval in conducted sinus beats.
- VA conduction during junctional rhythm may be noted even if there is no VA conduction during ventricular pacing.
- Isorhythmic AV dissociation may mimic intact VA conduction. In the presence of poor fast pathway conduction VA conduction during junctional rhythm may occur and is not a reliable indicator of potential AV block.
- To monitor for intact AV conduction atrial pacing at the fastest rate associated with 1 : 1 conduction should be performed while observing for the prolongation of the PR interval.
- Isorhythmic AV dissociation may occur during atrial pacing and RF application should be discontinued.
- 40–50% of patients may demonstrate residual slow pathway function, as evidenced by single echo beats, even after successful ablation of AVNRT.
- AVNRT may reoccur in 3–5% of patients. Most of the recurrences are reported in the first three months after ablation.
- Following a slow pathway ablation the fast pathway effective refractory period shortens.
- RF ablation should be considered for patients with frequent episodes of symptomatic tachycardia. Slow pathway ablation can be performed in the presence of prolonged PR interval. Atypical AVNRT can be successfully eliminated by slow pathway ablation.
- The alternative to RF energy is cryothermal energy. The long-term success rate is 90–94%.

- It has the following advantages over the sources of energy that results in thermal injury to the tissue:[70]
  1 The ability to reversibly demonstrate loss of tissue function with cooling. During cryomapping 90% of the lesions are reversible.
  2 It preserves the endothelial lining and tissue architecture with minimal thrombus formation, unlike the hyperthermic injury produced by RF.
  3 Less likely to produce pulmonary vein stenosis, if used for AF ablation.
  4 It is a reasonable strategy in patients with AVNRT who may be at high risk (preexisting prolonged PR interval) of anteroseptal or midseptal bypass tracts in whom the risk of damage to the AVN might be high with RF energy.
- Patients who have clinically documented SVT and dual AVN physiology but do not have inducible AVNRT at the time of electrophysiologic study may benefit from empirical slow pathway ablation.
- There is increased incidence of catheter-induced RV perforation in elderly women. RV catheter manipulation should be minimized.

5.6 AV REENTRANT TACHYCARDIA
Atrio-ventricular Reentry Tachycardia (AVRT)[60–64]

- 30% of all supraventricular tachycardia (SVT) are due to AVRT, 10% due to atrial tachycardia (AT) and the rest due to atrio-ventricular node reentry tachycardia (AVNRT).
- Atria, AVN, His Purkinje system (HPS), and ventricles comprise the circuit.
- Ventricles and HPS are not necessary for AVNRT.
- Accessory pathway (AP) connection can occur anywhere along the mitral and tricuspid annulus (TA) except in the region of the fibrous trigone where the mitral annulus joins the aorta.
- AP is capable of antegrade or retrograde conduction.
- The presence of antegrade conduction results in a short PR interval, slurring on the initial component of the QRS called delta wave and an increase in the duration of the QRS. These electrocardiographic features are due to preexcitation of the ventricles and if accompanied by tachycardia are characteristic of WPW syndrome (Fig. 5.18).
- AP with intermittent preexcitation is incapable of rapid antegrade conduction.
- Concealed AP is capable of only retrograde conduction; there is no preexcitation at any time. Retrograde conduction is more reliable as it is easier to activate smaller atrium.
- If AP is located in the lateral wall of the annulus, the presence of rapid AVN conduction may mask preexcitation. This can be uncovered by rapid atrial pacing.
- Slowing of AVN conduction may accentuate preexcitation.

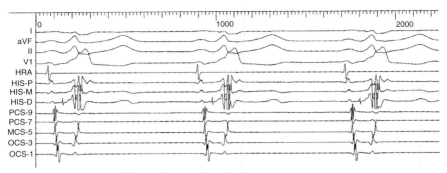

Fig 5.18 Preexcitation: surface and intracardiac electrograms.

- During orthodromic AV reentrant tachycardia antegrade conduction is through the AVN and retrograde conduction through AP, resulting in narrow QRS complex tachycardia.
- Antegrade conduction through AP and retrograde conduction through the AVN results in antidromic (wide complex, preexcited) tachycardia.
- During AT, atrial flutter or AVNRT antegrade conduction may occur through bystander AP. These entities will present with wide complex preexcited tachycardia. AP is not a part of the reentrant circuit.
- Atriofascicular tachycardia or the tachycardia utilizing two APs, one for antegrade and the other for retrograde conduction, will also present as wide complex preexcited tachycardia.

Clinical presentation
- Common symptoms during tachycardia are palpitations, chest discomfort, shortness of breath, dizziness, or near syncope.
- Tachycardia may be exercise induced.
- Patients have no structural heart disease.

Electrocardiogram
- EKG shows regular narrow complex tachycardia. Functional right or left bundle branch block may occur.
- Changes in tachycardia cycle length (CL) depend on AVN conduction, which may vary according to autonomic tone.
- AVN blocking agents terminate the tachycardia in AVN resulting in P as a last complex, followed by no QRS complex.
- The P wave is located within the ST segment. This would be characterized as short RP tachycardia. Lewis lead may help in identification of the P wave.
- In typical AVNRT, the P wave is within the QRS complex.
- Other tachycardias associated with short RP are atypical AVNRT or AT with prolonged PR interval.
- Occurrence of AV block during the tachycardia excludes the diagnosis of AVRT.

- Morphology of the P wave during the tachycardia may help identify the insertion site of the retrogradely conducting AP.
- Prolongation of tachycardia CL or ventriculoatrial (VA) conduction with bundle branch block suggests that the mechanism of the tachycardia is AVRT and that AP is located ipsilateral to the type of bundle branch block. These changes are not seen in septal AP or if bundle branch occurs in the ventricle contralateral to the location of the AP.
- Electrical alternans of the QRS is not helpful in making the diagnosis of AVRT.
- During preexcited tachycardia QRS morphology/axis is similar to delta wave seen in sinus rhythm.
- Preexcited tachycardia may mimic ventricular tachycardia. Structurally normal heart in a young patient and preexcitation during sinus rhythm exclude the diagnosis of VT. The presence of AV dissociation during tachycardia suggests the diagnosis of VT.
- Location of the AP can be determined by the morphology and the vector of delta wave from the surface EKG (Fig. 5.21).

Electrophysiologic features of AVRT

- Electrophysiologic study should be performed in a systematic and diligent manner. Attention should be paid to the following points:
  1 Onset and termination of the tachycardia.
  2 Changes in the morphology of the QRS.
  3 Changes in CL and its effect on the relationship of various electrograms and intervals.
  4 Zone of transition of the QRS.
  5 Changes in conduction intervals with BBB.
  6 Atrial activation sequence.
  7 AV relation.
  8 Ventricular activation sequence.
  9 Identification of His electrogram and its relation to atrial and ventricular electrogram.
  10 Assessment of HV, VA and HA relationship and intervals.
  11 Deliver premature ventricular contraction (PVC) during narrow complex tachycardia and deliver premature atrial contractions (PACs) during wide complex tachycardia.
  12 Parahisian pacing.
  13 Intracardiac electrograms should be assessed in the light of fluoroscopic location of the recording electrodes.
  14 Effects of various vagal maneuvers and administration of pharmacologic agents such as adenosine or isoproterenol.
- AVRT is a narrow QRS tachycardia with a normal HV interval preceding each QRS.
- There may be functional bundle branch block during the tachycardia.
- AV block is not compatible with AVRT.

- AH interval may change resulting in variation of CL. The VA interval remains constant unless there are two AP responsible for retrograde conduction during tachycardia.
- AVRT can be induced by PAC that blocks antegradely in AP and conducts antegradely through the AVN with prolonged AH interval and arrives retrogradely at AP. This initiates the tachycardia.
- Shortening of the AVN refractory period by atropine or isoproterenol may facilitate the induction of tachycardia.
- PVC may induce AVRT by producing retrograde block in HPS and conduction over AP.
- The shortest VA interval during AVRT is generally greater than 60 milliseconds and QRS to HRA interval of at least 95 milliseconds.
- In the presence of septal AP the VA interval during RV pacing tends to be similar to the VA interval during AVRT.
- In AVNRT VA during RV pacing tends to be longer than during tachycardia. In AVNRT there is simultaneous antegrade and retrograde conduction from the AVN, resulting in a short VA interval.
- Atrial activation is eccentric in the presence of lateral AP. AVRT utilizing septal AP demonstrates caudo-cranial atrial activation in the septal region.
- Earliest retrograde atrial activation during AVRT or during ventricular pacing defines the site of AP insertion. Atrial activation during V pacing is identical to the sequence of atrial activation during SVT (Fig. 5.19).
- If the occurrence of bundle branch block during AVRT results in VA prolongation by 30 milliseconds, it suggests the presence of ipsilateral AP. VA prolongation with LBBB will suggest left lateral AP.
- PVC delivered from RV, during AVRT, is likely to induce functional left bundle branch block because of delayed retrograde activation of LB.
- His catheter may be used to induce right bundle branch block.

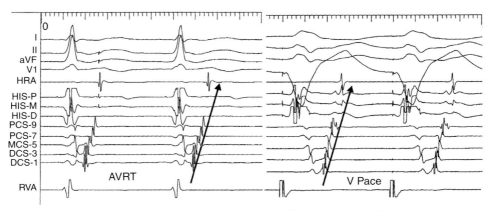

Fig 5.19 During tachycardia atrial activation is eccentric and earliest in DCS. During V pacing retrograde activation is identical to one during tachycardia.

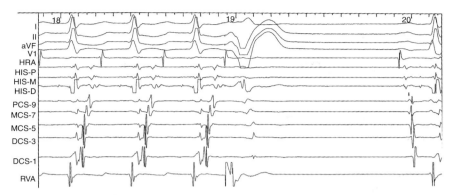

Fig 5.20 Termination of the tachycardia with His synchronous PVC without activation of the atrium.

- If PVC delivered during SVT, when His bundle is refractory, advances the atrial electrogram would suggest the presence of AP. AVN delay in the next beat may prevent the advancement of the whole tachycardia circuit.
- If PVC delivered during SVT, when His bundle is refractory, terminates the tachycardia without retrograde activation of the atrium, it is suggestive of AVRT utilizing AP (Fig. 5.20).
- Left-sided pathway, due to the distance from the RV pacing site, may not show atrial preexcitation.
- PVC delivered from the base of the heart or close to the AP is more likely to show atrial preexcitation. Atrial preexcitation may reveal multiple AP.
- The preexcitation index is defined as the difference between tachycardia CL and the longest coupling interval of RV PVC that results in atrial preexcitation.
- An index of 75 milliseconds or more suggests the presence of left lateral AP. Septal pathways demonstrate an index of less than 45 milliseconds.
- In septal and right-sided AP the VA interval during tachycardia remains the same as during RV pacing.
- If the pathway is located on the left side the VA during RV pacing tends to be longer than the VA during tachycardia.
- VA block during V pacing at CL longer than the tachycardia CL excludes AVRT.
- Administration of adenosine during V pacing may result in transient retrograde AVN block and unmask retrograde conduction through AP.
- If retrograde conduction is through septal AP the VA interval will be shorter with basal than apical pacing site. The opposite will occur if conduction is through His Purkinje AVN because the right bundle inserts into the RV apex.
- A change in atrial activation, during decremental RV pacing, from concentric to eccentric suggests the presence of AP.
- A change in atrial activation could also be due to a shift in conduction from retrograde fast to retrograde slow pathway.

- HA during V pacing at tachycardia CL minus HA during SVT of less than −10 milliseconds (for example of −20 to −30 milliseconds) is highly suggestive of AVRT utilizing septal bypass tract. This criterion may be helpful in distinguishing AVNRT from AVRT utilizing septal bypass tract. Although sensitive it may be difficult to utilize if retrograde His during V pacing cannot be recorded.
- Lack of decrement in the VA interval with decremental V pacing suggests the presence of AP.
- V pacing at a slower rate at which HPS refractoriness increases more than that of AP may allow conduction over concealed AP.
- In the absence of AP, the VA interval during RV apex pacing will be shorter than VA during RV base pacing.
- During parahisian pacing a constant VA interval with or without capture of the His is suggestive of AP.
- On termination of the tachycardia if the last electrogram is A then AT is unlikely. The likely diagnosis includes AVNRT or AVRT that blocks in AVN.
- CL variation during SVT depends on antegrade conduction over the AVN. In AVRT the AH interval may vary depending on whether the antegrade conduction is utilizing fast or slow pathway. The HA (or VA) interval will be constant.
- Variation in the VA interval could be due to ipsilateral BBB or multiple retrogradely conducting AP or decremental retrograde conduction through AP.
- Changes in the HH interval preceding or predicting changes in the AA interval are suggestive of AVN participation in the tachycardia circuit and will not occur in AT.
- Constant VA in spite of variability of the rate excludes AT.
- If A to A interval follows changes in the AH interval then AT is unlikely.
- During PAC if atrial echo beat occurs following His activation, it suggests that AVN is part of the tachycardia mechanism.
- During tachycardia (orthodromic or antidromic) to differentiate if the retrograde limb is fast pathway or septal AP, late PVC should be delivered near His. If this advances the next A, it indicates the presence of septal AP.

Differential diagnosis
- Differential diagnosis of orthodromic reentrant tachycardia includes AT or AVNRT. The following criteria may be useful in differentiating the mechanisms (Table 5.1).
- Left AT may be mistaken for AVRT utilizing a left lateral AP. However in left AT, the earliest atrial activation will be away from the mitral annulus and His synchronous PVC will not advance atrial electrogram.
- During tachycardia, with lengthening of the AH interval, if there is shortening of the VA interval, it is suggestive of AT and excludes AVRT or AVNRT.
- On termination of the wide complex tachycardia, if atrial pacing at the tachycardia CL results in AV block then SVT with aberrant conduction is unlikely.

Table 5.2 Differential diagnostic features of AVRT, AVNRT and atrial tachycardia

AVRT	AVNRT	Atrial tachycardia	Atypical AVNRT
Features that suggest			
Preexcitation on baseline EKG	Induction dependent on critical AH interval	AV block during SVT	AV block during tachycardia
Increase VA >20 milliseconds with BBB	Dual AVN physiology	Earliest atrial activation away from AV groove	HA V pace minus HA SVT of >−10 milliseconds
Eccentric atrial activation during SVT	Septal VA <70 milliseconds	VA dissociation during rapid V pacing	VA dissociation during SVT with rapid V pacing
Extranodal response to His pacing	Concentric activation of A during SVT	A activation during V pacing different then SVT	Earliest retrograde A in atrial septum
On cessation of A pacing first VA same as subsequent VA	On cessation of A pacing first VA same as subsequent VA	On cessation of A pacing first VA variable	On cessation of A pacing first VA same as subsequent VA
Eccentric activation of A during V pacing same as SVT	Concentric activation of A during V pacing same as SVT	VA block CL during V pacing longer than SVT CL	SA-VA >85 milliseconds
			PPI-TCL >115 milliseconds*
AV response on termination of V pacing	AV response on termination of V pacing	AAV response on cessation of V pacing**	AV response on termination of V pacing
Atrial preexcitation with PVC when His refractory	No atrial preexcitation with PVC when His refractory	No atrial preexcitation with PVC when His refractory	No atrial preexcitation with PVC when His refractory
SVT terminates with A	SVT terminates with A	Tachycardia terminates with V not A	SVT terminates with A
HA is constant during tachycardia	HA is constant during tachycardia	HA may be variable during tachycardia	HA may be variable during tachycardia
Termination by PVC when His is refractory without retrograde A	Shortening of VA with BBB if HV prolongs	Shortening of VA with BBB if HV prolongs	AH during A pacing >40 milliseconds longer than AH SVT
Features that exclude			
Septal VA <70 milliseconds	Increase VA <70 milliseconds	Termination with AV block	Increase VA with BBB
AV block during SVT	Termination by PVC when His refractory	Induction dependent on critical AH interval	Termination by PVC when His refractory
No VA conduction at baseline	Earliest atrial activation away from AV groove	Atrial preexcitation with PVC when His refractory	Earliest atrial activation away from AV groove
VA block CL during V pacing longer than SVT CL	Atrial preexcitation with PVC when His refractory	On cessation of A pacing first VA same as subsequent VA	Atrial preexcitation with PVC when His refractory
A activation different during V pacing then SVT	Eccentric activation of A during V pacing same as SVT	Termination by PVC when His refractory without atrial activation	Eccentric activation of A during V pacing same as SVT
AAV response on cessation of V pacing	AAV response on cessation of V pacing	Eccentric activation of A during V pacing same as SVT	AAV response on cessation of V pacing

* Entrainment of AVNRT during RV pacing SA is measured from last pacing stimulus to last retrogradely entrained HRA electrogram. VA, VA interval during tachycardia. PPI (post pacing interval) is measured from last pacing stimulus to first return cycle RV electrogram. TCL, tachycardia cycle length.

** First of the two atrial complexes is accelerated to V pacing CL. Pseudo VAAV response may be seen in slowly conducting septal pathway or slow AVNRT.

Differential diagnosis of long RP tachycardia includes

1 Atypical AVNRT.
2 AV reentrant tachycardia utilizing slowly conducting retrograde AP.
3 AT.

- Comparison of the AH interval (in His electrograms) during tachycardia and atrial pacing may help in differentiation. The AH interval during atrial pacing is 40 milliseconds longer than the AH during tachycardia in patients with atypical AVNRT. In patients with AVRT or AT the difference in AH A pace and AH tachycardia is less than 20 and 10 milliseconds respectively.
- On termination of V pacing during tachycardia stimulus to A minus VA interval of >85 milliseconds and post pacing interval minus tachycardia CL interval of >115 milliseconds are suggestive of atypical AVNRT (Fig. 5.12).

Wolf, Parkinson and White (WPW) syndrome

- The incidence of new cases appears to be 4/100,000/year. The prevalence of a WPW electrocardiographic pattern is 0.1–0.3%.
- A missense mutation of the gene that encodes a subunit of the adenosine monophosphate-activated protein kinase (*PRKAG2*) is associated with the Wolff–Parkinson–White syndrome, conduction abnormalities, and apparent left ventricular hypertrophy. This condition is due to glycogen accumulation within myocytes and should be regarded as a metabolic storage disease rather than a HCM.
- The term WPW syndrome describes electrocardiographic preexcitation accompanied by symptoms of tachycardia. In the absence of symptoms it should be described as WPW pattern.
- The occurrence of tachycardia in the absence of preexcitation which during electrophysiologic study is determined to be due to AP is labeled as concealed.
- APs are myocardial muscle fibers bridging over the annulus and providing electrical continuity between the atrium and the ventricle.
- Conduction over AP is rate independent. In a small number of patients (7%) AP may demonstrate decremental conduction.
- Antegrade decremental conduction is commonly seen over right-sided pathways.
- APs are classified according to their location on the AV annulus.
- The left free wall location of AP is seen in 50–60%, posteroseptal location in 20–30%, right free wall in 10–20%, and anteroseptal is least common.
- Identification of AP potential helps in localization of the pathway.
- Antegrade or retrograde conduction block in left lateral and posteroseptal AP occurs on the ventricular insertion side.
- For right-sided and septal AP, the site of block appears to be the atrium.
- AP may cross the annulus obliquely.
- Multiple APs are found in 10–20% of patients. These are commonly seen in patients with Ebstein anomaly and in those who have been resuscitated from VF.
- Combination of the posteroseptal and right free wall AP is common.
- Not all pathways, found histologically, are functional.

Clinical and electrocardiographic findings in WPW

- Asymptomatic patients with WPW pattern have a benign course.
- 25% of the patients lack retrograde conduction over AP and are incapable of producing AVRT.
- 1/3 of patients lose antegrade conduction over AP.
- Once the tachycardia occurs in adulthood, it does not spontaneously resolve.
- Symptoms include palpitations. Syncope does not carry poor prognosis.
- The incidence of sudden death appears to be 1 per 1000 patient years due to AF.
- The degree of preexcitation depends on relative conduction over AVN and AP. It also depends on the distance of the SA Node from the AP and conduction time.
- Minimal preexcitation is often seen in left lateral AP.
- Intermittent preexcitation (PE) implies slow conduction over AP and low risk of sudden death from AF and rapid conduction.
- An increase in sympathetic tone or a decrease in vagal tone may enhance AVN conduction and mask preexcitation. In these patients AP may still be capable of rapid conduction.
- Preexcitation due to LLAP produces negative delta waves in LI, aVL, or V6 and RBBB morphology in V1.
- Activation by right anteroseptal AP produces positive delta waves in L II, L III, aVF with inferior axis, and QS patterns in V1–V3.
- Posteroseptal AP produces superior axis, negative delta waves in inferior leads and rapid transition from V1 to V3.
- Right free wall AP produces positive delta wave in L1, aVL, LBBB pattern, and positive delta wave in V1 and left axis (Fig. 5.21).

Electrophysiologic features of preexcitation

- Decremental pacing from atrium and coronary sinus (CS) will determine the antegrade refractory period of the AP. The stimulus to delta interval will be shorter closest to the insertion site of the AP, while ventricular pacing will demonstrate retrograde activation and refractory period of AP.
- For septal AP differential RV pacing from the RV apex and from the AP insertion site and parahisian pacing may help differentiate conduction over AVN versus AP.
- During parahisian pacing a constant VA during capture and non capture of the His suggests the presence of AP.
- If retrograde conduction is through AVN myocardial capture will show longer VA than His capture.
- Atrial preexcitation, during SVT, with PVC delivered when His bundle is refractory suggests the presence of AP.

There are two types of involvement of AP in tachycardia:

1 AP is an obligatory part of the circuit:
   a Orthodromic and antidromic AV reentrant tachycardia.
   b Reciprocating tachycardia using multiple APs.

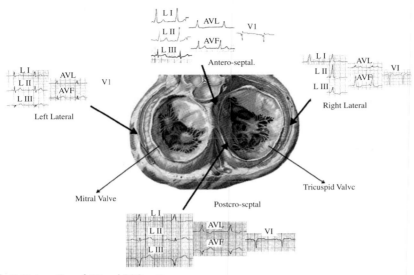

Fig 5.21 Location of AP and ECG pattern.

2 AP as a bystander:
  i AT, Atrial flutter
  ii AVNRT.
  iii VT.

• During AVRT antegrade conduction is over the AVN and retrograde conduction is over AP. This results in a narrow QRS complex. QRS alternans may be present.

• Functional bundle branch block during tachycardia may prolong CL and the VA interval if the AP is ipsilateral.

• ST segment depression during tachycardia is common but it is not related to coronary artery disease.

• Retrograde P wave morphology may help identify the location of AP. Retrograde conduction through posteroseptal AP produces negative P waves in L11, L111, and AVF. Retrograde conduction over left lateral AP produces negative P waves in L1 and aVL.

• Participation of the AVN in tachycardia allows the use of vagal maneuvers or AVN blocking agents to terminate the tachycardia. Minor fluctuations in tachycardia CL are due to variation in AVN conduction.

• Preexcitation of the atrium by PVC that is delivered when His bundle is refractory is suggestive of conduction over AP. This does not prove that AP is an obligatory participant in the tachycardia. The greater the distance from PVC site to AP, the more premature PVC has to be to produce atrial preexcitation.

• An abnormal pattern of retrograde activation during tachycardia or during ventricular pacing suggests the presence of AP.

• Atypical AVNRT may resemble AVRT on surface EKG 15% of patients with preexcitation may have dual AV nodal physiology.

- During AVNRT retrograde conduction will be concentric. Retrograde conduction through bystander concealed AP during AVNRT may result in atrial fusion.
- During AVNRT the VA interval in His electrograms tends to be less than 50 milliseconds and His synchronous PVCs do not preexcite the atrium.
- Differential ventricular pacing and parahisian pacing may help differentiate retrograde conduction over slow pathway and posteroseptal AP.
- RV apex pacing should yield a shorter VA interval if retrograde conduction is through slow pathway while pacing from the base will result in a shorter VA if the conduction is through septal pathway.
- 30% of patients with AP may present with AF. Initial arrhythmia may be AVRT, which may regress to AF. After ablation of AP spontaneous AF may decrease.
- During AF the presence of multiple preexcited QRS morphologies suggests that multiple AP may exist.
- The shortest preexcited RR of less than 250 milliseconds may predispose one to VF.
- The risk of sudden death is minimal in patients with concealed AP or intermittent preexcitation.
- Recent data suggests that electrophysiologic study and ablation may be indicated in asymptomatic patients. Lifestyle or occupation may also necessitate risk stratification by electrophysiologic study.
- In patients with preexcitation digitalis and verapamil should not be used as these drugs are known to accelerate conduction over AP.
- Ablation is the treatment of choice for high risk and/or symptomatic patients.

Antidromic tachycardia
- Antegrade conduction is through AP and retrograde conduction is through AVN.
- It occurs in 5% of WPW patients. It is rarely seen in patients with septal AP.
- Abrupt lengthening of CL during tachycardia may occur due to bundle branch block in the retrograde limb of the circuit.
- It may be difficult to differentiate preexcited tachycardia from VT and antegrade conduction over bystander AP during atrial flutter and AVNRT.
- Atrial pacing from the AP site will reproduce the QRS morphology identical to tachycardia and will also identify the location of AP.
- AV dissociation during tachycardia will exclude antidromic AVRT.
- Retrograde atrial activation should be through AVN unless antegrade and retrograde conduction are both through AP. Multiple AP may present with preexcited tachycardia.
- AVN blocking agents and maneuvers will terminate antidromic tachycardia.
- QRS is preexcited and is identical to that during atrial pacing with conduction over AP.
- There is no His electrogram preceding each QRS. Retrograde His after QRS may be recorded. The HA interval during antidromic tachycardia will be similar to the HA interval during V pacing.

- Atrial activation is concentric (retrograde conduction through AVN).
- Ventricular activation can be advanced by PAC without involving the AVN. PAC could be delivered near the atrial insertion site of AP.
- If PAC delivered near the AVN simultaneously with atrial activation advances the ventricular electrogram it suggests the antegrade conduction is through the AP.
- It may resemble VT. If decremental atrial pacing during sinus rhythm reproduces preexcitation similar to tachycardia, VT is excluded.
- If atrial pacing during tachycardia advances the QRS without a change in morphology it is likely to exclude VT.
- Decremental atrial pacing may produce preexcitation and as the antegrade refractory period of AP is reached, it may result in normalization of the QRS if antegrade conduction continues through the AVN (Fig. 5.22).
- Atrial tachycardia or atrial flutter with 1:1 antegrade conduction through AP should be differentiated from antidromic reentrant tachycardia where the earliest retrograde activation is in low septal area and is similar to the activation during ventricular pacing if retrograde conduction is through AVN.
- In AT the site of earliest atrial activation depends on the site of origin of the tachycardia.
- Adenosine may terminate the tachycardia by blocking retrograde conduction in AVN, resulting in QRS that is not followed by A.

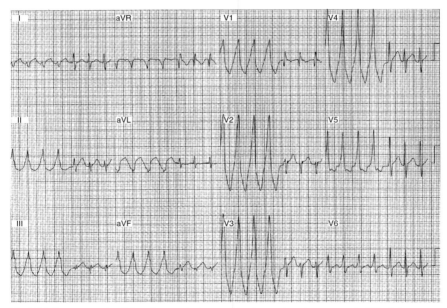

Fig 5.22 Decremental atrial pacing results in preexcitation and as the antegrade ERP of the accessory pathway is reached, it results in normalization of the QRS, the antegrade conduction continues through AV node.

- AVNRT with antegrade conduction through bystander AP may result in wide complex preexcited tachycardia. PVC delivered at the site of antegrade conduction of the AP will block antegrade conduction through AP; however, AVNRT will continue with narrow complex morphology.
- The HA interval will be shorter during AVNRT with preexcited QRS due to bystander AP as opposed to the HA interval during antidromic tachycardia in the same patient.
- Normalization of the QRS with His extrasystole suggests the presence of preexcitation.
- During bystander preexcitation the ventricles can be dissociated from the tachycardia.
- In the presence of preexcitation if there is no retrograde conduction during V pacing, orthodromic tachycardia is unlikely to occur. Antegrade conduction through the AP during atrial pacing and AF should be assessed.
- In pathway to pathway tachycardia:
  1 Atrium and ventricle are an obligatory part of the circuit.
  2 Atrial activation is eccentric.
  3 QRS is preexcited.

Electrophysiologic differential diagnosis of wide complex tachycardia

SVT Aberrancy	VT	Antidromic tachycardia	V preexcitation due to bystander AP
HV same as in SR	No H preceding QRS	No H preceding QRS	HV shorter than SR
		PAC preexcites V no change in QRS morphology and no change in His A–A	PAC preexcites V but does not affect septal A–A excludes Nodoventricular reentry
Bifascicular block pattern unusual	If VT morphology changes from RB to LB without change in H–H interval or CL BB reentry unlikely. Suggests myocardial VT with penetration of His.	A pacing reproduces QRS morphology	PAC preexcites V and advances next A excludes AVNRT or AT utilizing bystander AP
	QRS morphology similar during sinus rhythm and during tachycardia but AV dissociation is present suggestive of BB reentry or fascicular or His tachycardia.	In atriofascicular tachycardia earliest V at RV apex (RB). No retrograde conduction through atriofascicular pathway	Variable VA with constant AV

Management

- Vagal maneuvers such as valsalva or carotid sinus massage and AVN blocking drugs such as adenosine β-blockers or calcium channel blockers are effective in acute termination of tachycardia.
- Drugs that prolong the refractory period and conduction over AP such as Procainamide, Disopyramide, and Quinidine and drugs that prolong refractoriness in AVN and AP such as Flecainide, Propafenone, Sotalol, and Amiodarone can be used for chronic treatment of tachycardia.
- Digitalis decreases the refractory period of the AP and should be avoided in the presence of preexcitation.
- Antiarrhythmic drugs may suppress PACs and PVCs thus preventing induction of the tachycardia.
- Adenosine is the drug of choice in acute management of the AVRT. It can be used in patients with hypotension and left ventricular dysfunction. Its half-life is 10 seconds. Its effectiveness is diminished by Theophylline and caffeine.
- Adenosine shortens the atrial refractory period and facilitates the occurrence of atrial fibrillation (AP) in 10% of patients.
- Intravenous Verapamil may take 5–10 minutes to terminate the tachycardia.
- AVN blocking agents should not be used in AF with preexcitation.
- Infrequent episodes of orthodromic tachycardia can be treated by oral dose of Verapamil at the time of occurrence.
- Patients with AF and preexcited RR interval of less than 250 milliseconds could develop hemodynamic collapse.
- Intermittent preexcitation implies poor antegrade conduction through the AP.
- Drug therapy may increase the frequency of the AVRT if it prolongs the antegrade refractory period of the AP without affecting the retrograde conduction or refractoriness.

RF ablation for AVRT

- Most APs travel from the atrium to the ventricle across the AV ring.
- In symptomatic patients radiofrequency ablation of AP is the treatment of choice.
- The TA differs from the mitral annulus as outlined below.
  1 The TA is displaced apically.
  2 Larger circumference.
  3 Less fibrous skeleton.
  4 Absence of venous structure along the annulus to map epicardium.
- The AV annulus is identified by the amplitude of the atrial and ventricular electrogram recorded from the mapping/ablation catheter.
- RF ablation could be performed during V pacing. Pathway potentials should be identified (Fig 5.23).
- Left-sided AP is approached using transseptal puncture.
- Minimum beat-to-beat variation in the amplitude of the electrogram indicates firm contact with the tissue.

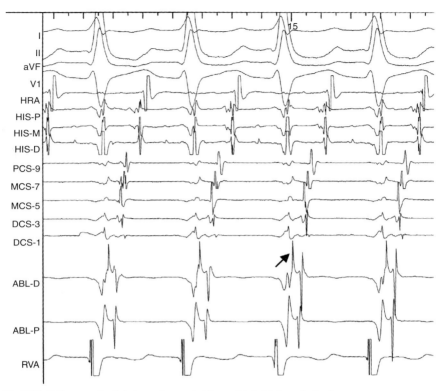

Fig 5.23 Pathway potentials (arrow) recorded from distal ablation electrode.

- Ablation catheter tends to be less stable along the TA and may require the use of the preshaped sheath for optimum tissue contact.
- The location of the pathway is identified by the shortest local AV (preexcited) or VA interval and by recording pathway potentials. Ventricular or atrial insertion sites can be identified by ventricular and atrial pacing and earliest atrial or ventricular activation (Fig. 5.23).
- Ebstein's anomaly is characterized by apical displacement of the septal leaflet of the tricuspid valve. This results in atrialization of a part of the right ventricle.
- 25–30% of the patients with Ebstein's anomaly may have AP mediated tachycardia. These patients are likely to have multiple AP.
- Mapping through the right coronary artery may be necessary to localize AP.
- Anteroseptal AP are located in the proximity of the His bundle and are best ablated from the ventricular side (large V and small A with bypass potential).
- During ablation of anteroseptal AP, pathway potentials should be prominent and sharper than His.

- Midseptal pathways are located between His electrode anteriorly and the CS ostium (os) catheter posteriorly. Ablation is performed close to the ventricular aspect of the TA after identifying the pathway potential.
- Right posteroseptal APs are located between CS os and TA. Subepicardial left posteroseptal APs are located in the proximal CS or in the cardiac vein structures. Subendocardial pathways are located along the mitral annulus in the posterior septum.
- Epicardially located pathways produce smaller pathway potentials.
- There may be atrial appendage to ventricular connections. During tachycardia earliest atrial activation is several millimeters away from the annulus.
- Left anterior AP is located at the superior medial aspect of the mitral annulus and are best ablated by the retrograde transaortic approach.
- 5% of patients may have multiple APs. These patients tend to have right-sided APs.
- Reoccurrence of tachycardia after ablation may occur in 6–10% of patients. Complication during procedure may occur in 2–4% of patient.

Atriofascicular (Nodofascicular) pathways[63]

- First described by Mahaim and Winston as connections between the AVN and the bundle branch or ventricular myocardium.
- These are characterized by
  1 Subtle preexcitation with left bundle morphology and left axis suggestive of right-sided connection.
  2 The pathway demonstrates anterograde conduction only.
  3 PAC or atrial pacing increases the AH or the A-delta interval and enhances preexcitation.
  4 During tachycardia antegrade conduction is over AP and retrograde conduction over AVN.
  5 Earliest activation occurs at the RV apex rather than at the base near the TA.
  6 Demonstration of VA dissociation during tachycardia.

Fasciculoventricular connections (FVC)

- Fasciculoventricular connections are "true Mahaim" fibers and atriofascicular/atrioventricular connections are "pseudo-Mahaim" or "Mahaim-like" fibers. These are two different entities.
- Fasciculoventricular fibers connect the fascicle (or, in rare cases, the most distal part of the AVN) with the ventricular septum and are responsible for ventricular preexcitation.
- Decremental properties of AV conduction are always preserved, and a constant degree of preexcitation is observed at any heart rate.
- Fasciculoventricular pathways cannot sustain reentry and do not cause reciprocating tachycardia, although they can be activated as bystanders in different SVTs.
- It produces minimally preexcited QRS and a short and fixed HV interval.

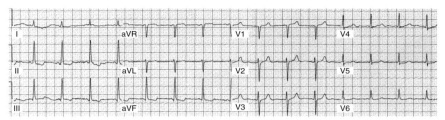

Fig 5.24 ECG in fasciculoventricular connection.

- Baseline HV (H-delta) interval during sinus rhythm is less than 35 milliseconds. During decremental atrial pacing the HV interval does not change.
- Atrial premature beats cause progressive prolongation of the AH interval without any change in the HV interval and QRS configuration. If a closely coupled PAC blocks the fasciculoventricular pathway, it results in a normal HV interval and a narrow QRS complex.
- The response to adenosine triphosphate suggests the presence of FVC when prolongation of the PR interval (AH interval) does not change the degree of preexcitation or complete AV block is nodal and not infra nodal and conducted atrial beats always show preexcitation .

ECG in Fasciculoventricular connection
- The delta wave is positive in the inferior leads and in V5 and V6. The delta wave is flat or negative in V1, consistent with a right ventricular insertion.
- The mean PR interval is 0.10 ± 0.01 seconds (Fig. 5.24).
- The QRS width tends to be narrower in FVC when compared with the preexcited QRS in the presence of midseptal and anteroseptal bypass tracts.
- Fasciculoventricular pathways may be involved as bystander during AVNRT or AVRT.
- During AVNRT with bystander activation of FVC, a constant degree of preexcitation is present, His-bundle is activated in an anterograde fashion. During ventricular pacing retrograde conduction is over the fast AV node pathway.
- Preexcitation due to fasciculoventricular pathways is benign and requires no therapy.

Permanent form of junctional reciprocating tachycardia (PJRT)
- PJRT is an incessant long RP tachycardia.
- It may result in tachycardia mediated cardiomyopathy.
- The Electrocardiogram shows negative P waves in inferior lead. Each QRS is preceded by a P wave.
- There is no preexcitation on surface ECG.
- It is an AVRT utilizing slowly conducting posteroseptal AP.

- The antegrade limb is the AVN and the retrograde limb is the slowly conducting posteroseptal AP which demonstrates retrograde decremental conduction and is sensitive to vagal maneuvers β-blockers and calcium channel blockers.
- The long serpiginous course and fiber orientation of the pathway may contribute to slow conduction.
- Slowly conducting left free wall AP may demonstrate similar features.

Electrophysiologic features
- Electrocardiographic features include board and negative P waves in L11 L111 AVF, long RP interval, and transient termination occurs in retrograde limb.
- CL may change due to modulation of the PR and RP interval.
- Premature beats are not required for initiation of tachycardia.
- Earliest activation, during tachycardia, occurs in the posteroseptal region near CS os. Retrograde AVN conduction is nonexistent.
- The incessant nature of the tachycardia is due to unidirectional block in limbs, slow conduction, and balanced refractoriness.
- It must be differentiated from atypical AVNRT and AT.
- If PVC, delivered when His is refractory, advances atrial activation, it suggests the presence of AP.
- Tachycardia occurs spontaneously at a critical sinus CL without PACs or PVCs. RP interval is longer than the PR interval.
- QRS complexes are narrow and are preceded by His electrogram and normal HV interval.
- Late coupled PVC may terminate tachycardia by retrograde block in AP.
- Differential diagnosis includes AT arising from the posteroseptal region or atypical AVNRT (Table 5.1).
- These pathways are sensitive to adenosine and may not help in differentiating from other tachycardia.
- If a PVC delivered when His bundle is refractory (His synchronous) results in termination of the tachycardia without atrial activation, it excludes the possibility of AVNRT and AT.
- Retrograde conduction through AP is facilitated by isoproterenol.
- PVC may delay atrial activation (post excitation phenomenon). This occurs if the delay in retrograde conduction exceeds the coupling interval of the PVC, resulting in delayed atrial activation longer than the tachycardia CL.
- Drug therapy is ineffective. Ablation is the treatment of choice.
- Ablation is guided by earliest atrial activation, during tachycardia, which precedes the onset of the P wave and an AP potential that precedes atrial activation.

PJRT is characterized by:
1 Narrow complex tachycardia.
2 Initiation of the tachycardia is not preceded by prolongation of the PR or AH interval.

3 1 : 1 Av relation.

4 RP longer than PR interval.

5 Negative P waves in L2, L3 and aVF.

6 Extra nodal slow and decrementally conducting AP forms the retrograde limb of the circuit.

7 The atrial insertion site is close to or inside the CS os.

The following features suggest the presence of PJRT and make atypical AVNRT less likely.

1 During tachycardia, PVC delivered when His bundle is refractory results in atrial preexcitation without any change in the activation sequence.

2 PVC may terminate tachycardia without atrial activation.

3 Prolongation of the local VA interval.

Ablation is targeted at the earliest atrial activation site during tachycardia.

Complications of ablation and recurrences of tachycardia

- Tachycardia may reoccur in 5% of the patients.
- Complications include cardiac tamponade, thromboembolic events, AV block and hematomas and may occur in 2–3% of the patients undergoing procedure.
- Fluoroscopic exposure related radiation may pose an increased risk of malignancies.

Atriofascicular reentrant tachycardia[64]

- During tachycardia antegrade conduction is through atriofascicular fibers (also known as Mahaim fibers) and retrograde conduction is through AVN (antidromic).
- These fibers are capable of only antegrade conduction and have decremental conduction properties.
- The atrial insertion site is in the right posterolateral, lateral, or anterolateral free wall near the TA.
- The distal insertion site is the right bundle branch.
- Conduction over these fibers during tachycardia produces ventricular preexcitation with left bundle morphology.
- Right ventricular apical activation is earlier than basal.
- His Purkinje activation occurs retrogradely as demonstrated by the RB electrogram preceding His electrogram. Impulse from RB must travel retrogradely to His and antegradely to the ventricle simultaneously. This results in simultaneous activation of His and onset of ventricular activation.
- During atrial pacing, progressive AV and AH interval prolongation coupled with a decreasing HV interval results in a greater degree of ventricular preexcitation with a left bundle branch-like morphology.
- The occurrence of retrograde right bundle branch block during tachycardia will shift His activation to late in the QRS.

- PAC delivered during tachycardia, in the RA lateral wall, will advance V and His without activating the AVN.
- AP potential can be recorded from the right AV groove and successful ablation can be performed from this site.
- Right-sided AP with antegrade conduction will produce ventricle activation at the base of the right ventricle as opposed to apical activation that occurs with atriofascicular fibers.
- PACs or PVCs can induce atriofascicular tachycardia.
- During tachycardia a 1 : 1 atrium and ventricle relationship must be present.
- QRS complexes demonstrate left bundle morphology.
- During sinus rhythm QRS morphology is normal.
- Atriofascicular tachycardia can be differentiated from right ventricular tachycardia by atrial pacing during which QRS morphology will be similar to atriofascicular tachycardia.
- Dual AVN physiology is common in patients with atriofascicular fibers.
- Antidromic AVRT can be distinguished from AT and AVNRT with bystander AP activation by recording retrograde activation of HPS where RB electrogram precedes His bundle electrogram during tachycardia.
- Termination of the tachycardia by single PVC without atrial activation excludes AT.
- Adenosine administration may terminate tachycardia by antegrade block in atriofascicular fibers.
- The following characteristics are noted during electrophysiologic evaluation:
  1 Tachycardia is characterized by LBBB morphology.
  2 Late right atrial extrastimulus delivered during preexcited tachycardia advances ventricular activation without affecting low right atrial septal activation.
  3 Tachycardia can be entrained from the right atrium.
  4 Right atrial pacing from the free wall close to the TA results in ventricular preexcitation.
  5 Stimulus to QRS duration is shortest when pacing from TA. This is not a very reliable criterion.
  6 Recording of pathway potentials along the TA.
  7 The pathway demonstrates decremental conduction on right atrial pacing with prolongation of the A to AP potential.
  8 The ventricular insertion site is identified by earliest ventricular activation during preexcited tachycardia

Differential diagnosis
Atriofascicular pathway
- During preexcited tachycardia, there is a short V–H interval, early activation of the right ventricular (RV) apex, and late activation at the annulus. The atrial insertion is located by finding the AP potential.

Short-decremental AV pathways
- During preexcited tachycardia, there is a long V–H interval, early ventricular activation at the TA, and late activation at the RV apex.

Long decremental right superior AV pathways
- During preexcited tachycardia, there is late activation of the RV apex and late activation at the TA.
- 12-lead ECG shows normal QRS frontal plane axis between +30 and +60. There is no left-axis deviation.
- Atrial insertion can be located by finding the AP potential at the right superior area at the TA.

Treatment
- Tachycardia may respond to AVN blocking drugs or it can be ablated at the atrial insertion site.
- Earliest atrial activation is at the retrograde exit site of the AVN. Earliest ventricular activation is not near the AV groove. These markers cannot help locate the atrial insertion site.
- Identification of pathway potential along the AV groove and delivery of energy at that site appears to be the most promising ablation technique.
- Damage to RB may make tachycardia incessant.

References

1 Bernstein NE. Sandler DA. Goh M. Feigenblum DY. Why a sawtooth? Inferences on the generation of the flutter wave during typical atrial flutter drawn from radiofrequency ablation. *Ann Noninvasive Electrocardiol.* 9:358–61, 2004.
2 Wellens HJJ. Contemporary management of atrial flutter. *Circulation.* 106:649, 2002.
3 Hongo RH. Themistoclakis S. Raviele A. et al. Use of ibutilide in cardioversion of patients with atrial fibrillation or atrial flutter treated with class IC agents. *J Am Coll Cardiol.* 44:864–8, 2004.
4 Mead GE. Flapan AD. Elder AT. Electrical cardioversion for atrial fibrillation and flutter. *Cochrane Database Syst Rev.* 1:CD002903, 2002.
5 Khan IA. Nair CK. Singh N. Gowda RM. Acute ventricular rate control in atrial fibrillation and atrial flutter. *Int J Cardiol.* 97(1):7–13, 2004.
6 Ghali WA. Wasil BI. Brant R. Exner DV. Cornuz J. Atrial flutter and the risk of thromboembolism: A systematic review and meta-analysis. *Am J Med.* 118:101–7, 2005.
7 Feld GK. Radiofrequency ablation of atrial flutter using large-tip electrode catheters. *J Cardiovasc Electrophysiol.* 15 (10 Suppl):S18–23, 2004.
8 Okishige K. Kawabata M. Yamashiro K. et al. Clinical study regarding the anatomical structures of the right atrial isthmus using intra-cardiac echocardiography: Implications for catheter ablation of common atrial flutter. *J Interv Card Electrophysiol.* 12 (1):9–12, 2005.
9 Chen SA. Higa S. The roles of anatomy, image, and electrogram voltage in ablation of cavotricuspid isthmus. *J Interv Card Electrophysiol.* 12:13–15, 2005.

10 Husser D. Bollmann A. Kang S. Effectiveness of catheter ablation for coexisting atrial fibrillation and atrial flutter. *Am J Cardiol.* 94(5):666–8, 2004.

11 Bottoni N. Donateo P. Quartieri F. Outcome after cavo-tricuspid isthmus ablation in patients with recurrent atrial fibrillation and drug-related typical atrial flutter. *Am J Cardiol.* 94:504–8, 2004.

12 Saoudi N. Cosio F. Waldo A. et al. Classification of atrial flutter and regular atrial tachycardia according to electrophysiology mechanism and anatomical bases: A statement from a joint expert group from the Working Group of Arrhythmias of the European Society of Cardiology and the North American Society of Pacing and Electrophysiology. *Eur Heart J.* 22:1162–82, 2001; *J Cardiovasc Electrophysiol.* 12:852–66, 2001.

13 Lin YJ. Tai CT. Liu TY. et al. Electrophysiological mechanisms and catheter ablation of complex atrial arrhythmias from crista terminalis. *Pacing Clin Electrophysiol.* 27(9):1231–9, 2004.

14 Strickberger SA. Ip J. Saksena S. Curry K. Relationship between atrial tachyarrhythmias and symptoms. *Heart Rhythm.* 2:125–31, 2005.

15 Yame T. Shah DC. Peng J-T. et al. Morphological characteristics of P waves during selective pulmonary vein pacing. *J Am Coll Cardiol.* 38:1505–10, 2001.

16 Ouyang F. Ernst S. Vogtmann T. et al. Characterization of reentrant circuits in left atrial macroreentrant tachycardia: Critical isthmus block can prevent atrial tachycardia recurrence. *Circulation.* 105:1934–42, 2002.

17 Jais P. Shah DC. Haissaguerre M. et al. Mapping and ablation of left atrial flutters. *Circulation.* 101:2928–34, 2000.

18 Morton JB. Sanders P. Deen V. et al. Sensitivity and specificity of concealed entrainment for the identification of a critical isthmus in the atrium: Relationship to rate, anatomic location and antidromic penetration. *J Am Coll Cardiol.* 39:896–906, 2002.

19 Yang J. Cheng J. Bochoeyer A. et al. Atypical right atrial flutter patterns. *Circulation.* 103:3092–8, 2001.

20 Lukac P. Pedersen AK. Mortensen PT. Ablation of atrial tachycardia after surgery for congenital and acquired heart disease using an electroanatomic mapping system: Which circuits to expect in which substrate? *Heart Rhythm.* 2:64–72, 2005.

21 Stevenson IH. Kistler PM. Spence SJ. Scar-related right atrial macroreentrant tachycardia in patients without prior atrial surgery: Electroanatomic characterization and ablation outcome. *Heart Rhythm.* 2:594–601, 2005.

22 Tanner H. Lukac P. Schwick N. Irrigated-tip catheter ablation of intraatrial reentrant tachycardia in patients late after surgery of congenital heart disease. *Heart Rhythm.* 1:268–75, 2004.

23 Ikeguchi S. Peters NS. Novel use of postpacing interval mapping to guide radiofrequency ablation of focal atrial tachycardia with long intra-atrial conduction time. *Heart Rhythm.* 1:88–93, 2004.

24 Dong J. Zrenner B. Schreieck J. Catheter ablation of left atrial focal tachycardia guided by electroanatomic mapping and new insights into interatrial electrical conduction. *Heart Rhythm.* 2:578–91, 2005.

25 Miyazaki H. Stevenson WG. Stephenson K. et al. Entrainment mapping for rapid distinction of left and right atrial tachycardias. *Heart Rhythm.* 3:516–23, 2006.

26 Abedin Z. Conner R. Interpretation of Cardiac Arrhythmias: Self Assessment Approach. Norwell, Mass.: Kluwer, 2000.

27 Chen SA. Pathophysiology of the pulmonary vein as an atrial fibrillation initiator. *Pacing Clin Electrophysiol.* 26:1576–82, 2003.

28 Beyerbach DM. Zipes DP. Mortality as an endpoint in atrial fibrillation. *Heart Rhythm.* 1(Suppl.):8–19, 2004.

29 Reiffel JA. Drug choices in the treatment of atrial fibrillation. *Am J Cardiol.* 85:2D, 2000.

30 Stroke Prevention in Atrial Fibrillation Investigators. Stroke prevention in atrial fibrillation study: Final results. *Circulation.* 84:527, 1991.

31 Peterson P. Boysen G. Godtfredsen J. et al. Placebo-controlled randomized trial of warfarin and aspirin for prevention of thromboembolic complications in chronic atrial fibrillation: The Copenhagen AFASAK study. *Lancet.* 1(8631):175–9, 1989.

32 Boston Area Anticoagulation Trial for Atrial Fibrillation Investigators. The effect of low dose warfarin on the risk of stroke in patients with nonrheumatic atrial fibrillation. *N Engl J Med.* 323:1505, 1990.

33 Stroke Prevention in Atrial Fibrillation Investigators. Warfarin versus aspirin for prevention of thromboembolism in atrial fibrillation: SPAF II study. *Lancet.* 343:687, 1994.

34 SPAF III Writing Committee for the Stroke Prevention in Atrial Fibrillation Investigators. Patients with nonvalvular atrial fibrillation at low risk of stroke during treatment with aspirin: SPAF III study. *JAMA.* 279:1273, 1998.

35 The Atrial Fibrillation Follow-up Investigation of Rhythm Management (AFFIRM) Investigators. A comparison of rate control with rhythm control in patients with atrial fibrillation. *N Engl J Med.* 347:1825, 2002.

36 Van Gelder IC. Hagens VE. Bosker HA. et al. A comparison of rate control and rhythm control in patients with recurrent persistent atrial fibrillation. *N Engl J Med.* 347:1834, 2002.

37 Tamariz LJ. Pharmacological rate control of atrial fibrillation.*Cardiol Clin.* 22(1):35–45, 2004.

38 Klein AL. Grimm RA. Daniel Murray R. et al. Use of transesophageal echocardiography to guide cardioversion in patients with atrial fibrillation. *N Engl J Med.* 344:1411, 2001.

39 Page RL. Kerber RE. Russell JK. et al. Biphasic versus monophasic shock waveform for conversion of atrial fibrillation: The results of an international randomized, double-blind multicenter trial. *J Am Coll Cardiol.* 39:1956, 2002.

40 Mead GE. Flapan AD. Elder AT. Electrical cardioversion for atrial fibrillation and flutter. *Cochrane Database Syst Rev.* 1:CD002903, 2002.

41 Roy D. Talajic M. Dorian P. et al. Amiodarone to prevent recurrence of atrial fibrillation. *N Engl J Med.* 342:913, 2000.

42 Torp-Pedersen C. Møller M. Bloch-Thomsen PE. et al. Dofetilide in patients with congestive heart failure and left ventricular dysfunction. *N Engl J Med.* 341:857, 1999.

43 Khan IA. Nair CK. Singh N. Gowda RM. Nair RC. Acute ventricular rate control in atrial fibrillation and atrial flutter. *Int J Cardiol.* 97:7–13, 2004.

44 Camm AJ. Savelieva I. Advances in antiarrhythmic drug treatment of atrial fibrillation: Where do we stand now? *Heart Rhythm.* 1:244–6, 2004.

45 Bottoni N. Donateo P. Quartieri F. Outcome after cavo-tricuspid isthmus ablation in patients with recurrent atrial fibrillation and drug-related typical atrial flutter. *Am J Cardiol.* 94(4):504–8, 2004.

46 Saad EB. Marrouche EF. Natale A. Ablation of focal atrial fibrillation. *Card Electrophysiol Rev.* 6:389, 2002.

47 Finta B. Catheter ablation therapy for atrial fibrillation.*Cardiol Clin.* 22(1):127–45, 2004.

48 Husser D. Bollmann A. Kang S. Effectiveness of catheter ablation for coexisting atrial fibrillation and atrial flutter. *Am J Cardiol.* 94(5):666–8, 2004.

49 Chugh A. Oral H. Lemola K. Prevalence, mechanisms, and clinical significance of macroreentrant atrial tachycardia during and following left atrial ablation for atrial fibrillation. *Heart Rhythm*. 2:464–71, 2005.

50 Kobza R. Hindricks G. Tanner H. et al. Late recurrent arrhythmias after ablation of atrial fibrillation: Incidence, mechanisms, and treatment. *Heart Rhythm*. 1:676–83, 2004.

51 Olshansky B. Is the approach to atrial fibrillation ablation becoming more complex and fractionated? *Heart Rhythm*. 3:35–6, 2006.

52 Ozcan C. Jahangir A. Friedman PA. et al. Long-term survival after ablation of the atrioventricular node and implantation of permanent pacemaker in patients with atrial fibrillation. *N Engl J Med*. 344:1043, 2001.

53 Gilbert CJ. Common supraventricular tachycardias: Mechanisms and management. *AACN Clin Iss*. 12:100–13, 2001.

54 Scherlag BJ. Patterson E. Nakagawa H. et al. Changing concept of A-V nodal conduction: Basic and clinical correlations. *Prim Cardiol*. 21:13–24, 1995.

55 Morady F. Radio-frequency ablation as treatment for cardiac arrhythmias. *N Engl J Med*. 340:534–44, 1999.

56 Estes NAM. Catheter cryoablation of supraventricular tachycardia: Quo vadis? *Heart Rhythm*. 1:139–40, 2004.

57 Michaud GF. Tada H. Chough S. Baker R. et al. Differentiation of atypical atrioventricular node re-entrant tachycardia from orthodromic reciprocating tachycardia using a septal accessory pathway by the response to ventricular pacing. *J Am Coll Cardiol*. 38:1163–7, 2001.

58 Knight BP. Zivin A. Souza J. Flemming M. et al. A technique for the rapid diagnosis of atrial tachycardia in the electrophysiology laboratory. *J Am Coll Cardiol*. 33:775–8, 1999.

59 Katritsis DG. Becker AE. Ellenbogen KA. et al. Right and left inferior extensions of the atrioventricular node may represent the anatomic substrate of the slow pathway in humans. *Heart Rhythm*. 1:582–6, 2004.

60 Kerr C. Gallaghar JJ. German L. Changes in ventriculoatrial intervals with bundle branch block aberration during reciprocating tachycardia in patients with accessory atrioventricular pathways. *Circulation*. 66:196, 1982.

61 Sternick EB. Cruz FES. Timmermans C. Sosa EA. et al. Electrocardiogram during tachycardia in patients with anterograde conduction over a Mahaim fiber: Old criteria revisited. *Heart Rhythm*. 1:406–13, 2004.

62 Tan HL. Wittkampf FHM. Nakagawa H. Derksen R. Atriofascicular accessory pathway. *J Cardiovasc Electrophysiol*. 15: 118, 2004.

63 Tchou P. Lehmann MH. Jazayeri M. Akhtar M. Atriofascicular connection or a nodoventricular Mahaim fiber? Electrophysiologic elucidation of the pathway and associated reentrant circuit. *Circulation*. 77:837–48, 1988.

64 McClelland JH. Wang X. Beckman KJ. Hazlitt HA. et al. Radiofrequency catheter ablation of right atriofascicular (Mahaim) accessory pathways guided by accessory pathway activation potentials. *Circulation*. 89:2655–66, 1994.

6 Differential Diagnosis of Wide Complex Tachycardia

Self-Assessment Questions

1 A 52-year-old man, who suffered from uncomplicated inferior wall myocardial infarction 3 years ago, became aware of the palpitations 4 months ago. Palpitations would last for several hours during which he has no other symptoms. During one such episode he came to the emergency room. Palpitations had persisted for 3 hours.

   BP was 106/70. The patient was alert and in no distress. ECG strip is shown.

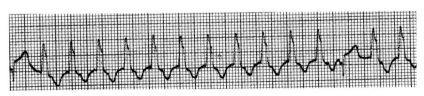

   What will be the next step?
   A IV adenosine
   B 200 mg of PO flecainide and continue maintenance dose
   C Cardioversion
   D Valsalva maneuver

2 A 67-year-old female whose baseline ECG shows prolonged PR interval, LBBB presents to ER with palpitations. A 12 lead ECG is shown on page 128.
   What is the likely diagnosis?
   A SVT with aberrant conduction
   B VT
   C Preexcited tachycardia
   D SVT bystander accessory pathway conduction

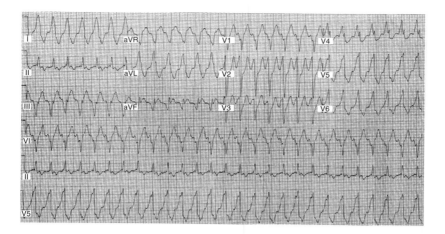

Causes of wide complex tachycardia (WCT)

- Ventricular tachycardia (VT): 80% of all WCT are due to VT.
- Supraventricular tachycardia (SVT): in the presence of functional or persistent bundle branch block (BBB), electrolyte abnormalities and antiarrhythmic drugs.
- Preexcited tachycardia with positive concordant pattern in precordial leads.
- Ventricular paced rhythm.

Differential diagnosis (Table 6.1)

Clinical features

WCT in the presence of previous myocardial infarction (MI) is likely to be due to VT.

Electrocardiographic features

- In lead V1 triphasic complex with RBBB morphology and the initial portion of the QRS similar to sinus rhythm is suggestive of SVT. Broad monophasic complexes are suggestive of VT.
- In lead V1 with LBB morphology if the QRS demonstrates narrow (<30 milliseconds) initial *r* and sharp smooth descent it is likely to be due to SVT with aberrant conduction.
- Notching in the down slope of the QRS and an interval of 60 milliseconds from the onset of the QRS to the nadir of the S wave is suggestive of VT.
- LBBB morphology with right axis deviation is invariably due to VT.
- RBBB morphology with normal axis is suggestive of SVT (uncommon in VT).
- Concordance pattern is uncommon in SVT. Positive concordance may be present in preexcited tachycardia.
- Negative concordance in limb leads L1, L11, and L111 is suggestive of VT (Northwest Axis).
- Presence or preserved Q waves during WCT is suggestive of VT. Pseudo Q waves may be seen in AVNRT.
- Absence of RS complex in precordial leads (concordant pattern) is suggestive of VT. If the RS pattern is present, the interval from the onset of R wave to the nadir of S wave of >100 milliseconds is suggestive of VT.
- If the QRS duration during tachycardia is narrower than the QRS duration during sinus rhythm, it is suggestive of VT.
- Occurrence of contralateral BBB during WCT is highly suggestive of VT. If RBBB was present during sinus rhythm and LBBB developed during SVT, it will result in CHB unless the BBB pattern is due to peripheral conduction delay.
- QRS alternans does not help in differentiating WCT.
- Some of the criteria may not be reliable in the presence of preexisting BBB during sinus rhythm.

Table 6.1 Differential diagnosis of WCT[1]

Clinical features	SVT with AC	VT
History of MI	Less likely	More likely
Canon Waves, Variable S1		If present suggest AV dissociation
Carotid sinus pressure Valsalva, Adenosine	Terminates tachycardia	Produces AV dissociation
ECG Features		
QRS Duration	<140 milliseconds	>140 milliseconds
QRS Axis frontal plane	Normal	Right Superior
RBBB morphology		
QRS in V1	Triphasic	Mono or Biphasic
QRS in V6	R/S ratio >1	R/S ratio <1
LBBB morphology		
QRS in V1	Narrow r, sharp descent	Notching, R to S >60 milliseconds
QRS V6	RS	QR QS
LBBB RAD	Less likely	Likely to be VT
RBBB normal axis	Likely SVT	Less Likely
Other features		
Concordance pattern V lead	Uncommon	Common
Preserved Q during WCT	Unlikely	Common
AV dissociation, fusion, capture. Number of V > A	Unlikely	Diagnostic of VT
If RS pattern present in V leads	RS less than 100 milliseconds	RS >100 milliseconds
QRS narrower during tachycardia than in SR	Unlikely	Likely
Contralateral BBB during WCT	Unlikely	Suggestive of VT
Change in axis from SR	<40°	>40°
QRS similar during SR and WCT	Suggestive of SVT	Uncommon

AC = Aberrant conduction.

- In the presence of preexisting RBBB, AV dissociation, precordial concordance, right superior axis and monophasic R wave in V1 are highly suggestive of VT.
- If the WCT does not conform to any patterns of aberration it is likely to be due to VT.

Exceptions to VT criteria
- Bundle branch reentry tachycardia may mimic SVT with aberration of LB morphology. The presence of AV dissociation will help in making the correct diagnosis.
- VT can be irregular during the first 30 seconds.

- Narrow complex VT is likely to originate from the septum or the fascicle.
- Fusion complexes may occur with two ventricular ectopic foci.
- AV dissociation can be present in junctional tachycardia.

Reference

1 Wellens HJ. Electrophysiology: Ventricular tachycardia: diagnosis of broad QRS complex tachycardia. Heart. 86(5):579–85, 2001.

7 Ventricular Tachycardia and Ventricular Fibrillation

Self-Assessment Questions

1 Which one of the following is not a risk factor for SCD?
   A Deafness
   B Left ventricular hypertrophy
   C Na, Ca, and K channel abnormalities
   D Autonomic dysfunction such as an increase in sympathetic tone and a decrease in parasympathetic tone

7.1 VENTRICULAR TACHYCARDIA IN THE PRESENCE OF CORONARY ARTERY DISEASE

1 An 83-year-old man is brought to the emergency department because of palpitations that began 4 hours ago. He denies chest pain or dyspnea. He is alert and anxious. Blood pressure is 120/70 mm Hg. He suffered from a myocardial infarction 7 years ago.

   Electrocardiogram is shown below.

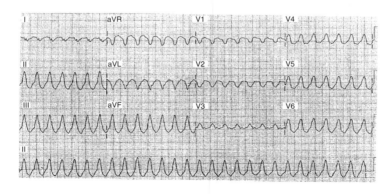

   Which of the following is the most likely diagnosis?
   A Atrial flutter with 1 : 1 AV aberrant conduction
   B Ventricular tachycardia
   C AV reentrant tachycardia using an atriofascicular pathway
   D Antidromic tachycardia utilizing left-sided accessory pathway

2 Eight months ago, a 52-year-old man, who had a history of skipping of heart beats for several years, had an inferoposterior myocardial infarction. No clinical evidence of heart failure was noted during recovery.

Echocardiogram showed inferior akinesis and estimated left ventricular ejection fraction of 42%. Ambulatory electrocardiographic monitoring revealed frequent episodes of three-beat nonsustained monomorphic ventricular tachycardia.

The patient has no cardiovascular symptoms. His only medication is aspirin, 81 mg daily.

Which of the following is most appropriate at this time?

A Electrophysiologic study

B Amiodarone

C A β-adrenergic blocking agent

D An implantable cardioverter-defibrillator

3 A 56-year-old man, undergoing cardiac rehabilitation, complained of palpitations. He had a myocardial infarction 6 weeks ago. He has no history of angina pectoris, or syncope. Echocardiogram shows left ventricular ejection fraction of 30%.

Which of the following is the most appropriate next step?

A Observation

B 24-hour ambulatory electrocardiography

C An implantable cardioverter-defibrillator

D Electrophysiologic study

7.2 ARRHYTHMOGENIC RIGHT VENTRICULAR DYSPLASIA/CARDIOMYOPATHY ARVD/C

1 A 17-year-old male presents to the emergency room with a history of syncope. Cardiac monitoring reveals frequent PVCs but no ventricular tachycardia. Echocardiogram revealed mild RV dilatation. Cardiac MRI revealed fatty myocardial infiltration. The next step will be (choose more than one):

A Myocardial Biopsy

B Head up tilt test

C RV angiogram

D Signal average ECG

2 What will be your recommendation?

A ICD implant

B Sotalol

C Amiodarone

D None of the above

3 A 40-year-old sales representative presents with progressively increasing dyspnea, fatigue, and severe swelling around the ankles. Five years ago he had recurrent episodes of ventricular tachycardia. A diagnosis of ARVD/C was made. An ICD was implanted in the left pectoral region. At the time of the initial implant R wave amplitude was 6 mV and the pacing threshold was 0.6 V at 0.5 milliseconds pulse width. On today's evaluation R wave amplitude was 1.5 mV and the pacing threshold was 2.5 V at 0.5 pulse width. In the last 4 weeks four pleural taps were performed and each time 700–1000 ml of fluid was removed. Echocardiogram shows enlarged and hypokinetic RV.

The patient has not had ventricular arrhythmias in the last 14 months. What will be your recommendation?

A Implant new ICD on the right side

B Start Sotalol

C Consider cardiac transplant

D Surgically isolate RV

4 Which of the following findings is most likely to be present in arrhythmogenic right ventricular dysplasia?

A Areas of fatty infiltration without fibrosis in the myocardium

B Normal cardiac evaluations of family members

C Late potentials on signal-averaged electrocardiography

D No inducible arrhythmias on programmed electrical stimulation

7.3 VENTRICULAR ARRHYTHMIA IN HYPERTROPHIC AND DILATED CARDIOMYOPATHY

1 Which one of the following is the risk factor for SCD in patients with IHSS?

A Age >50 years

B History of frequent PVCs

C Gene Mutation coding for Troponin and Tropomyosin

D LV wall thickness of 15 mm

2 You are asked to provide an opinion regarding a younger brother of a 28-year-old asymptomatic athlete who was found to have IHSS on an echocardiogram. This 21-year-old man is asymptomatic and his echocardiogram is normal. The 12-lead ECG showed ST-T changes.

What will be your recommendations?

A This could be suggestive of carrier or preclinical state

B This is perhaps a juvenile pattern

C The patient should not be allowed to participate in sports

D Coronary angiogram should be performed as these changes could be due to anomalous origin of the coronary arteries

3 In which of the following conditions are echocardiographic findings suggestive of IHSS are unlikely to be present?
A Friedreich ataxia
B Noonan syndrome
C Amyloidosis
D Addison's disease

4 You are asked to evaluate a 17-year-old high school student who has been diagnosed to have IHSS. His main symptoms are palpitations and occasional non exertional chest pain. 24-hour ambulatory ECG monitoring revealed frequent PVCs and 3–4 beat nonsustained VT. There is no history of syncope or sustained VT. To further risk stratify what will be your recommendations?
A Electrophysiologic study
B Signal average ECG
C Stress test
D Cardiac catheterization and angiography

5 This patient expresses the desire to participate in the high school football team. What will be your therapeutic recommendations?
A Start β blockers and allow him to participate in contact sports
B Start Disopyramide and allow him to participate in contact sports
C Start Digoxin and allow him to participate in contact sports
D The patient should refrain from participating in contact sports

7.4 LONG QT SYNDROME AND TORSADE DE POINTE

1 A 22-year-old female, without deafness, presents with history of seizures. During EEG recording she has a brief seizure. At that time the following rhythm strip is recorded. Serum potassium was 3.6 mEq. The echocardiogram was normal.

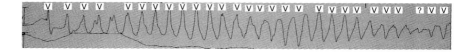

What will be your recommendation?
A Dilantin
B Mexiletine
C Keep serum potassium level >4.0 mEq
D Implant ICD

2 Which of the following channel/current activity will prolong the APD?
   A Increase in I_{to}
   B Block of I_{Na}
   C Decrease in I_{Kr}
   D Block of K_{ATP}

3 Which one of the following agents is least likely to prolong the QT interval?
   A Cefepime HCL
   B Ketoconazole
   C Haloperidol
   D Trimethoprim-sulfa

4 A 46-year-old male was treated for hypertension with hydrochlorothiazide and Felodipine and for diabetes with long acting insulin. He developed low grade fever and cough. He was prescribed erythromycin and benadryl. Two days later he developed transient loss of consciousness lasting for 30–40 seconds, during which tonic and clonic movements were noted. Serum potassium was 3.7 mEq. Blood sugar was normal. Electrocardiogram done 3 weeks earlier was normal. Echocardiogram was normal.
   What is the most likely cause of this event?
   A Hypoglycemia
   B TDP
   C Neurocardiogenic syncope
   D Seizure disorder

5 You are asked to evaluate a 19-year-old woman who was found to have a QT_c of 480 milliseconds. Three months ago, her 25-year-old maternal aunt, who was recently diagnosed to have congenital long Q-T syndrome, died suddenly. The patient has no history of syncope or other cardiac symptoms. Her mother and 15-year-old brother are asymptomatic. There is no family history of deafness.
   What will be your recommendations?
   A Permanent pacemaker implant
   B Initiate β blockers
   C Implant ICD
   D Observation

6 A 27-year-old female, on routine evaluation, had ECG (shown below). She is asymptomatic. There is no family history of syncope, sudden cardiac death, deafness or prolonged QT interval. Her echocardiogram is normal. Serum potassium is 4.0 mEq. She is not receiving any medications.

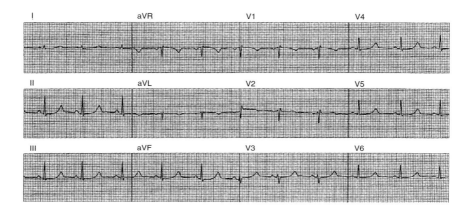

What will be your recommendation?

A Observation
B β blockers
C Electrophysiologic study
D Permanent pacemaker implant

7.5 BRUGADA SYNDROME

1 As a volunteer physician for doctors without borders you are posted in Cambodia. You are asked to evaluate a 17-year-old male who had one episode of syncope. There is family history of sudden cardiac death. ECG shows type 1 Brugada pattern.

What will be your recommendation?

A Flecainide
B Quinidine
C β blockers
D Close observation, no antiarrhythmics

2 A 24-year-old asymptomatic subject presents with ECG diagnosis of Brugada syndrome. Family history is unremarkable. What will be your recommendation?

A ICD implant
B EPS
C Observation
D β blockers

7.6 VENTRICULAR TACHYCARDIA IN STRUCTURALLY NORMAL HEART

1 A 50-year-old physician comes to the emergency department because of rapid palpitations that began 1 hour ago. He has had multiple episodes in the past year. The patient is in no distress. The pulse rate is 180 per minute, and blood pressure is 110/70 mm Hg. Electrocardiogram is shown.

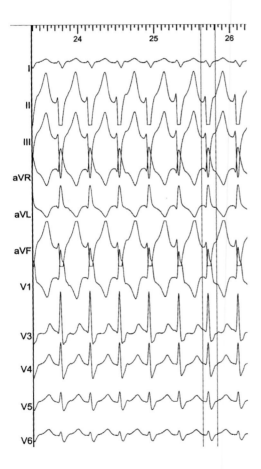

Adenosine, 6 mg intravenously, is administered, without any effect. Tachycardia terminates spontaneously 15 minutes later. The complete blood count, serum electrolytes and thyroid-stimulating hormone, chest radiograph, echocardiogram, and cardiac magnetic resonance imaging scan are normal. Cardiac perfusion studies are normal.

Which of the following statements regarding this patient's tachycardia is most likely correct?

A It originates from the left ventricular outflow tract

B It originates from the right ventricular outflow tract

C It originates from the Purkinje system of the apical left ventricular septum

D It uses a left lateral AV accessory pathway

2 An 18-year-old woman is brought to the emergency room for a painful and swollen right knee that she suffered while playing tennis. In the ER the following ECG was recorded.

She denies any palpitations, chest pain, or syncope. The physical examination is normal. Serum electrolytes and blood count are within normal limits. Echocardiogram and cardiac MRI are normal.

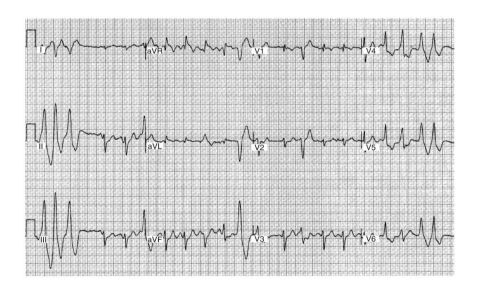

What will be your recommendations?

A Lidocaine 50 mg IV bolus and drip at 2 mg/minute

B Begin oral flecainide

C Admit the patient and schedule for electrophysiologic study

D Observation reassurance without further diagnostic and therapeutic intervention

3 A 36-year-old man seeks your advice regarding frequent palpitations. Last week he was in the emergency room with one such episode. Electrocardiogram recorded during that episode is shown.

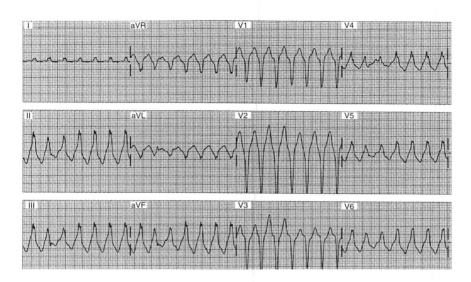

Ablation at which of the following sites is most likely to resolve the arrhythmias.

A Posterior free wall of the right ventricular outflow tract
B Left septal wall of the right ventricular outflow tract
C Lateral wall of the LV outflow tract
D Left ventricular basal-septum

4 A previously healthy 30-year-old man has sudden onset of palpitations and lightheadedness while playing soccer. The pulse rate was 190 per minute, and blood pressure is 100/58 mm Hg. The arrhythmia terminates spontaneously, and he is brought to the hospital.

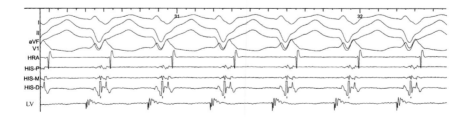

Cardiac enzymes, electrocardiogram, echocardiogram, and treadmill exercise electrocardiogram are normal. Recordings obtained during electrophysiologic study are shown below.

Which of the following statements is most likely correct regarding this condition?

A Intravenous administration of verapamil may result in hemodynamic collapse

B The tachycardia originates in the region of the left posterior fascicle

C Left lateral accessory pathway ablation will terminate the tachycardia

D An identical pace map is required for successful radiofrequency catheter ablation

7.7 BUNDLE BRANCH REENTRY VENTRICULAR TACHYCARDIA

1 During electrophysiologic study a wide complex tachycardia is induced. The tracing is shown below.

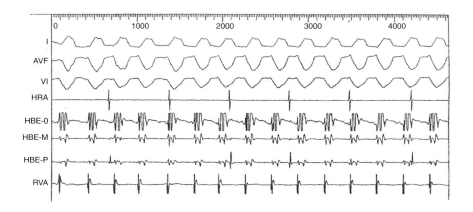

Which one of the following is likely to terminate and render tachycardia noninducible?

A AVN ablation

B Ablation of the focus in RVOT

C Ablation of the right bundle

D Ablation of the atriofascicular pathway

2 Which one of the following conditions is unlikely to present with BBR-VT?
A Myotonic dystrophy
B Hypertrophic cardiomyopathy
C Ebstein anomaly
D Brugada syndrome

3 Which one of the following observations is unlikely to be present in BBR-VT?
A A short HV interval during VT when compared with HV in sinus rhythm as measured from the onset of surface QRS.
B Conduction abnormality of HPS during sinus rhythm
C VT with LB morphology
D His electrogram precedes RB electrogram.

7.8 CATECHOLAMINERGIC POLYMORPHIC VENTRICULAR TACHYCARDIA

1 A 21-year-old male presents to ER with palpitations. Cardiac examination is normal. Echocardiogram is normal. ECG shows bidirectional ventricular tachycardia. Which one of the following is least likely to be effective?
A Digoxin antibodies
B β blockers
C Flecainide
D Potassium replacement

2 A 16-year-old male presents to the emergency department with abdominal pain. Diagnosis of acute appendicitis is made and surgery is recommended.

There is no history of palpitations, syncope, or seizures. His uncle had died suddenly at the age of 19.

The patient's mother reported that the patient was found to be a carrier for RyR2 mutation. Her concern is that general anesthesia may induce malignant hyperthermia.

Cardiac examination and echocardiogram are normal.

What will be your recommendations?
A The patient can safely undergo surgery under general anesthesia
B ICD should be implanted prior to surgical intervention
C IV amiodarone should be started prior to surgery and should be continued after surgery
D Electrophysiologic study should be performed to assess the risk of inducible ventricular arrhythmias

7.9 MISCELLANEOUS FORMS OF VENTRICULAR ARRHYTHMIAS

1 Which one of the following conditions is least likely to present with bidirectional VT?

   A Digitalis toxicity

   B Herbal aconite poisoning

   C Familial hypokalemic periodic paralysis

   D Hypocalcemia

Ventricular arrhythmias

- Cardiovascular disease remains a major cause of sudden cardiac death (SCD).
- 50% of all cardiac deaths are sudden. The majority of SCD are caused by ventricular arrhythmias. Its incidence increases with age.
- The high-risk subgroup includes patients with low ejection fraction (EF), history of heart failure, resuscitated out-of-hospital cardiac arrest, and previous myocardial infarction.
- Ventricular arrhythmias generate a high percentage of SCD but absolute numbers are low.
- In the general population the incidence of SCD is low, 0.1–0.2%, but absolute numbers are high, 300,000 SCD per year.
- A large number of patients in the general population will have to be treated to avoid the small number of deaths.
- The risk of sudden death is highest in the first 6–18 months after an index event such as myocardial infarction or a recent onset of heart failure. The risk of sudden death is proportionate to the increasing number of CAD risk factors.
- Structural abnormalities of the heart such as myocardial infarction, dilatation due to myopathy and left ventricular hypertrophy predispose to the genesis of ventricular life-threatening arrhythmias. Use of these risk factors in identifying individuals at risk of sudden cardiac death is limited.
- The incidence of ventricular arrhythmia induced SCD, as a percentage of total mortality tends to be high in patients with congestive heart failure (CHF) in functional class II and III; however in patients with functional class IV bradyarrhythmias, asystole and pulseless electrical activity appear to be the cause of death.

Risk factors for SCD

1 Myocardial ischemia.
2 Left ventricular hypertrophy.
3 Na, Ca, and K channel abnormalities.
4 Metabolic abnormalities such as hypokalemia, acidosis, and stretch-related modulations of ion channels.
5 Autonomic dysfunction such as increase in sympathetic and decrease in parasympathetic tone.
6 Drugs that could alter repolarization and cause Torsade de pointes (TDP).

In 80% of SCD victims no acute myocardial infarction (MI) is found. The triggering mechanism appears to be ischemia.

Ventricular fibrillation (VF)[1]

- VF is a common arrhythmia noted in patients with out-of-hospital cardiac arrest.
- Slowing of the VF rate after initial rapid onset may be due to ischemia and acid/base, electrolyte abnormality.

- Coronary artery disease is the most common substrate in patients with VF. Acute MI is found in 20% of patients with VF cardiac arrest and recurrence is less than 2% in one year in these patients. Recurrence is 30% if VF occurs in the absence of acute MI.
- Slowing of conduction may occur in the scar tissue of the healed MI predisposing to reentrant VT/VF.
- 25% of patients with cardiomyopathy may develop VF cardiac arrest in the first year.
- Identification of the high-risk patients is difficult. In patients with hypertrophic cardiomyopathy, risk factors such as family history of sudden death and inducible VT during EPS may identify the high risk group. An ejection fraction of less than 35% remains a major risk factor for patients with ischemic or nonischemic cardiomyopathy although the sensitivity of these markers is low.
- During metabolic acidosis the VF threshold is decreased and the reverse is likely in metabolic alkalosis.
- Alkalization of the serum may retard class I antiarrhythmic related proarrhythmias.
- Prophylactic Lidocaine should not be used in post-MI patients.
- Defibrillator implant is the treatment of choice.
- Mortality remains 40% in five years irrespective of the treatment chosen.

7.1 VENTRICULAR TACHYCARDIA IN THE PRESENCE OF CORONARY ARTERY DISEASE

Ventricular tachycardia

- Occurrence of the arrhythmias is facilitated by the presence of **substrate** such as slowing of conduction (scar, anisotropy), dispersion of refractoriness, electrical **triggers** such as PVCs and physiologic **modulating factors** such as ischemia, electrolyte abnormalities, hypoxia, and proarrhythmic drugs.
- Sustained monomorphic VT arises from the scar of healed myocardial infarction.
- Classification/definitions of VT are outlined in Fig. 7.1.

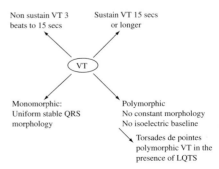

Fig 7.1 Classification/definitions of VT.

Factors associated with development of ventricular arrhythmias

1 Large MI
2 Septal involvement in MI
3 Left ventricular dysfunction
4 Hypotension during evolving MI
5 Ventricular fibrillation during early stages of MI
6 Conduction abnormalities

- Patients with hemodynamically stable sustained VT tend to have scars from MI, left ventricular aneurysm, and left ventricular dysfunction when compared with patients whose first presentation is SCD.

Clinical manifestations during VT

- Heart rate during VT is a major determinant of homodynamic status.
- Other factors include systolic and diastolic dysfunction, ischemia, and degree of mitral insufficiency.
- Electrocardiographic features of VT are described in Chapter 6.

Electrocardiographic features

When attempting to localize the origin of the VT following points should be considered:

1 **QRS width**: QRS duration in septal VTs is less than the VTs originating from the free wall.
2 **QRS axis**: Right superior-axis suggests that the VT is arising from apical septal or apical lateral region. QS pattern is seen in leads I, II, and III and QS or rS in V5 and V6.
  Presence of QS complexes in inferior leads are due to spread of activation from inferior wall. QS pattern in precordial leads suggests activation moving away from the anterior wall.
  VT with Inferior-axis arises from the basal areas, right ventricular outflow tract, superior left ventricular septum, or basal lateral wall of the left ventricle. The inferior axis will point to left if VT is arising from the superior right free wall or superior left ventricular septum.
  Left-axis deviation is present when in the presence of inferior infarction the VT exit site is near the septum. The axis moves to the right and superior as the site of the origin of the VT moves postero-laterally.
3 **Bundle branch block pattern**: The bundle branch block pattern is a result of the sequence of right and left ventricular activation. Left bundle branch block morphology is present in VTs arising from right ventricle or from LV side of septum.
4 **Concordance**: Positive concordance is present when the direction of the activation is anterior and apical and is generally present in VTs arising from the posterior basal area of the heart.

VT arising from the scar of inferior infarction, activation is from posterior to anterior resulting in R wave in precordial leads (V2 to V4). In the presence of RBBB this pattern may persist up to V6.

Negative concordance is seen in VTs arising from apical septum as a sequel of anteroapical MI.

5 **Presence of QS or QR complexes**: Presence of QS complexes in V4–V6 suggests apical origin of the VT.

- Frontal plane axis and QRS morphology may help localize the exit site and location of the VT circuit (Fig. 7.2a).

Electrophysiologic features

- His bundle deflection preceding a QRS complex is usually absent. If His electrogram is present the HV interval is shorter than the HV interval during sinus rhythm.
- Changing the AH interval in the presence of the constant but shorter HV interval indicates that the His is engaged retrogradely by VT.
- If His is retrogradely activated during VT, RB potential will precede His potential (Fig. 7.2b).
- If His is engaged by an antegrade impulse His electrogram will precede the RB electrogram.
- If atrial pacing during WCT (wide complex tachycardia) entrains the tachycardia with normal HV and QRS then it is highly suggestive of VT (Fig. 7.3).
- The HV interval during VT should be compared with the HV interval during sinus rhythm. The HV during VT may appear normal but will be shorter than the HV in sinus rhythm.
- The occurrence of HV interval that is shorter than the HV in sinus rhythm implies retrograde activation of the His with a conduction time to His being shorter than the antegrade conduction time to the rest of the ventricular myocardium. It also implies that the site of origin is in proximity to the Purkinje system.

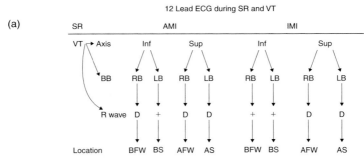

Fig 7.2a ECG algorithm for identifying the site of origin of VT. SR, sinus rhythm; AMI, anterior MI; IMI, inferior MI; BB, bundle branch block; RB, right bundle branch block morphology; LB, left bundle branch block morphology; D, delayed R progression; +, R wave present across precordial leads; −, R wave absent; BFW, basal free wall; BS, basal septum; AFW, apex free wall; and AS, apex septum.

(b)

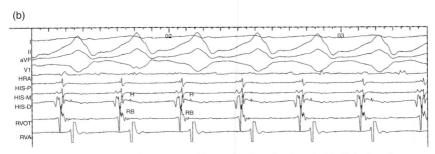

Fig 7.2b (b) VT originating in the septum with retrograde activation of HPS. Right bundle precedes His electrograms. The underlying atrial rhythm is AF.

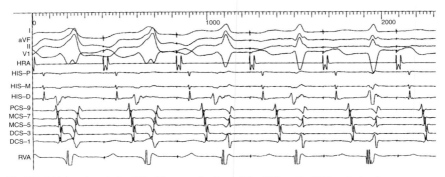

Fig 7.3 Atrial pacing during VT with normalization of the QRS as the VT is entrained.

- During BB reentry tachycardia HV during VT may be the same or longer than the HV during sinus rhythm (Figs 7.15 and 7.16).
- In BB reentry retrograde conduction occurs over the LB and antegrade conduction over the right bundle, the His electrogram precedes the RB electrogram.
- In BB reentry tachycardia changes in V to V interval follow the changes in H to H interval. RV activation precedes left ventricular activation.
- Electrophysiologic study has low yield in patients who present with VF cardiac arrest due to ischemia.
- Ventricular tachycardia arise from surviving myocytes within the scar; conduction through these tissues is slow and inhomogeneous, resulting in low amplitude (<0.5 mV) and fractionated potentials (lasting for >130 milliseconds) that precede the onset of the surface QRS.
- Substrate for ventricular tachycardia after myocardial infarction develops in the first two weeks but persists indefinitely.
- If a ventricular tachycardia is induced two weeks after myocardial infarction it remains reproducible one year later.
- The risk of developing ventricular tachycardia is greatest (3–5%) in the first year after a MI but may occur 15–20 years later. Progression of

coronary artery disease and worsening of the left ventricular function may act as a trigger.

Mechanisms

- The mechanism of the scar-related VT is reentry, which can be initiated and terminated by programmed stimulation.
- 95% of spontaneously occurring ventricular tachycardia are inducible.
- 54% of the patients with CAD and SCD have inducible VT and 30% have inducible sustained polymorphic VT.
- 20% of all VT are induced from RVOT when apical stimulation fails.
- The inverse relation between the extra stimulus coupling interval and the interval to the first beat of VT suggest the presence of slow conduction.
- The presence of mid-diastolic or presystolic potentials is suggestive of slow conduction.
- To avoid nonspecific and nonclinical responses, during programmed electrical stimulation, a coupling interval of extra stimulus of less than 200 milliseconds should be avoided.
- The use of three extra stimuli at two different RV endocardial sites and at two different cycle lengths is considered adequate. This protocol provides optimum sensitivity and specificity.
- The use of increasing current (5–10 mA) may result in nonspecific responses without increasing the yield.
- During programmed stimulation demonstration of resetting and concealed entrainment are suggestive of reentry.
- Reentrant VT can be terminated by overdrive RV pacing. Pacing stimuli should be synchronized to the VT complexes.

Electrophysiologic criteria for selecting ablation site[2]

Activation time

- Endocardial activation time is defined as the interval from the local earliest fractionated ventricular electrogram, continuous or isolated potential, of the mapping catheter to the onset of the QRS complex. Activation time of >-70 msec suggest proximity of the mapping/ablation catheter to area of slow conduction.

Resetting has the following characteristics:

1 Extra stimulus delivered during VT results in a less than compensatory pause.
2 The first VT beat (return cycle) after the extrastimulus is morphologically identical to subsequent VT beats.
3 The return cycle, measured from the extrastimulus to the onset of the first VT beat, is the same as the tachycardia cycle length.

- Resetting occurs in more than 85% of stable VT (CL more than 270).
- Extrastimulus encounters an excitable gap within the VT circuit. It collides retrogradely with the previous tachycardia beat and continues antegradely, thus advancing the next tachycardia beat by the duration of its prematurity.

- The ability to demonstrate resetting does not prove reentry; automatic and triggered activity can also be reset.
- Triggered rhythms show constant return cycle length, 100–110% of the VT cycle length.
- Resetting with fusion is suggestive of reentry. This phenomenon is not seen in triggered activity.
- Resetting does not help in identifying the site of successful ablation.

Post pacing interval

- On termination of the pacing, that entrained the tachycardia, the interval from the last pacing stimulus to first spontaneous depolarization at pacing site is called the post pacing interval (PPI). If the pacing site is within the reentrant circuit then the PPI will equal the tachycardia cycle length (TCL). Pacing from the bystander sites will result in PPI longer than TCL. PPI should not be the sole criteria for selecting the ablation target.
- For PPI to be identical to TCL one has to speculate that the pacing site is identical to the recording site, and the revolution of last pacing stimulus around the reentrant circuit is identical the to a spontaneous revolution during VT. It may be difficult to precisely determine local activation time in the presence of broad, fractionated electrograms.

Concealed entrainment

- Entrainment utilizes the same physiology as resetting when overdrive pacing is used during tachycardia.
- During entrainment first paced beat interacts with tachycardia circuit however subsequent paced beats interact with previously reset tachycardia circuit.
- Continuous resetting of the circuit by pacing at a rate faster than VT cycle length results in acceleration of the tachycardia to pacing cycle length and resumption of the tachycardia on terminating the pacing fulfills the criteria for entrainment.
- Entrainment without evidence of surface or intracardiac electrogram fusion is called concealed entrainment. This generally occurs when pacing is performed from the isthmus of a tachycardia circuit.
- During concealed entrainment stimulus to QRS interval will be short if the pacing site is close to the exit of the isthmus and longest at the proximal entry site.
- Concealed entrainment suggests that the pacing is being performed from the isthmus of the VT circuit. However the predictive value for identifying the site for successful ablation is approximately 50%.

Stimulus to QRS and Electrogram to QRS interval

- At sites with concealed entrainment, less than 30 ms difference between stimulus–QRS and electrogram–QRS interval identifies the most useful criterion for successful ablation. Identical stimulus–QRS and electrogram–QRS intervals suggest that the catheter is in contact with an area of slow conduction within the reentrant circuit.

Isolated potentials
- Low frequency fragmented continuous or isolated electrograms are often recorded from the tip of the mapping catheter.
- Isolated potential that can not be dissociated from VT also identifies the area likely to be a successful site for ablation.

Termination of VT without global capture
- Termination of the VT by a pacing stimulus that does not produce QRS suggests that the pacing stimulus was delivered in the reentrant circuit.
- Ablation at a site where ventricular pacing or extrastimulus results in termination of VT without global capture is likely to yield positive results. This phenomenon indicates that the extrastimulus collided with orthodromically conducting reentrant beat within the VT circuit and terminated the tachycardia.
- Multiple morphologies of VTs may be inducible however intent is to ablate clinically documented VT.
- qS pattern in unfiltered unipolar electrogram indicates electrode is in close proximity of the origin of focal VT. Unipolar electrograms are not helpful in mapping scar related VT. Closely spaced bipolar electrograms are used to record low amplitude fractionated signal from the scar tissue.
- Pacing from the mapping/ablation catheter is performed for pace mapping and entrainment mapping. Unipolar pacing provides more accurate information but large pacing artifact distorts the QRS complex.
- Pace mapping is performed during sinus rhythm form the site of focal VT. This produces QRS complex identical to VT. Pace mapping is not helpful for mapping scar related VT but may help identify general area of interest where more precise mapping should be performed.
- Electrograms from the area of slow conduction are fragmented and can be recorded during sinus rhythm or during VT.
- During sinus rhythm these electrograms are recorded at the end of the QRS complex and during diastole or presystolic phase during scar related VT. These electrograms can occur at bystander site and are not reliable indicators of the ablation target unless they can be associated with VT.
- In focal VT local electrograms may precede QRS complex by 15–30 msec.
- Concealed entrainment, stimulus to QRS interval same as electrogram (isolated diastolic potentials) to QRS and PPI same as VT cycle length increases the likelihood of successful VT ablation.[4]

Treatment
- Hemodynamically unstable patients should be cardioverted.
- I.V. Procainamide appears to be superior to Lidocaine.
- Patients with incessant or recurrent VT may respond to IV Amiodarone. 30-day mortality remains high in this group (30–50%).
- Long-term treatment of choice is ICD.

- In AVID trial patients with hemodynamically stable VT and EF of greater than 40% were excluded from the trial but were followed in a registry. Mortality risks were found to be lower in this group.[3]
- In patients with previous myocardial infarction, EF of 35%, spontaneous NSVT and inducible VT ICD implant improved survival by 20% in one year.
- Patients with a low ejection fraction irrespective of nonsustained VT or inducibility during electrophysiologic study have been shown to derive survival benefit from prophylactic ICD implant.

Catheter ablation of the VT[2,4]

- Hemodynamically stable monomorphic VT can be considered for RF ablation (Table 7.1).
- The circuit of scar-related VT has an area of slow conduction and isthmus. Travel of electrical impulse through the isthmus is not detected on surface ECG. Exit of electrical impulse from this isthmus inscribes the onset of the QRS. Electrical impulse returns to the entry site of the loop. There may be multiple bystander loops.
- Radiofrequency application interrupts the slowly conduting isthmus.
- Rapid initial upstroke of the QRS suggests that the VT may be arising from normal myocardium. Slurring of the initial forces is seen when the tachycardia arises from an area of scar or from the epicardium.
- Low amplitude complexes are seen in the presence of diseased heart.
- Notching of the QRS is seen in scar-related VT.
- QR or qR or Qr complexes are seen in the presence of an infarct.
- Frontal plane axis and QRS morphology may help localize the exit site and location of the VT circuit.
- Radiofrequency application interrupts the slowly conducting isthmus.
- Multiple morphologies of VTs may be inducible, however, the intent is to ablate clinically documented VTs.

Table 7.1 Ventricular tachycardia likely to be considered for RF ablation

Site of origin of VT	QRS morphology
RVOT VT	LBBB inferior axis
LV idiopathic VT	RBBB superior left or right axis
Bundle branch reentry VT	LBBB occasionally RB
Scar related VT	
RV dysplasia	LBBB
Fallot tetralogy	LBBB
Prior MI	
Sarcoidosis	
Chagas disease	

- qS pattern in unfiltered unipolar electrogram indicates that the electrode is in close proximity to the origin of focal VT. Unipolar electrograms are not helpful in mapping scar-related VT. Closely spaced bipolar electrograms are used to record low amplitude fractionated signals from the scar tissue.
- Pacing from the mapping/ablation catheter is performed for pace mapping and entrainment mapping. Unipolar pacing provides more accurate information but large pacing artifact distorts the QRS complex.
- Pace mapping is performed during sinus rhythm from the site of focal VT. This produces QRS complex identical to VT. Pace mapping is not helpful for mapping scar-related VT but may help identify the general area of interest where more precise mapping should be performed.
- Electrograms from the area of slow conduction are fragmented and can be recorded during sinus rhythm or during VT.
- During sinus rhythm these electrograms are recorded at the end of the QRS complex and during diastole or presystolic phase during scar-related VT. These electrograms can occur at bystander sites and are not reliable indicators of the ablation target unless they can be associated with VT.
- In focal VT local electrograms may precede QRS complex by 15–30 milliseconds.
- Following an inferior wall myocardial infarction the reentrant circuit is located in the basal region near the mitral annulus. Surviving myocardium beneath the mitral annulus forms the critical corridor that maintains the reentrant circuit.
- Ablation of clinical VT can be considered if it results in frequent ICD shocks.
- In RV dysplasia reentrant circuits may be located in RVOT or near the tricuspid annulus. Recurrences are high.
- VT following tetralogy repair can be successfully ablated.
- LV mapping and ablation should be avoided if thrombus is present. A retrograde or transseptal approach can be used.
- The recurrence rate is 15% if the VT is not inducible after ablation and is higher if modified or clinical VT is still inducible.
- Warfarin aspirin should be continued after ablation.
- Complications include mortality, cerebral ischemia or infarction, cardiac perforation, and AV block.

7.2 ARRHYTHMOGENIC RIGHT VENTRICULAR DYSPLASIA/CARDIOMYOPATHY ARVD/C

Incidence and prevalence[5–10]

- The prevalence of the disease in the general population is estimated at 0.02–0.1% or 1 in 5000. The male/female ratio is 2.7/1.0.
- In Italy (Padua, Venice) and Greece (Island of Naxos), prevalence of 0.4–0.8% has been reported.

- Occurrence of ARVD/C in the Veneto region of Italy, in some clusters of families, has earned the term Venetian cardiomyopathy.

Genetics/classification of ARVD/C
- Transmission is autosomal dominant.

The type of ARVD and its chromosome location is shown in the following table.

ARVD Type	ARVD1	ARVD2	ARVD3	ARVD4	ARVD5	ARVD6	ARVD7	ARVD8
Chromosome location	14q23–q24	1q42–q43	14q12–q22	2q32	3p23	10p12–14	10q22, 6p24	12p11

- An autosomal recessive variant of ARVD/C that is associated with palmoplantar keratosis and woolly hair ("Naxos disease") has been mapped on chromosome 17q21 which controls plakoglobin.[5]
- Plakoglobin participates in cell-to-cell junctions. The absence of plakoglobin may result in inadequate cell adherence and injury to cardiac cell membranes. This may result in cell death and fibrofatty replacement.
- Mutations in the desmosomal protein plakophilin-2 are common in ARVD/C patients. Abnormalities of cardiac Ryanodine receptor gene, which is responsible for catecholamine-related ventricular tachycardia, may be present in ARVD/C.
- Fifty percent of the ARVD/C families do not show any linkage with the identified chromosomal loci.

Pathological features
- There is patchy loss of right ventricular myocytes with replacement by fibrofatty tissue and persistence of normal myocardial tissue in between. This may result in an area of slow conduction that initiates reentrant ventricular arrhythmias.
- There is thinning of the right ventricular wall.
- Fibrosis contributes to slowing of conduction and provides the substrate for arrhythmias.
- Fibrofatty replacement begins in the subepicardium or midmural layers and progresses to the subendocardium. It involves the right ventricular outflow tract, apex, and infundibulum.
- It might also affect the interventricular septum and the posteroseptal and posterolateral wall of the left ventricle.
- The left ventricular involvement rarely appears first.
- Inflammatory changes with lymphocyte infiltration may be noted.

Diagnosis
- The diagnosis of ARVD is based on the presence of major and minor diagnostic criteria as suggested by the international task force.
- The diagnosis is established by the presence of two major criteria or one major and two minor criteria or four minor criteria.

Table 7.2 Task force criteria for diagnosis of arrhythmogenic right ventricular dysplasia

Major	Minor
Severe RV dilation, reduction of RV ejection fraction, localized RV aneurysms	Mild RV dilatation and/or reduced ejection fraction
Fibrofatty replacement of myocardium as proven by biopsy	T-wave inversion in leads V1–V3 or beyond
Epsilon waves or localized QRS prolongation (>110 ms) in leads V1–V3	Late potentials on signal-averaged ECG
Familial disease confirmed at necropsy or surgery	Left bundle branch block-type ventricular tachycardia (sustained and nonsustained) or frequent PVCs (>1000/24 h)
	Familial history of premature sudden death (<35 years) or clinical diagnosis based on present criteria

- A definite diagnosis of ARVD is made when all the full criteria are met. A diagnosis of probable ARVD is made when fewer criteria are present such as one major and one minor or three minor criteria (Table 7.2).

- Task force recommendations do not incorporate the findings of imaging such as MRI, angiography and echocardiogram, nor does it specify which imaging technique should be preferred to examine and grade right ventricular morphology and function.

Electrocardiogram
- ECG shows a regular sinus rhythm.
- QRS duration is >110 milliseconds in lead V1, a terminal deflection within or at the end of the QRS complex called epsilon wave may be present in lead V1–V3 in 30% of patients.
- QRS duration may be longer over right precordial leads (V1–V3) compared with lead V6.
- T-waves inversion in the right precordial leads is noted in 50% of patients.
- Signal average EKG tends to be abnormal.
- Holter monitor may show frequent PVCs and nonsustained ventricular tachycardia.
- During a stress test there may be ST segment changes over the right precordial leads.
- During electrophysiologic study VT may be inducible by programmed stimulation.

Myocardial biopsy
- It lacks sensitivity as the tissue is obtained from the interventricular septum, whereas pathological changes are more noticeable in the free wall of the right ventricle.

RV angiogram
- It shows dyskinetic bulging, localized in the outflow tract, apex, and infundibulum, the anatomic triangle of dysplasia, and the presence of hypertrophic trabeculae in other areas.

Echocardiography
- It shows right ventricular dilatation, enlargement of the right atrium, isolated dilatation of the right ventricular outflow tract, increased reflectivity of the moderator band, localized aneurysms, and decreased fractional shortening of the RV. There is dyskinesis of the inferior wall and the right ventricular apex.
- In obese patients and in patients with pulmonary emphysema, transesophageal echocardiography is the preferred approach to visualize the right ventricle.
- Radionuclide angiography may demonstrate abnormal right ventricular function, but it is not an optimum imaging technique for ARVD/C.

Computed tomography
- It may demonstrate a dilated hypokinetic right ventricle, abundant epicardial fat, intramyocardial fat deposits and conspicuous trabeculation with low attenuation.
- Multislice computed tomography may be helpful in serial evaluation of ARVD/C patients with an implantable cardioverter defibrillator.

Cardiovascular magnetic resonance imaging
- It demonstrates intramyocardial fat deposits characterized by high-signal intensity areas indicating the substitution of myocardium by fat, focal wall thinning and wall hypertrophy, trabecular disarray, right ventricular outflow tract enlargement and ectasia, right ventricular aneurysms characterized dyskinetic bulges, diminished RV function, and enlargement of the right atrium.
- Sole reliance on fatty infiltrate may result in inappropriate overdiagnosis of ARVD/C/C.
- Fibrosis may be more specific than intramyocardial fat deposit. Contrast enhanced signal acquisition is capable of demonstrating fibrosis.
- Cardiovascular MRI remains normal in idiopathic right ventricular outflow tract tachycardia.
- If fatty infiltration is demonstrated, the diagnosis of ARVD/C should be confirmed by demonstrating other RV morphological and functional abnormalities. These findings should be confirmed by other imaging techniques such as echocardiography or angiography.

- The diagnosis of ARVD/C and therapeutic decisions must be made on the basis of Task Force criteria rather than structural abnormalities alone.
- Echocardiography should be the initial diagnostic approach.

Differential diagnosis

- Uhl's disease is characterized by a paper thin right ventricle. There is loss of myocardial muscle fibers due to the apoptotic process.
- In Uhl's disease there is no gender difference (male/female ratio 1.3) or family history of SCD. It presents in early childhood, usually with congestive heart failure as the first symptom.
- Myocarditis and idiopathic cardiomyopathy should also be considered in differential diagnosis.
- VT with LB morphology and inferior axis may occur in ARVD/C and may be mistaken for idiopathic RVOT-VT, sarcoidosis and congenital heart disease.
- In contrast to RVOT-VT, VT in ARVD/C demonstrates reentry multiple morphologies, and fragmented potentials.

High risk group[10]

- Patients with the following characteristics are considered to be at high risk for ventricular arrhythmias and SCD:
    - i Definite ARVD/C as defined by task force criteria.
    - ii Severe structural right ventricular disease, diffuse right ventricular involvement.
    - iii Increased QRS duration and T-wave inversion in leads V1–V3.
    - iv Nonsustained or sustained VT.
    - v Syncope.
    - vi Family history of SCD.
    - vii Inducible sustained ventricular arrhythmia during electrophysiologic study.
- Patients with probable ARVD and negative electrophysiology study could be considered to be low risk group.
- ICD therapy plays an important role in primary prevention of sudden cardiac death in patients with ARVD/C.
- Known causes of autosomal-dominant ARVC include mutations in the cardiac ryanodine receptor (*RYR2*) and desmoplakin genes.
- Other autosomal-dominant ARVD/C loci include regions on chromosomes 2, 3, 10, and 14.
- ARVC is a genetically heterogeneous group of diseases with phenotypic overlap.
- ARVC linked to 3p25 is a malignant disease, particularly in males, who frequently die suddenly in early adulthood.
- SCD may be the first symptom in those at high risk.
- ICD should be considered as a primary prevention therapy in familial ARVC linked to 3p25.

Clinical presentation

- Patients with ARVD/C typically present between the second and fifth decades of life with symptoms of palpitation, syncope or SCD associated with ventricular tachycardia.
- These patients may also present with nonspecific chest pain.
- In a concealed form of ARVD/C sudden death, usually during exercise, could be the first clinical presentation.
- Symptomatic ventricular arrhythmias may occur during exercise. 50–60% of patients present with monomorphic ventricular tachycardia with LBBB morphology.
- VT with multiple morphologies may occur.
- An inferior QRS axis during ventricular tachycardia reflects the right ventricular outflow tract as the site of origin, while a superior axis reflects the right ventricular inferior wall as the site of origin.
- The occurrence of arrhythmic cardiac arrest due to ARVD/C is significantly increased in athletes. Patients with established diagnosis of ARVD/C should not be allowed to participate in competitive sports and/or moderate-to-high intensity level recreational activities.
- In certain parts of Italy, ARVD/C has been shown to be the most frequent cause of exercise-induced cardiac death in athletes.
- Patients with advanced disease may present with right ventricular failure with or without arrhythmias. These patients may be eligible for cardiac transplant.

Prognosis

- Both sexes have similar mortality risk with peak occurring in the fourth decade.
- ARVD/C may account for up to 5% of sudden deaths in young adults in the United States and 25% of exercise-related deaths in the Veneto region of Italy.
- In the absence of SCD progressive impairment of cardiac function may result in right or biventricular heart failure, usually in four to eight years.

Treatment
Antiarrhythmic agents

- There are no data to support the use of antiarrhythmic agents for prevention of SCD.
- Sotalol Amiodarone and beta-blockers could be used to reduce the arrhythmia burden and recurrent shocks from the defibrillator.

Radiofrequency ablation

- Radiofrequency ablation can be considered if antiarrhythmic agents are ineffective or produce side-effects.
- There are no data to suggest that the ablation alone will be effective in preventing SCD.

- Three-dimensional mapping system and endocardial electrograms demonstrating low amplitude fractionated and earliest electrogram are effective in targeting the site of origin of VT.
- The long-term success of the ablation is low because of the progressive and diffuse nature of the disease, resulting in multiple arrhythmogenic foci and multiple morphologies of the VT, which may be difficult to abolish.
- The initial success of ablation is 60–80%, with a recurrence rate of approximately 30%.
- The commonest complication during ablation is cardiac perforation (10%) probably due to thinning of the RV walls.

ICD implant[10,11]

- It is the treatment of choice for patients who had syncope, family history of SCD, sustained VT, or aborted cardiac arrest.
- Patients who receive ICD for secondary prevention have a higher rate of appropriate ICD therapies.
- Electrophysiologic study may not be able to predict, in a primary prevention group, who will receive appropriate shock.
- ICD therapy plays an important role in primary prevention of sudden cardiac death in patients with ARVD/C.
- Possible problems with the use of ICD in patients with ARVD/C include right ventricular perforation during lead implant or during follow-up and increase in pacing threshold due to fibrosis at the tip of the pace sense electrode. This may also result in a decrease in R wave amplitude and poor detection of the arrhythmia.
- There may be an increase in defibrillation energy requirements.
- As the disease progresses and involves the left ventricle, CHF may occur. Its treatment with diuretics, ace inhibitors and β-blockers should be considered.
- Intractable heart failure may require cardiac transplant.

7.3 VENTRICULAR ARRHYTHMIAS IN HYPERTROPHIC AND DILATED ARDIOMYOPATHY

Heart failure and hypertrophy

- Mortality is 40% in four years. Half of it is due to sudden death.
- Fibrosis, apoptosis, hypertrophy, dispersion of refractoriness, neuroendocrine activation, electrolytes abnormalities, and drugs are the common factors that may precipitate arrhythmias.
- In LVH action potential prolongation is due to a decrease in I_{to}. This results in nonhomogeneous repolarization and propensity for EAD.
- Hypertrophied myocytes may produce DAD due to an increase in Ca load.
- Abnormal pacemaker current (I_f) has been reported in LVH. Intensity of I_f current increases with beta adrenergic stimulation.

- In LVH the density of I_{to} is reduced. The density of I_{CaL} and I_K is unchanged and density of I_f is increased.
- Hemodynamic overload may re-express fetal channel proteins such as T-type calcium channel.
- I_{K1} (inward rectifier) is reduced by 40% in a failing heart. I_{K1} contributes to the final phase of repolarization and sets resting membrane potential. Its reduction results in prolongation of the terminal phase of repolarization.

SAC – Stretch activated ion channels

- Stretch may activate the chloride channel and I_{Ks}.
- Stretch decreases the resting potential and induces premature depolarization by activating inward depolarizing sodium current.
- A sustained increase in preload causes shortening of APD and refractoriness.
- SAC can be blocked by gadolinium, streptomycin, and spider venom peptides.
- Unlike intraventricular pressure which is equally distributed throughout the left ventricle, wall stress may differ according to regional differences in the circumference, wall thickness, and compliance. This could explain heterogeneous shortening of APD.
- Shortening of refractoriness and the presence of slow conduction favors VF.
- Dilatation of the heart, which shortens refractoriness and hypokalemia, which decreases conduction velocity, when combined can cause serious arrhythmias.
- Ventricular dilatation causes shortening of refractoriness at rapid heart rate and not at slow heart rates. Shortening of refractoriness may predispose to arrhythmia.
- The beneficial effects of the beta-blockers in CHF may be due to slowing of the heart rate and restoring of the refractoriness.
- I_{Ks} is increased by mechanical stretch. This may cause abbreviation of APD in a rate dependent manner and decrease refractoriness.
- Dilatation may result in an increase in defibrillation threshold.

Tachycardia induced myocardial changes

- Changes in ERP and calcium loading occur earlier than autonomic changes, which may take several weeks.
- Tachycardia induced low intracellular magnesium in ventricular myocytes may contribute to abnormal repolarization in congestive heart failure.
- Tachycardia also reduces repolarizing potassium currents.
- Heterogeneity of sympathetic stimulation of the myocardium due to reduction of β-receptors may result in arrhythmias.
- Short-term tachycardia results in activation of the I_{KATP} channel, which may contribute to shortening of APD after tachycardia.
- Rapid pacing decreases I_{to}.
- A prolonged increase or decrease in cytosolic calcium increases or decreases sodium current respectively.

Ventricular arrhythmias in patients with heart failure

- Incidence of congestive heart failure increases with the patient's age. Mortality approaches 50% in patients with class IV CHF. With increasing severity of heart failure the mechanism of death shifts from tachyarrhythmias to bradyarrhythmias.
- Mechanisms that increase the vulnerability of a failing heart to ventricular arrhythmias include:
    i Ischemia produces shortening of action potential and slowing conduction in the ischemic zone and predisposes to reentry.
    ii Left ventricular hypertrophy results in an increase in APD.
    iii Changes in Ion channels and currents may occur. In CHF increase in APD is due to reduced I_{to} and I_K. I_f current is increased, resulting in an increased automaticity. The activity of Na/K ATPases is decreased, thus increasing the susceptibility to digoxin induced arrhythmias.
    iv In CHF there is alteration in gap junction and decrease in density of Connexion 43, which results in slowing of conduction.
    v Homodynamic changes such as an increase in ventricular volume and stretching of myocytes shorten the refractory period, resulting in early and late-after depolarization.
    vi Increased sympathetic activation promotes automatic and reentrant arrhythmias. Elevated norepinephrine levels correlate with poor prognosis.
    vii Electrolyte abnormalities such as hypokalemia and hypomagnesemia may induce DAD.

Ventricular arrhythmias in hypertrophic cardiomyopathy (HCM)[12]

- Hypertrophic cardiomyopathy is caused by gene mutation of either β myosin heavy chain or α tropomyosin or cardiac troponin T and I or cardiac myosin binding protein C or regulatory myosin light chain (Table 7.3).
- 35–50 percent of the HCM patients have a mutation in cardiac MHC gene, 15–25 percent due to mutations of myosin-binding protein C, 15–20 percent due to mutations of the cardiac troponin T gene, less than 5% due to mutations of the tropomyosin gene.

Table 7.3 Chromosome location of the genes for cardiac proteins

Chromosomes	Encoding proteins
1q32	Troponin T
19p13	Troponin I
15q22	α-Tropomyosin
11p11	Myosin-binding protein C
3p21 and 12q23–p21	Myosin light chains
15q14	Actin

- Unexplained abnormalities of the electrocardiogram in first-degree relatives of patients with HCM may be suggestive of a carrier or preclinical state.
- Mutations of the troponin T gene results in mild to moderate hypertrophy; however, it is associated with poor prognosis and a high risk of sudden death.
- These mutations express in autosomal dominant fashion. Penetrance and expression may be variable and age related.
- Mutations result in abnormal force generation that causes hypertrophic response.
- Prevalence of HCM is low, about 0.2% in the general population.
- Hypertrophy usually occurs during adolescence and period of rapid somatic growth. It has also been noted to occur in the elderly.
- Myocardial hypertrophy is out of proportion to the hemodynamic load.
- Occurrence of sustained VT is uncommon, however, non-sustained VT is frequent.

Classification of the HCM based on imaging

1 Asymmetric septal hypertrophy (ASH): predominantly affects the septum.
2 Apical hypertrophy: Affects the apex of LV (Japanese type). It demonstrates a narrow apex during angiographic study, giant negative T waves in the precordial ECG leads; there is no intraventricular pressure gradient; symptoms are mild. It has a benign course with low mortality. Atrial fibrillation may occur.
3 Idiopathic subaortic stenosis (IHSS): Septal hypertrophy resulting in obstruction.
4 Hypertrophy and obstruction are localized to the mid-segment of the LV.

- Although the diagnosis of HCM is made on the basis of echocardiographic findings, a single normal echocardiogram does not exclude HCM in a child or adolescent.
  Cardiac hypertrophy suggestive of HCM may be seen in
1 Infants of diabetic mothers.
2 Hyperparathyroidism.
3 Neurofibromatosis.
4 Generalized lipodystrophy.
5 Lentiginosis.
6 Pheochromocytoma.
7 Friedreich ataxia.
8 Noonan syndrome.
9 Amyloid, glycogen storage disease, or tumor involvement of the septum may mimic HCM.

Risk factors for sustained ventricular arrhythmia and sudden death

- The incidence of sudden death in patients with HCM is approximately 2–4 %.
- Nonsustained VT is associated with increased risk of sudden cardiac death. The presence of nonsustained VT has low positive predictive value and high negative

predictive value. The absence of nonsustained ventricular tachycardia indicates a relatively good prognosis. The presence of nonsustained VT indicates a possible high risk group that may require further risk stratification.

- The absence of severe symptoms, malignant family history, nonsustained ventricular tachycardia, marked hypertrophy, marked left atrial dilation, and abnormal blood pressure response to exercise identifies a low-risk group.
- The commonest cause of SCD in HCM is VT.
- The mechanism of ventricular arrhythmia may be reentry due to (1) disarray of hypertrophied myocytes and fibrosis (2) ischemia.
- The major causes of ischemia are as follows:
  i Impaired vasodilator reserve due to thickness and narrowing of the intramural coronary arteries.
  ii Increased oxygen demand due to hypertrophy and outflow obstruction.
  iii Elevated filling pressures with resultant subendocardial ischemia.
- A higher incidence of accessory pathways has been reported.
- Adolescence is a vulnerable period for sudden death especially in males.
- 25% of HCM have abnormal blood pressure response during exercise. This may be due to inappropriate vasodilatation during exercise. These patients tend to have a small LV cavity. LV cavity C fiber or baroreceptor stimulation may contribute to inappropriate vasodilatation. Abnormal blood pressure response is associated with increased risk of sudden death.
- 40% of SCD occur during or immediately after exercise.
- Patients with LV wall thickness of more than 30 mm are at increased risk of SCD.
- Family history of sudden cardiac death is an important risk factor. This may be due to more malignant mutation in certain families.
- Exertion-related syncope is an ominous symptom in young patients with HCM.
- The presence of nonsustained VT may increase the risk of sudden death but the positive predictive value is low.
- A short PR interval is commonly seen in patients with HCM, which may reflect enhanced AV node conduction. This may facilitate rapid conduction during atrial arrhythmia.
- Conduction system disease and AV block may occur in HCM.
- QT dispersion, signal average ECG, heart rate variability, and programmed stimulation are not helpful in risk stratification because of low positive predictive value.
- History of sudden cardiac death and sustained VT are important risk factors.
- Low risk patients are characterized by lack of symptoms, absence of family history of SCD, normal blood pressure response to exercise, and no ventricular arrhythmias.
- Runs of nonsustained ventricular tachycardia on the Holter monitor and the signal-averaged electrocardiogram are not helpful in identifying patients at increased risk for sustained or lethal ventricular arrhythmia.
- Electrophysiologic study with programmed stimulation, as a means of identifying high risk patients, has been relinquished.

Risk factors for SCD in HCM

> A Syncope
> B Age <30 years
> C History of sustained ventricular arrhythmias
> D Family history of SCD
> E Abnormal blood pressure response to exercise
> F LV wall thickness >30 mm
> G Gene Mutation coding for Troponin and Tropomyosin

- Prognosis correlates with the degree of hypertrophy; in patients with severe hypertrophy (>30 mm) there is 2% risk per year of sudden death.

Atrial arrhythmias in HCM
- SVT and AF may occur in up to 30% of the patients and may be due to left atrial enlargement.
- Left atrial enlargement may be due to LV diastolic dysfunction, mitral regurgitation, or atrial muscle fibrosis.
- Patients with persistent or paroxysmal atrial fibrillation should be anticoagulated.
- Amiodarone or Sotalol can be used to maintain sinus rhythm. If that fails Ca channel blockers or beta-blockers can achieve rate control.

Treatment
- Strenuous physical activity should be prohibited in all patients with HCM even in the absence of symptoms.
- Unsuspected HCM is the most common finding at autopsy in young competitive athletes who die suddenly.
- Cardiovascular screening before participation in competitive sports may identify asymptomatic patients with silent HCM and may prevent unexpected sudden death.
- Digitalis should be avoided.
- The majority of patients with HCM require only medical management.
- Beta-blockers exert a negative chronotropic response and decrease myocardial oxygen consumption, thus alleviating ischemia.
- Verapamil, by depressing myocardial contractility, may decrease the LV outflow gradient and improve diastolic filling.
- Disopyramide, an antiarrhythmic drug that alters calcium kinetics, reduces contractility the may produce symptomatic improvement by reducing the pressure gradient.
- Prophylactic use of Amiodarone in high-risk patients may decrease the occurrence of SCD.
- Amiodarone is effective in the treatment of both supraventricular and ventricular tachyarrhythmias.

- Insertion of a dual-chamber DDD pacemaker may be useful in some patients, especially the elderly, with an outflow gradient and severe symptoms.
- Pacing for the treatment of medically refractory HCM is currently a class IIb indication by the ACC/AHA guidelines.
- When pacing is applied in the patient with HCM, AVI has to be short enough to result in ventricular depolarization by the paced event. However, the shortest AVI may not provide optimum hemodynamics. AV node ablation has been recommended to ensure paced ventricular depolarization.
- It may help 10% of HCM patients. Symptoms are improved and the gradient may be reduced by 20–25%.
- Surgical or chemical septal ablation could be considered in symptomatic patients with significant gradients.
- Complications of the percutaneous technique include (1)development of right bundle branch block and (2) complete heart block.
- ICD is the treatment of choice in high-risk patients[12,13].
- Five percent of the patients in the high risk group, who receive ICD for primary prevention of SCD, may experience appropriate discharge per year.
- Time to first appropriate shock after the initial ICD implant may be quite variable and may extend to 10 years.

Dilated cardiomyopathy

- Ventricular arrhythmias are common in dilated cardiomyopathy (DCM) irrespective of etiology.
- The causes of dilated cardiomyopathy include CAD, valvular or hypertensive heart disease, pregnancy, infections, or alcohol.
- 35% of the patients with DCM may have autosomal dominant familial disease.
- X-linked form of inheritance is seen in infants and children. It may be due to mutation in Lamin A/C gene. It is associated with conduction defects, variable skeletal muscle involvement, and reduced survival to adulthood. Female carriers may have a mild form of DCM.
- The gene responsible for this disorder codes for dystrophin, a cytoskeletal protein responsible for structural support to myocytes by producing a mesh of sarcolemma.
- Subendocardial scarring provides the substrate, and hypokalemia, hypomagnesemia, and circulating catecholamines may be the modulating factors for arrhythmias.
- Ejection fraction of less than 35% is the single most predictor of mortality.
- Other markers of mortality include low serum sodium, elevated plasma norepinephrine, renin, and BNP.
- The presence of LBBB and AV blocks are the markers of poor outcome.
- Ventricular arrhythmias are common but have low positive predictive value.
- Programmed electrical stimulation is not a reliable predictor of SCD in DCM.

Causes of mortality in DCM

- 50% of all deaths in DCM are sudden and the majority of those may be due to VT.
- In the majority of patients with advanced heart failure the cause of sudden death may be bradyarrhythmias and pulseless cardiac electrical activity, rather then tachyarrhythmias.
- Ischemia and MI may also be responsible for mortality in patients with DCM.

Predictors of Mortality

EF <35%
NYHA classification
Third heart sound
Syncope
Low serum sodium
Increased plasma norepinephrine
Increased plasma rennin
Elevated levels of natriuretic peptide
Presence of left bundle branch block, first and second-degree AV block and AF
Frequent PVCs, nonsustained VT

- The incidence of nonsustained ventricular tachycardia increases with worsening CHF.
- The role of programmed stimulation in risk stratification of patients with DCM is poorly defined. Even in patients who present with ventricular tachycardia or SCD programmed stimulation may fail to induce index arrhythmia. Polymorphic VT could be induced. It has no prognostic significance.
- Patients with DCM who present with decreased LVEF and syncope should be considered for prophylactic ICD insertion even if the electrophysiologic study is negative.
- Signal average electrocardiogram, heart rate variability, QT dispersion and T wave alternans are not helpful in predicting the outcome in patients with DCM.

Treatment

- The optimum pharmacologic treatment for CHF includes ACE inhibitors, adrenergic receptor blocking agents, digitalis, diuretics and aldosterone antagonists.
- The use of ace inhibitors and β-blockers may decrease the mortality by 30%.
- Identification and treatment of ischemia, electrolyte abnormalities should be considered.

- The use of Phosphodiesterase inhibitors, as an inotropic agent, increases mortality.
- Amiodarone may be effective in controlling symptomatic ventricular arrhythmias and decreasing SCD in patients with DCM. Efficacy and tolerance of Amiodarone decreases with decreasing EF and duration of the treatment.
- Biventricular pacing, by resynchronizing ventricular contraction and improving conduction, reduces diastolic mitral regurgitation, improves symptoms of LVF and may improve survival.
- Current indication for ICD in patients with DCM include cardiac arrest survivors, syncopal VT, or spontaneous sustained VT and EF <35.

7.4 LONG QT SYNDROME AND TORSADE DE POINTES

LQT1[14,15]

- It is due to mutation of gene KCNQ1 located on chromosome 11. It is the most common form of mutation. It is responsible for expression of the protein K_VLQT1. It codes for I_{Ks}, slowly activating delayed rectifier potassium current. In LQT1 T waves are broad-based (Fig. 7.4).
- Mutation in KvLQT1 and KCNE1 results in Jervell and Lange–Nielson (JLN) syndrome. It is accompanied by deafness. QT prolongation in this syndrome is autosomal dominant and deafness is transmitted as autosomal recessive disorder.
- Romano Ward syndrome presents as QT prolongation without deafness.
- JLN phenotype occurs when an offspring inherits mutant KvLQT1 gene from both parents and is therefore homozygous. This results in deafness. Parents are heterozygous and are not deaf.
- It is due to single residue substitution such as replacement of alanine by valine or glutamic acid. This results in amino acid change and loss of function.
- In patients with LQT1 sympathetic stimulation prolongs the QT interval and causes torsades de pointes. Sympathetic stimulation abbreviates APD in epicardium and endocardium but not in M cells causing transmural dispersion.
- Different responses of the three cell types to adrenergic stimulation is related to the level of augmentation of I_{Ks}, which is strong in epicardium and endocardium and weak in M cells.
- Augmented I_{Ks} in epicardium and endocardium abbreviates APD and causes dispersion of repolarization and broad-based T waves.
- Potassium channel openers improve the QT interval in LQT1.
- Beta-blockers may be useful for the treatment of patients with LQT1 because it inhibits isoproterenol induced transmural dispersion of repolarization.
  B blockers may help LQT2 but not LQT3 patients (Table 7.4).

Table 7.4 Classification of LQTS

LQTS	T wave pattern	Gene defect/ channel	Chromosome	Response to β blockers	Response to Na channel blockers	Response to K channel openers
LQT1	Broad base	KCNQ1 (KVLQT1) I_{Ks}	11p15.5	Effective	Somewhat effective	Shortens QT
LQT2	Bifid, Notched	KCNH2 (HERG) I_{Kr}	7q35–36	Effective	Effective	Shortens QT
LQT3	Late appearing	SCN5A I_{Na}	3p21–24	Not effective	Effective in shortening QT	No effect
LQT4	Unknown	ANK2	4q25–27	Unknown	Unknown	Unknown
LQT5	Same as LQT1	KCNE1 I_{Ks}	21q22.1–22.2	Unknown	Unknown	Unknown
LQT6	Same as LQT2	KCNE2 (MiRP1)/I_{Kr}	21q22.1–22.2	Unknown	Unknown	Unknown
LQT7	Same as LQT2	KCNJ2 I_{Kr2}		Unknown	Unknown	Unknown

LQT2

- It is due to mutation of gene KCNH2 located on chromosome 7. It is responsible for expression of the protein HERG. It codes for α subunit of the I_{Kr} channel, a rapidly activating delayed rectifier potassium current.
- LQT2 is characterized by low amplitude notched T waves.
- D-Sotalol, an I_{Kr} blocker, mimics LQT2 and acquired LQTS. It causes greater prolongation of APD in M cells and slows phase-3 repolarization in all the cell layers. This results in prolongation of the QT interval and low amplitude T waves.
- Hypokalemia and I_{Kr} block results in a marked slowing of repolarization and low amplitude notched T waves.
- The start of the T wave corresponds to the onset of the epicardial AP plateau. Final repolarization of epicardium causes the peak of the 2nd component of the T wave. Final repolarization of M cells defines the end of the T wave.
- Exogenous administration of potassium may correct the repolarization abnormality in LQT2 and in acquired LQTS.
- Nicorandil, a potassium channel opener, abbreviates the long QT interval and reduces transmural dispersion in LQT1 and LQT2 that are secondary to reduced I_{Ks} and I_{Kr} respectively.
- LQTS-related cardiac events, during a 40-week postpartum interval, may occur in women harboring mutations in KCNH2 (LQT-2).

- Members of the ether-a-go-go (ERG) K^+ channel family are expressed in endocrine cells and in the nervous system. Anterior pituitary cells express ERG channels, and block of these channels by the class III antiarrhythmic agent E-4031 leads to cell membrane depolarization and increased excitability, which, in turn, may perturb prolactin secretion by these cells.[16]

LQTS3

- The mutation is in cardiac sodium channel gene, SCN5A, located on chromosome 3. This mutation results in sustained inward current during repolarization, resulting in gain of function and prolongation of APD in M cells, increase in the QT interval and late appearing T waves. M cells have large late sodium current.
- Mutation in the same sodium channel without gain of function causes Brugada syndrome.
- Single amino acid substitution of SCN5A at residue 1623 causes LQT3; however, similar mutation at position 1620 causes Brugada syndrome.
- Mexiletine causes I_{Na} block in M cells, resulting in abbreviation of APD and QT interval in LQT3. This effect may be of value in the treatment of LQT1, LQT2, and LQT3.
- Pacemaker, by increasing the heart rate, will abbreviate the slow kinetic of late Na current and shorten the QT interval in LQT3.
- Bradycardia, either spontaneous (during sleep) or drug induced (beta blockers), will prolong APD and QT interval in LQT3 patients. β-Blockers should not be used in LQT3 patients.

LQT4

- It is caused by mutation in gene ANK2, which is located on chromosome 4. This results in abnormality of the anchoring protein Ankyrin B. Details of its phenotype expression are unknown.

LQT5

- It is caused by mutation of gene KCNE1 located on chromosome 21. This gene is responsible for expression of the protein MinK which co assembles with protein KvLQT1 to form IKs.

LQTS6

- It is due to mutation of the gene KCNE2 located on chromosome 21. It is responsible for the expression of the protein MiRP1. It codes for the β subunit of the I_{Kr} channel. Defect results in faster deactivation of the current.

Andersen–Tawil syndrome (ATS) LQTS7

- It is characterized by periodic paralysis, ventricular ectopy, dysmorphic features, and prolongation of the QT interval.
- Inheritance of Anderson–Tawil syndrome is autosomal dominant.

- Mutations in the K^+ channel gene *KCNJ2* have been identified as one cause of ATS.
- It results in disorder of both cardiac and skeletal muscle excitability. ATS is unique among ion channelopathies, implying a defect in an ion channel expressed in both tissues.
- *KCNJ2* encodes the inward rectifier K^+ channel Kir 2.1, a component of the inward rectifier current I_{K1}. I_{K1} provides substantial repolarizing current during the terminal repolarization phase of the cardiac action potential and is the primary conductance controlling the diastolic membrane potential.
- Variable expressivity is typical of ATS with individual *KCNJ2* mutation carriers manifesting any or none of the classic triad features. Likewise, cardiac manifestations are also variable and include LQT, frequent premature ventricular contractions (PVCs), bigeminy, multifocal PVCs, prominent U waves, polymorphic ventricular tachycardia (VT), and bidirectional VT.
- Symptoms such as syncope and sudden cardiac death are rare.
- Despite frequent episodes of polymorphic and bidirectional VT, ATS patients are often asymptomatic and unaware of their underlying rhythm disturbance.
- Pharmacological therapy is not effective in reducing the frequency of ventricular ectopy.
- Many ATS patients are asymptomatic in the face of a large tachycardia burden; some are at risk for life-threatening events. These patients may benefit from ICD implant.

Clinical presentation

- 1 in 7000 to 10,000 persons is a carrier of the LQTS gene. 60% of gene carriers may present with syncope in their early teen years. Three to four thousand children and young adults may succumb to sudden death each year.[15]
- Recurrent syncope and resuscitated cardiac arrest are the hallmark of high-risk patients. Sudden death may be the first manifestation of the LQTS.
- During follow-up, 30% cardiac arrest survivors may have recurrence and 19% of patients who present with syncope may continue to have symptoms in spite of β-blockers.[15]
- Some gene carriers may have normal QTc yet may suffer from syncope or cardiac arrest.
- 10% of family members of LQTS patients who have a QT interval of less than 440 may present with cardiac arrest.
- Patients may present with syncope or cardiac arrest due to Tdp. There is usually a family history of syncope, long QT or sudden death. 30% of the LQTS cases are sporadic without family history.
- Sudden infant death (SID) could be due to LQTS.
- In patients with LQTS1, SCD may occur during increased sympathetic activity such as fright, anger, sudden awakening or physical activity such as exercise or emotional stress; however, in patients with LQTS3 it may occur during sleep.

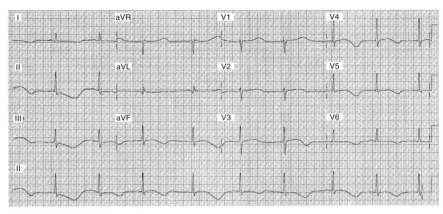

Fig 7.4 ECG LQTS1 T wave alternans.

- Symptoms may be caused or aggravated by QT prolonging drugs and hypokalemia.
- Occurrence of cardiac events at rest or during sleep is commonly seen in LQT2 and LQT3.
- LQTS1 and LQTS2 are likely to be symptomatic. LQTS3 is more likely to be lethal. LQT4 patients may have paroxysmal AF.
- Homozygous KVLQT1 and KCNE1 mutations are associated with congenital deafness (Jarvell and Lange–Nielsen syndrome).

Electrocardiographic features
- Electrocardiographic changes consist of prolongation of the QT interval corrected for the heart rate and measured in LII.
- In patients with LQTS1 T waves tend to be smooth and broad (Fig. 7.4); however, it tends to be low amplitude and notched in LQTS2. Late onset but normal appearing T waves are seen in LQTS3.
- The QT interval, corrected for the heart rate, of 440 milliseconds in males and 460 milliseconds in females is considered abnormal. The QT interval becomes longer after puberty in females.
- The extent of QT prolongation does not correlate with symptoms. Marked prolongation of the QT interval (more than 600 milliseconds) may be associated with Tdp.
- T wave abnormalities are more noticeable in precordial leads.
- The appearance of notched T wave during the recovery phase of exercise is seen in LQTS patients but not in control subjects.
- QT dispersion is common in patients with LQTS.
- Dispersion of repolarization improves after anti-adrenergic therapy.
- The persistence of QT dispersion after beta-blocker therapy identifies high-risk patients.

- T wave alternans is a marker of electrical instability. It is generally seen during emotional or physical stress in patients with LQTS. It identifies high-risk patients.
- Patients with LQTS may have sinus pauses and bradycardia. These changes may precede the occurrence of Tdp.
- Echocardiogram may show an increased rate of thickening in the early phase of systole and slowing of thickening and plateau in the late phase.
- Verapamil may normalize contraction and may be due to a decrease in intracellular calcium and EAD.
- Paradoxical prolongation of the QT interval by >30 milliseconds, on infusion of the epinephrine at a rate of 0.025–0.3 mcg/kg/min for 5 minutes may identify patients who otherwise have borderline QT prolongation. Sensitivity and negative predictive value are high.[18]

Molecular genetics and risk stratification[17–19]

- Screening for gene mutation should be limited to patients and family members in whom the clinical diagnosis of LQTS is clear or suspected.[17]
- Abnormal gene test confirms the diagnosis; however, a negative test does not exclude LQTS.
- Screening of asymptomatic carriers may help in counseling about the use of certain drugs, anesthesia or prenatal planning.[18]
- Mexiletine, a sodium channel blocker, may shorten the QT interval in LQT3 and to a lesser extent in LQT1 and LQT2.
- 3% of LQT1 patients and 61% of the patients with LQT3 had cardiac events during sleep.
- 97% of patients with LQT1 had cardiac events during physical or emotional stress while 33% with LQT3 had such events.
- Patients with LQT2 behave more like LQT3. Both these groups have normal IKs.
- Among LQTS gene carriers only 14–33% may have phenotype expression.
- Silent carriers may have ventricular arrhythmias on exposure to certain triggers such as QT prolonging drugs or hypokalemia.
- The probability of successfully identifying genotype by the molecular method is 30–50% because of the lack of knowledge about all the possible genes involved in LQTS.
- Molecular diagnosis is 100% sensitive and specific for the affected family members of a genotype proband.
- Asymptomatic gene carriers may need counseling about the reproductive risks and the risk of exposure to certain drugs.
- Syncope or cardiac arrest is the presenting symptom in the majority of the probands.
- LQTS is common among females.
- Diagnosis of LQTS can be made by assigning a score to abnormal ECG and clinical history findings (Table 7.5).

Table 7.5 LQTS diagnostic criteria

Clinical findings	Points
Syncope with stress	2
Syncope without stress	1
Congenital deafness	0.5
Family history	
LQTS among family members	1
Unexplained SCD among immediate family members age <30 years	0.5
Electrocardiographic findings	
QT_c > 480 ms	3
QT_c 460–470 ms	2
QT_c 450 ms (Male)	1
Torsade de pointes	2
T wave alternans	1
Notched T waves in three leads	1
Bradycardia	0.5

A score of 1 or less is regarded as low probability of LQTS.

A score between 2 and 3 is regarded as intermediate probability of LQTS.

A score of 4 points or more is considered a high probability of LQTS.

In intermediate group assessment of T wave abnormalities during the recovery phase of the stress test, QT dispersion and echocardiographic abnormalities of wall thickness and relaxation may help in diagnostic decisions.

Therapeutic options in LQTS[20–22]

Gene specific therapy for LQTS (Table 7.4)

- Potassium channel openers shorten the QT interval in LQT1.
- β-Blockers reduce the incidence of syncope and sudden cardiac death in patients with congenital LQTS1 by inhibiting adrenergic induced transmural dispersion of repolarization.[20]
- LQT1 events occur during exercise and emotion, beta-blockers are likely to be effective in this group.
- Exogenous administration of potassium and an increase in extracellular potassium may correct repolarization abnormality in LQT2 and acquired LQTS.
- β-Blockers may be useful in treating patients with LQTS2 but not those with LQTS3.
- Nicorandil, a potassium channel opener, abbreviates long QT intervals and reduces transmural dispersion in LQT1 and LQT2, which are secondary to reduced I_{Ks} and I_{Kr} respectively.
- There is no need to limit physical activity if QT shortens during an exercise test.
- Na channel blocker Mexiletine, which suppresses the late reopening of the sodium channel, shortens the QT interval in LQT3.

- There are data to indicate that shortening of the QT interval will confer protection from life-threatening arrhythmias.
- M cells have a large late I_{Na}. Mexiletine causes I_{Na} block in M cells, resulting in abbreviation of APD. This effect may be of value in the treatment of LQT1, LQT2 and LQT3.
- Pacemakers are likely to be effective in LQT3, as a faster heart rate will abbreviate the slow kinetic of late Na current and shorten the QT interval. A permanent pacemaker may be helpful in preventing bradycardia during rest and sleep.
- These patients may be at a lesser risk of syncope during exercise. β-Blockers are likely to be less effective or even contraindicated in LQT3.
- Mortality in untreated patients is 20% in the first year and 50% in five years. Those patients who were treated with β-blockers had yearly mortality of 0.9%.
- The incidence of sudden cardiac death as a first event is 7%.
- Propranolol, 2–3 mg/kg, remains the initial choice of therapy in symptomatic patients.
- Nadolol, because of its longer half-life, could also be used effectively in LQTS patients.
- Patients with spontaneous (LQTS3) or drug-induced bradycardia may benefit from pacemaker insertion.
- In patients who present with cardiac arrest there may be 13% reoccurrence in spite of treatment with β-blockers. These patients may benefit from ICD.
- Patients who have reoccurrence of syncope in spite of β-blockers should be considered for ICD.
- A pacemaker should be considered in patients with bradycardia; however, it should never be regarded as a sole therapy for LQTS and must be used in conjunction with β-blockers.
- Patients with LQT3 who have bradycardia at rest may benefit from a pacemaker.
- 20% of patients with LQTS may need a pacemaker.
- ICD should be programmed with a long detection interval to avoid recurrent shocks for self-terminating TDP. Rate smoothing features may prevent pauses.[16]
- Post-shock pacing should be programmed at a faster rate to avoid pauses and bradycardia that might reinduce TDP.

Management of asymptomatic patients with LQTS (Table 7.6)
- Sudden death may be the first manifestation in 7–9% of patients with LQTS. This risk tends to be higher in LQT3 than in LQT1.
- All the patients with LQTS should be treated with β-blockers.
- β-Blockers should be strongly considered in patients with LQTS and congenital deafness, neonates and infants in their first year, history of sudden death in a sibling, T wave alternans, QT_c greater than 600 ms, and a request from family members.
- Family should be educated about CPR.

Table 7.6 Treatment options in LQTS

Electrocardiogram	Symptoms	Family history	Treatment
Prolong QT$_c$	None	None	None
Prolong QT$_c$	None	SCD, Syncope due to LQTS	Beta-blockers
Prolong QT$_c$	Syncope	SCD, Syncope due to LQTS	Beta-blockers, ICD
Prolong QT$_c$	SCD		Beta-blockers, ICD

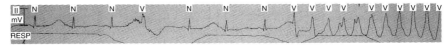

Fig 7.5 This ECG strip demonstrates prolonged QT interval, T wave alternans, and pause-dependent TDP.

- Patients should be provided with a list of drugs that could prolong the QT interval.
- All symptomatic patients and asymptomatic children with LQTS1 and LQTS2 should be treated with beta-blockers but not those with LQTS3.
- Raising the serum potassium level may shorten the QT interval in LQTS2.
- Patients with LQTS3 may benefit from the Na channel blocker Mexiletine.

Torsade de Pointes (TDP)

First described by Dessertenne as twisting of the QRS morphology around an imaginary axis.

- Torsade de Pointes (TDP) is a polymorphic VT associated with LQTS (Fig. 7.5).
- Quinidine and Hypokalemia produce EAD and triggered activity resulting in TDP.
- The initial event in TDP is EAD-induced triggered activity.
- TDP often occurs following a short–long–short cycle length.
- The term TDP should be reserved for polymorphic VT associated with LQTS.
- In the absence of LQTS, the term polymorphic VT should be used.
- In addition to twisting of the QRS complexes there may be a change in the amplitude.
- LQTS is due to abnormality of potassium and sodium currents. This results in prolongation and dispersion of repolarization, which lead to EAD-induced triggered activity in HPS.
- The balance between inward (Na, Ca, and Na/Ca exchange) and outward (K) currents determines the duration of repolarization.
- Acquired LQTS can be due to the following mechanisms[21] (Table 7.7 and 7.8):

Table 7.7 Drugs causing Long QT and TDP[23]

Antiarrhythmics	Disopyramide, Procainamide, Quinidine, Amiodarone, Bretylium, Sotalol
Antimicrobial	Erythromycin, Trimethoprim-sulfa
Antihistamine	Astemizole, Terfenadine
Antifungal	Fluconazole, Itraconazole, ketoconazole
Antiprotozoal	Chloroquine, Pentamidine, quinine, Mefloquine, Halofantrine
Psychotropic	Chloral hydrate, Haloperidol, Lithium, Phenothiazines, pimozide, Tricyclic antidepressants
GI prokinetic	Cisapride
Other	Indapamide, probucol, amantadine, tacrolimus, vasopressin
HypoK Hypo Mg induced by	Diuretics, Steroids, Cathartics, Liquid protein diet

Table 7.8 Drugs interfering with cytochrome P-450 enzyme

Antifungal	Fluconazole, Itraconazole, ketoconazole, metronidazole
Serotonin reuptake inhibitors	Fluoxetine, fluvoxamine, sertraline
HIV protease inhibitors	Indinavir, ritonavir, saquinavir
Dihydropyridine	Felodipine, Nicardipine, Nifedipine
Antimicrobial	Erythromycin
Others	Grapefruit juice. Hepatic dysfunction

    i I_{ks} or I_{kr} channel block by Quinidine, Procainamide, Sotalol, Cesium, and Bretylium. These actions can be reversed by potassium channel openers such as Pinacidil and Cromakalin.

    ii Suppression of I_{to} channel in M cells.

    iii Increase in I_{Ca} activity.

    iv Continuous activation of I_{Na} during repolarization will also result in prolongation of the QT interval. This can be blocked by Lidocaine.

- More than one mechanism may be responsible for prolongation of the QT interval.
- Bradycardia and low serum potassium have synergistic effect on prolonging repolarization and inducing TDP.
- High plasma levels of the drugs either due to high doses or lack of clearance may increase the risk of initiating TDP. Reduced clearance may be due to inhibition of the cytochrome P-450 enzyme.
- Bradycardia, short–long cycle length, T wave alternans, and hypertrophy result in dispersion of refractoriness and thus may predispose to TDP.

Polymorphic VT and normal QT interval
- It occurs in the presence of structural heart disease and ischemia and normal QT interval.

- Polymorphic VT may occur in the absence of structural heart disease such as in Brugada Syndrome, which is characterized by RBB pattern, ST segment elevation in V1–V3, normal QT interval.
- Genetic abnormality includes mutations in Na channel SCN5A, resulting in rapid recovery of sodium channel function from inactivation (opposite of LQT3) or in a nonfunctional sodium channel.

Acquired LQTS

- Bradycardia, hypokalemia, and QT prolonging drugs may precipitate TDP.
- The initiating event in TDP is EAD in the presence of dispersion of repolarization.
- IV magnesium sulfate, increase heart rate by pharmacological agents or by pacing suppresses polymorphic VT.

Short QT syndrome (SQTS)[24]

- Short QT syndrome is manifested by QT_C, of 300 milliseconds or less.
- Ventricular arrhythmias may result in sudden cardiac death in patients with SQTS.
- Gain of function in SCN5A, the gene that encodes for the subunit of the cardiac sodium channel, is associated with the LQT3, whereas a decrease in function of the same channel is associated with Brugada syndrome and familial conduction disease.
- Increase in the I_{Ks} current, caused by a mutation in the subunit KCNQ1, is linked to familial atrial fibrillation.
- SQTS is due to gain of function in KCNH2 encoding for I_{Kr}.
- SQTS is more common in men. Males tend to have a lower heart rate and shorter QT_C than females.
- QT duration is influenced by the autonomic nervous system, circulating catecholamines, and hormones.
- The T peak–T end interval may be a more reliable measure of repolarization. It is increased in LQT1, and may be shortened in SQTS.

7.5 BRUGADA SYNDROME[25,26]

- Its mode of transmission is autosomal dominant.
- Brugada syndrome is due to mutation of the sodium ion channel SCN5A alpha subunit located on chromosome 3. This mutation results in loss of function.
- Single amino acid substitution of SCN5A at residue 1623 causes LQT3; however similar mutation at position 1620 causes Brugada syndrome.
- Loss of AP dome (Plateau) in epicardium but not in endocardium causes ST elevation or early repolarization pattern seen in Brugada syndrome.
- Loss of the dome results in contractile dysfunction because the entry of calcium into the cells is greatly diminished and sarcoplasmic reticulum calcium stores are depleted.

- Delayed activation may be responsible for recording of late potentials.
- Abbreviation of APD occurs due to strong outward currents during the plateau phase due to decrease in I_{Na}, inhibition of the I_{Ca} or activation of I_{to} at the end of phase 1.
- Acetylcholine facilitates shortening of plateau by suppressing I_{Ca} or augmenting I_{to}. β-Adrenergic agonists restore these changes by increasing I_{Ca}.
- Sodium channel blockers facilitate shortening of plateau by shifting the voltage at which phase 1 begins.
- Loss of Na channel function by mutation or by blockade using drugs may reduce inward currents and leave outward currents unopposed, resulting in shortening of APD.
- Increased ST elevation in Brugada syndrome by vagal maneuvers or class I agents and reduction in ST elevation with β-adrenergic agonist is consistent with the above observations.
- Occurrence of ST elevation in right precordial leads is due to shortening of the plateau phase over the right ventricular epicardium where I_{to} is most prominent. These changes are also responsible for ST elevation, phase 2 reentry and episodes of VF in Brugada syndrome.
- Agents that inhibit I_{to} such as 4 amiopyridine (4 AP), Quinidine, and Disopyramide, restore the AP plateau phase and electrical homogeneity and abolish arrhythmias.
- Class IA agents such as Procainamide and Ajmaline that block I_{Na} but not I_{to} exacerbate the electrophysiologic abnormalities of Brugada syndrome.
- Lithium has been shown to be potent Na channel blocker and may unmask Brugada ECG changes.
- Gene mutations that increase the intensity and kinetic of I_{to}, I_{Katp} or decrease the intensity and kinetic of I_{Ca} during the early phase of AP will result in electrocardiographic changes suggestive of Brugada syndrome.
- Abnormal expression of the genes that modulate autonomic receptor and I_{Katp} may also produce Brugada like changes.

Clinical features
- The Brugada syndrome is characterized by ST-segment elevation in the right precordial leads.
- There is a high incidence of sudden death usually at a mean age of 40 years. These patients have structurally normal hearts. 20% of SCD in patients with structurally normal hearts are due to Brugada syndrome.
- Prevalence is estimated to be 5/10,000.
- Sudden death usually occurs at rest and at night.
- Hypokalemia may contribute to SCD. In certain oriental countries large carbohydrate meals may contribute to hypokalemia. Glucose insulin infusion may unmask Brugada-type ECG pattern[27].
- Elevated temperature is known to prematurely inactivate SCN5A. Febrile illness and use of hot tubs may precipitate VF[28].

- Approximately 20% of patients with Brugada syndrome may develop supra-ventricular arrhythmias, including AF. These arrhythmias may result in inappropriate ICD shocks.

Electrocardiographic features
- Type 1 ECG changes manifest as coved ST-segment elevation of >2 mm (0.2 mV) followed by a negative T wave in precordial leads (V1–V3).
- Other ECG abnormalities include prolongation of PR, QRS, and P duration, and presence of S waves in leads I, II, and III.
- There may be prolongation of the QT interval more in the right precordial leads. This may be due to selective prolongation of action potential duration in right ventricular epicardium.
- Concealed ECG manifestations can be unmasked by sodium channel blockers, during a febrile illness or with vagotonic agents.
- Asymptomatic patients with type I ECG changes do not require drug challenge.
- Diagnosis of Brugada syndrome should be considered if Type 1 ST-segment elevation with or without sodium channel blocking agent and one of the following are present:
  - i Documented ventricular fibrillation and/or polymorphic ventricular tachycardia.
  - ii Inducible VT with programmed electrical stimulation.
  - iii Syncope.
  - iv Nocturnal agonal respiration.
  - v Family history of sudden cardiac death at a young age (<45 years).
  - vi ST elevation T inversion in precordial leads of family members.
- Type 2 ECG changes are characterized by saddleback type ST-segment elevation of more than 2 mm, a trough and a positive or biphasic T wave.
- Type 3 ECG pattern is considered when saddleback or coved type of ST-segment elevation of <1 mm is present.
- Type 2 and type 3 ECG patterns are not diagnostic of Brugada syndrome.
- Serial ECGs from the same patient may show all three patterns, at different times, spontaneously or after the administration of specific drugs.
- Diagnosis of Brugada syndrome should be considered when a type 2 or type 3 ECG pattern changes to a type I pattern after administration of a sodium channel blocker.
- One or more of the clinical criteria described above should be present.
- Change from a type 3 to a type 2 pattern, after administration of Na channel blockers, is considered inconclusive for a diagnosis of Brugada syndrome.
- Recording right precordial leads from the second intercostal space may improve the detection of the Brugada-type ECG changes.

- Rounded or upsloping ST elevation or early repolarization pattern are not suggestive of Brugada syndrome.

Provocative test to unmask Brugada ECG pattern[29,30]
- The test is performed by giving one of the Na channel blockers, Procainamide 10 mg/kg IV over 10 min, or Flecainide 2 mg/kg IV over 10'min, or 400 mg, PO, or Ajmaline 1 mg/kg IV over 5'min, or Pilsicainide 1 mg/kg IV over 10 min.
- The test should be monitored with a continuous ECG recording and should be terminated when the diagnostic type1 Brugada ECG changes become evident, premature ventricular beats or other arrhythmias develop, or QRS widens to >130% of baseline.
- Patients with an underlying conduction defect may develop AV block.
- Elderly patients or those with preexisting conduction defects (prolong P, PR, QRS) may benefit by a temporary pacemaker prior to initiating the test.
- Isoproterenol and sodium lactate may be used to neutralize the effects of Na channel blockers.

Differential diagnosis
- The majority of patients with Brugada syndrome have structurally normal heart.
- Some patients with arrhythmogenic RV dysplasia may demonstrate ST changes suggestive of Brugada syndrome (Table 7.9).

Table 7.9 Differentiating features between ARVD/C and Brugada syndrome

	Brugada Syndrome	ARVD/C
Genetic characteristics	Defect in SCN5A	3 genes on 10 locations
ECG changes	1. Dynamic 2. Induced by Na channel blockers	Persistent and progressive 1. T wave inversion 2. Epsilon waves 3. ↓ R amplitude 4. Unaffected by Na channel blockers
RV imaging	No structural abnormality Wall motion abnormality due to conduction defect may be present	Structural and wall motion abnormalities are present
Ventricular arrhythmias	1. Polymorphic VT 2. Facilitated by vagotonic agents, β-blockers 3. Occur during sleep	1. Monomorphic VT with LBB morphology 2. Facilitated by catecholamines 3. Occur during exercise

The following conditions may mimic the ECG pattern of Brugada syndrome[31-32]

Acute myocardial ischemia or infarction
Acute pericarditis
Arrhythmogenic right ventricular dysplasia
Atypical right bundle-branch block
Central and autonomic nervous system abnormalities
Dissecting aortic aneurysm
Duchenne muscular dystrophy
Early repolarization
Hypercalcemia
Hyperkalemia
Hypothermia
Large pericardial effusions
Left ventricular hypertrophy
Mediastinal tumor compressing on RVOT
Pectus excavatum
Prinzmetal angina
Pulmonary embolism
Thiamin deficiency

Drugs responsible for Brugada-like ECG pattern[33]

1 Antiarrhythmic drugs: Flecainide, Propafenone, Ajmaline, procainamide, disopyramide
2 Calcium channel blockers: Verapamil Nifedipine, diltiazem
3 Blockers: Propranolol, Nadolol
4 Nitrates: Isosorbide dinitrate, nitroglycerine
5 Potassium channel openers: Nicorandil
6 Tricyclic antidepressants: Amitriptyline, nortriptyline, desipramine, clomipramine
7 Tetracyclic antidepressants: Maprotiline
8 Phenothiazines: Perphenazine, cyamemazine
9 Selective serotonin reuptake inhibitors: Fluoxetine
10 Miscellaneous: Cocaine, alcohol abuse

Risk stratification[34,35]

Following characteristics identify high risk patient:
1 Aborted sudden cardiac death.
2 Spontaneous and persistent Type 1 ST changes. Eightfold increase in SCD.
3 Inducible VT/VF. Eightfold increase in risk of aborted SCD.[33]
4 Syncope.
5 Male gender. Fivefold increase in SCD.

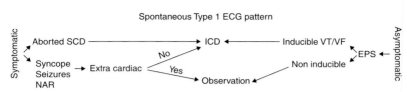

Fig 7.6 Approach to spontaneous type 1 ECG pattern. NAR nocturnal agonal respiration.

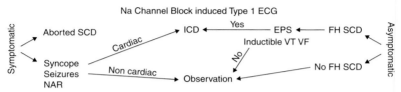

Fig 7.7 Approach to Na channel block induced type 1 ECG pattern (FH = Family history).

Treatment

- ICD is the only proven and effective therapy for Brugada syndrome.
- Recommendations for ICD implant in symptomatic patients are outlined in Fig. 7.6.
- Recommendations for ICD implant in patients with Na channel block induced Type 1 pattern are outlined in Fig. 7.7.
- Although the arrhythmias and sudden cardiac death are associated with bradycardia, the role of chronotropic agents and pacemakers remains undefined.
- Ablation of the ventricular premature beats that trigger VT/VF in Brugada syndrome may decrease the frequency of the arrhythmias and ICD shocks.
- Quinidine and tedisamil (Class 1 antiarrhythmic drugs) block I_{to}, thus restoring APD and provide therapeutic effect.
- Quinidine has been shown to restore the epicardial action potential dome, thus normalizing the ST segment and preventing phase-2 reentry and polymorphic VT. Large doses of 1200–1500 mg are recommended.[36]
- Catecholamines, by enhancing L type I_{Ca}, may also restore the action potential dome.
- I_{to} blockers and I_{Ca} enhancers have been shown to normalize ST-segment elevation and control recurrent ventricular arrhythmias (electrical storms) in patients with Brugada syndrome.
- Phosphodiesterase III inhibitor, Cilostazol may normalize the ST segment by enhancing calcium current (I_{Ca}) and by reducing I_{to} due to its chronotropic effect.
- Tedisamil is a potent I_{to} blocker. Unlike quinidine it does not block inward currents.

7.6 VENTRICULAR TACHYCARDIA IN STRUCTURALLY NORMAL HEART

Idiopathic VTs

- These VTs occur in the absence of structural heart disease.
- Idiopathic VT can be classified on the basis of the following:
  i Anatomic origin: RVOT or LVOT VT, LV VT, Fascicular VT.
  ii Response to pharmacologic agents: Adenosine or Verapamil sensitive.
  iii Morphologic features: Bundle branch pattern, QRS morphology.
  iv Mechanistic features: Triggered activity, Reentry, Automaticity.
  v Response to exercise: RVOT VT, LVOT VT, LV VT.
- Multiple characteristics may be present in a given VT. Description on the basis of anatomic location best describes the clinical features and therapeutic options for a given VT.

RVOTVT[37–40]

- The majority of the VTs in the absence of structural heart disease arise from the right ventricular outflow tract (RVOT).
- It arises from the RVOT. It is adenosine sensitive, exercise induced LBB morphology and inferior axis VT.
- It could present as nonsustain repetitive monomorphic VT (Gallavardin VT).
- It is caused by cAMP mediated triggered activity (DAD). It is sensitive to (inhibited by) adenosine. Response to adenosine is specific for catecholamine mediated DAD.
- Verapamil is also effective in terminating triggered activity induced VT.
- Nicorandil, ATP sensitive potassium channel opener, may also suppress or terminate adenosine sensitive VT.
- Without preceding catecholamines stimulation adenosine has no effect on ion channels in ventricular myocardium.

Clinical features

- It is common in women.
- Age at onset varies from 10 to 70 years.
- The commonest symptom is palpitation; however, 10% of the patients may present with syncope.
- Prognosis is good and spontaneous resolution may occur in 20% of the patients.
- Electrocardiogram during sinus rhythm is normal, however, during tachycardia it shows LBBB and inferior axis (Fig. 7.8), Table 7.11.
- On the basis of the QRS morphology in standard leads and precordial transition, the site of the origin of the RVOT VT can be speculated (Table 7.10).
- Runs of nonsustain monomorphic VT may occur during increased sympathetic tone.
- Echocardiogram is usually normal. Rarely, it may show RV enlargement or PMV.

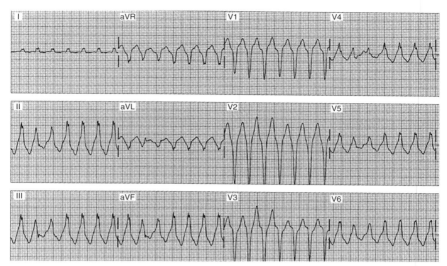

Fig 7.8 RVOT VT demonstrating LB morphology and inferior axis.

Table 7.10 Localization of the origin of RVOT VT from QRS morphology during VT or pace map

QRS morphology	Anterior septal	Posterior septal	Anterior free wall	Posterior free wall
Lead I	Negative QRS	Positive QRS	Negative QRS	Positive QRS
R wave Lead II, III and aVF	Tall and Narrow	Tall and narrow	Broader, shorter and notched	Broader, shorter and notched
Precordial transition	Early	Early	Late. R/S >1 by V4	Late. R/S >1 by V4
QRS duration	<140 ms	<140 ms	>140 ms	>140 ms

- Exercise may reproduce VT in 25–50% of the patients. Its induction is dependent on the critical heart rate.
- SAEGK, cardiac MRI, and RV biopsy are normal.

Electrophysiologic features
- Tachycardia can be initiated and terminated by programmed stimulation. It cannot be entrained. It can be induced by atrial pacing. Burst pacing is also effective in inducing the VT.
- Tachycardia is terminated with adenosine, valsalva maneuvers, carotid sinus pressure, edrophonium, Verapamil, and beta-blockers.

- Effects of vagal stimulation and acetylcholine are mediated by M2 muscarinic cholinergic receptors which produce the same cascade as adenosine.
- Isoproterenol, by increasing cAMP, atropine, by inhibiting the effects of acetylcholine, and aminophylline, by antagonizing the effects of adenosine, facilitate induction of the arrhythmias.
- Arrhythmias in the presence of arrhythmogenic right dysplasia (ARVD) morphologically may resemble RVOT VT. In patients with ARVD electrocardiogram may show conduction delay and ST-T wave changes in anterior precordial leads. MRI shows fatty infiltration in RV wall and wall motion abnormalities.

Treatment[41]

- No treatment required for asymptomatic patients.
- Beta-blockers, Ca channel blockers, and class I and class III antiarrhythmic drugs are found to be effective in half of the patients.
- Acute termination of the tachycardia can be achieved by vagal maneuvers, IV adenosine and IV Verapamil.
- For symptomatic patients the treatment of choice remains radiofrequency ablation.
- Ablation Focus is discrete. The commonest site of the origin for VT is the septal wall.
- Earliest activation during tachycardia at ablation site may precede by 20–40 milliseconds before the onset of the surface QRS.
- Identical match during pace map in 11 of the 12 leads is also helpful in identifying the suitable ablation site.
- Pace mapping is performed in sinus rhythm at VT cycle length.
- Unipolar electrograms demonstrate QS pattern at the site of earliest activation.
- Intracardiac echocardiogram may help delineate RVOT boundaries.
- Three-dimensional mapping has increased the success rate of the ablation.
- During ablation there may be acceleration of the tachycardia before termination.
- Successful ablation can be achieved in 90% of the patients. Recurrence rate is 10%.
- Complications include RBBB (2%), cardiac perforation and tamponade.

LVOT VT[42]

- Its presence is suggested by RBBB morphology in V1 or LBBB morphology with early transition in V2.
- LVOT ventricular tachycardia originates from the superior basal segment of the septum inferior to the AO valve. It may also originate from aorto-mitral continuity, medial aspect of mitral annulus, aortic coronary cusp (commonly from left coronary cusp) and epicardium along the anterior cardiac veins.
- The majority of septal outflow tract tachycardias arise from the right side, 10% may arise from the LV side of the septum.

Table 7.11 Causes and differentiating features of the tachycardia with LBBB morphology

	ECG	EP features	Entrainment	Adenosine sensitivity	Structural heart disease
RVOT VT	LB Inf axis	AVD No His	No	Yes	No
ARVD	LB Inf/Sup axis	AVD No His	Yes	No	Yes
Atriofascicular	LB Sup axis	His after V	Yes	Yes	No
BB reentry	LB Sup axis	Long HV	Yes	No	Yes
Septal VT in CAD	LB Inf/Sup axis	AVD No His	Yes	No	Yes
VT post repair of Fallot	LB Inf axis	AVD No His	Yes	No	Yes
SVT LBBB	LB Inf axis	Normal AH and HV	From atrium	Yes	No

AVD, AV dissociation.

- This tachycardia is sensitive to adenosine.
- Electrocardiogram shows dominate R in V1 V2, early R-wave progression and transition by lead V3.
- Axis is inferiorly directed.
- Later transitions at V3 and V4 are suggestive of VTs arising from the right ventricular outflow.
- LVOT VT arising from the epicardium demonstrates positive concordance in precordial leads and negative QRS complex in LI and aVL. Pace map tends to be suboptimal.
- Earliest electrogram potentials tend to be low amplitude and far field.
- Epicardial mapping from coronary venous system or pericardium may be required.
- Coronary artery angiograms must be performed to delineate the proximity of the ablation catheter to the artery.
- Left main coronary artery trauma may occur during ablation of LVOT VT originating from the left coronary sinus of Valsalva.
- Left coronary angiograms should be performed before and after the ablation. Location of the ostium of the left main coronary artery should be identified by placing a catheter or guide wire during ablation.

LV VT (intrafascicular tachycardia)
- It originates near the left posterior fascicle in the region of the inferoposterior LV septum.

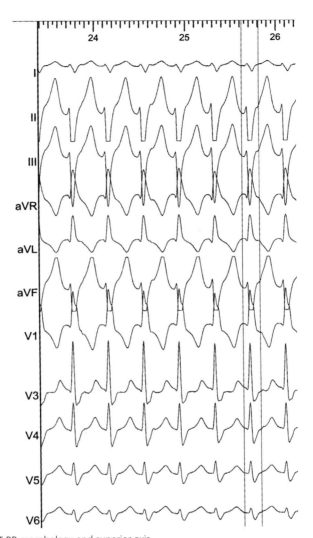

Fig 7.9 LV VT RB morphology and superior axis.

- It is common in men. There is no structural heart disease and baseline electrocardiogram tends to be normal.
- During tachycardia ECG shows RBBB morphology and superior axis (Fig. 7.9).
- It can be induced by atrial pacing. Tachycardia is Verapamil sensitive.
- Symptoms during tachycardia include palpitations, dizziness, and syncope.
- Tachycardia can be induced by exercise and emotional distress.
- It may originate from the superior fascicle in 5–10% of the patients. In these cases ECG shows RBBB morphology and right inferior axis.

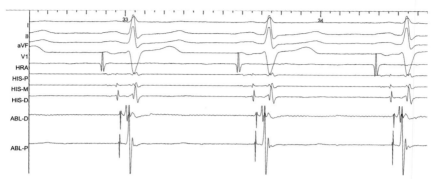

Fig 7.10 HPS potentials recorded from proximal and distal ablation catheter electrodes.

- The RS interval during VT is 60–80 milliseconds.
- QRS is relatively short and the morphology is sharp when compared with muscle or scar-related VT.
- SAECG tends to be normal.
- Tachycardia may originate from the false tendon.
- It does not result in SCD.

Electrophysiologic characteristics of the LV VT

- A short VH interval is recorded during the tachycardia. A sharp high frequency potential precedes earliest ventricular activation by 30–40 milliseconds during VT. These may represent Purkinje potentials.
- The HPS potential can be recorded during sinus rhythm (Fig. 7.10).
- The mechanism of the tachycardia is reentry. The antegrade limb appears to be slowly conducting verapamil sensitive Purkinje tissue and the retrograde limb is Purkinje tissue from the posterior fascicle.
- Antegrade His capture may occur during atrial pacing without affecting the VT cycle length. Sinus beats and PVCs can capture ventricle without resetting the tachycardia. These findings suggest a small reentrant circuit.
- His bundle is not a required component of VT circuit, because the retrograde His may be recorded 20–40 milliseconds after the earliest activation (Fig. 7.11).
- Tachycardia can be induced by pacing or programmed stimulation from the atrium or ventricle with or without isoproterenol infusion. The inverse relation between the initiating PVC and the first beat of the VT has been described.
- Continuous or mid-diastolic activity may be recorded from the ablation site.
- Fractionated electrograms may be recorded at the site of earliest activation (Fig. 7.12).
- The area of slow conduction in the VT zone depends on the inward calcium current. This may explain the sensitivity of the tachycardia to Verapamil but not to adenosine or Valsalva maneuvers.

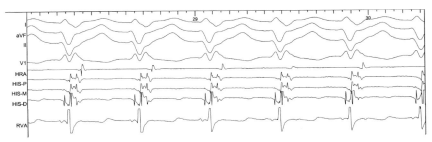

Fig 7.11 Retrograde activation of His during VT.

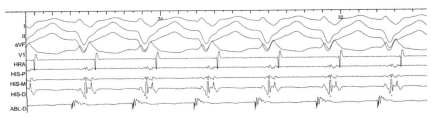

Fig 7.12 Fractionated electrograms recorded at the site of earliest activation from the distal electrodes of the ablation catheter.

- It may respond to adenosine if catecholamine stimulation is required to induce the tachycardia.
- Tachycardia can be entrained by pacing from RVOT.

Treatment
- IV Verapamil can be used for acute termination and oral Verapamil for chronic therapy of the LV VT.
- Ablation should be considered when antiarrhythmic therapy fails. A pace map may not be helpful in identifying the ablation site. The presence of earliest Purkinje potential is crucial for the success of the ablation and even more important than the earliest QRS activation site.
- Identification and ablation of Purkinje potentials during sinus rhythm, in patients in whom tachycardia cannot be induced, may provide a satisfactory outcome.
- Complications may include mitral and/or aortic regurgitation.

Interfascicular VT
- The reentrant circuit involves superior and inferior division of the left bundle.
- RBBB and anterior or posterior fascicular block is present during sinus rhythm.
- Tachycardia could present as RBBB and left posterior fascicular block if the antegrade conduction occurred over the left anterior fascicle and retrograde conduction over the left posterior fascicle. The presence of RBBB and left anterior fascicular block will occur if the circuit was reversed.

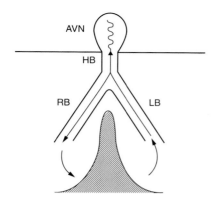

Fig 7.13 Schematic of BBR-VT antegrade conduction through RB and retrograde conduction through LB.

- RBBB morphology is similar during sinus rhythm and during tachycardia.
- During tachycardia there is a reversal in the activation sequence of His and the LB.
- HV interval is shorter during VT than in sinus rhythm.
- Variation in the LB to LB interval dictates the subsequent cycle length during the tachycardia.
- Block in either fascicle results in termination of the tachycardia.

7.7 BUNDLE BRANCH REENTRY VENTRICULAR TACHYCARDIA

- Tachycardia may present with LBBB or RBBB morphology depending on the antegrade conduction over the RB or the LB respectively. LBBB morphology is common.
- The introduction of RV premature beat at a short coupling interval results in retrograde block in RB. Transeptal delay and shorter refractory period of the LB allows the impulse to proceed over LB. If the RB recovers from its refractoriness, the impulse may conduct antegradely over RB and initiate reentrant tachycardia (Fig. 7.13).
- An inverse relationship exists between retrograde conduction delay in LB and recovery of the antegrade conduction over RB.
- Recording and analysis of His bundle and Bundle branch activation sequence during tachycardia is essential for the diagnosis of BB VT.
- Introduction of the premature beats with short to long cycle length changes the refractoriness of the HPS allowing the reentry to occur.
- BBRT commonly presents with LB morphology. Reverse reentry loop may occur if the LB refractoriness exceeds that of RB.
- LV pacing or extastimuli do not facilitate RB-type BBRT.
- In patients with structurally normal heart BBR tends to be self-limiting because of the spontaneous blocks in the retrograde limb (LB).

- The presence of conduction abnormalities in HPS facilitates BBR.
- BBRT commonly occurs in the presence of structural heart disease such as dilated cardiomyopathy with severe LV dysfunction and conduction abnormalities in the HPS.

Clinical manifestations[43–44]

- BBR-VT may result in syncope and sudden death.
- It is commonly associated with structural heart disease and low ejection fraction.
- This mechanism should be considered in VTs occurring in the presence of dilated cardiomyopathy.
- BBR VT may also be seen in:
  - i Myotonic dystrophy.
  - ii Hypertrophic cardiomyopathy.
  - iii Ebstein anomaly.
  - iv Following valvular surgery.
  - v Proarrhythmia due to Na channel blockers.

Electrophysiologic features

- The baseline electrocardiogram shows either sinus rhythm or AF. Nonspecific IVCD of the LBB type and prolonged PR interval are common findings.
- During tachycardia right or left bundle branch block pattern and AV dissociation are present (Fig. 7.14).
- Intracardiac electrograms reveal prolonged HV interval (average 80 ms).
- 6% of all inducible ventricular tachycardias have bundle branch reentry as their mechanism.

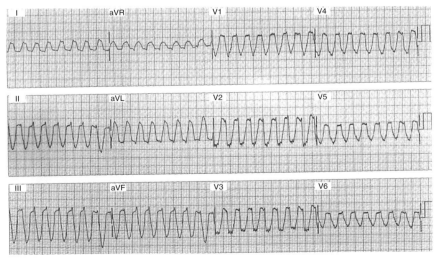

Fig 7.14 12 lead ECG of BBR-VT with LB morphology and left axis deviation.

- Tachycardia is induced by RV programmed stimulation. It may require introduction of short to long cycle length premature beats.
- Isoproterenol infusion may facilitate induction of the tachycardia.
- Infusion of procainamide may facilitate induction of tachycardia by increasing conduction delay in HPS.
- The HV interval during LBB morphology tachycardia tends to be similar or longer than the HV interval during sinus rhythm. During tachycardia the HV interval depends on the conduction characteristics of the contralateral bundle (Figs 7.15 and 7.16).
- The sequence of activation of His and bundle branch is essential in diagnosing the type of VT. During tachycardia with LBB morphology LB activation is followed by His and then RB activation. The sequence of activation is reversed in RBB morphology VT.

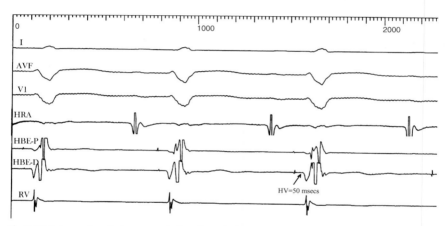

Fig 7.15 Intracardiac electrograms during sinus rhythm. LB morphology.

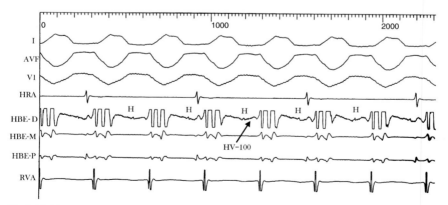

Fig 7.16 BBR-VT. H precedes each QRS. HV longer than HV in sinus rhythm.

- Tachycardia terminates with a block in His Purkinje tissue (No LB or His electrogram following last QRS).
- During tachycardia changes in the H to H interval precede the changes in the V to V interval. This helps to differentiate BBR-VT from myocardial origin VT with incidental HPS activation.
- The introduction of premature impulses during the tachycardia may reverse the circuit.
- The QRS morphology during entrainment by atrial pacing is identical to that of BBR VT. However, during RV pacing the QRS morphology is different.
- The difference between PPI and the tachycardia cycle length tends to be less than 30 milliseconds.

Electrophysiologic features of BBR-VT
1 During tachycardia QRS morphology is commonly LBBB type
2 His electrograms precede each V
3 HV interval during tachycardia >HV in baseline
4 Changes in V–V interval follow the changes in H–H
5 Delay in HPS conduction facilitates induction
6 Block in Bundle branches or HPS will terminate the tachycardia
7 Ablation of RB renders tachycardia noninducible

Differential diagnosis of BBR-VT

- VT of myocardial origin may present with incidental HPS activation preceding QRS, however, V to V cycle length variation dictates H to H variation. Often H cannot be discerned during this type of tachycardia.
- Supraventricular tachycardia with aberrancy may be mistaken for BBR-VT, especially if 1 : 1 retrograde conduction is present. His and BB activation is antegrade in SVT and resembles the activation during sinus.
- Atriofascicular reentry tachycardia presents with LBB morphology. However, RBB activation precedes His activation in this tachycardia and excludes BBR VT with LBB morphology. There is 1 : 1 AV relation and atrial premature beats preexcite the right ventricle.

Observations suggestive of BBR-VT

A Idiopathic dilated cardiomyopathy
B Conduction abnormality of HPS during sinus rhythm
C VT with LB morphology
D HV interval during VT same or longer than HV in sinus rhythm when measured from H to onset of QRS
E H electrogram precedes RB electrogram
F If entrained by A pacing, the QRS morphology is similar to QRS morphology during VT

Treatment

- The treatment of choice for BBR VT is ablation of the RB.[44]
- A permanent pacemaker should be implanted if the post-ablation HV interval is 100 mlliseconds or longer.
- ICD implant should be considered if myocardial VT occur spontaneously or are inducible or if EF is less than 35%.

7.8 CATECHOLAMINERGIC POLYMORPHIC VENTRICULAR TACHYCARDIA

- It is characterized by a reproducible form of polymorphic VT in the absence of heart disease or QT interval prolongation.
- It appears during exercise test, isoproterenol infusion, or other forms of adrenergic stimulation and can degenerate into ventricular fibrillation.

Genetic abnormalities[46-48]

- The causative genes are located on chromosome 1. Mutations of the cardiac ryanodine receptor gene (RyR2) have been implicated in the autosomal dominant type, while calsequestrin gene (CASQ2) mutations are seen in the recessive form.
- Ankyrin-B mutations have been identified in some cases of catecholaminergic polymorphic VT.
- Mutations in the Ankyrin-B gene were previously linked to the long-QT 4 phenotype.
- Cardiac RyR2 is located on the sarcoplasmic reticulum (SR) and controls intracellular Ca release and cardiac muscle contraction.
- RyR2 is responsible for calcium-induced calcium release from the SR.
- Skeletal muscle ryanodine receptor RyR1 mutation is responsible for malignant hyperthermia.
- Cardiac RyR2 receptors are also implicated in the cardiac arrhythmias associated with heart failure as these are mediated by sympathetic overactivity and catecholamine excess.
- Calstabin 2 is a stabilizing subunit of the RyR2 complex. Mutation may result in reduced calstabin 2 binding to RyR2, resulting in abnormal calcium release during exercise, which may trigger ventricular arrhythmias and sudden cardiac death.
- RyR2 mutations have also been identified in patients with a variant form of arrhythmogenic right ventricular dysplasia (ARVD2).
- Mutations in human cardiac CASQ2, a calcium-binding protein located in the SR, have been linked with a recessive form of catecholaminergic polymorphic VT.
- CASQ2 mutations impair sarcoplasmic calcium storing and calcium-induced calcium release. This may lead to delayed after-depolarizations (DADs).

- Ankyrin B is required for the assembly of the Na/Ca exchanger, Na/K ATPase, and inositol triphosphate (IP3) receptor in SR of cardiomyocytes.
- Mutations of ankyrin B may result in abnormal Ca dynamics, and catecholaminergic polymorphic VT.
- Ankyrin B gene mutations may be responsible for the LQTS4 phenotype.
- Thus there are four different genetic mutations that could express as catecholaminergic polymorphic VT:
  1 RyR2 Mutation.
  2 Calstabin 2 mutation.
  3 CASQ2 mutation.
  4 Ankyrin B mutation.

Clinical presentation
- Patients present with exercise or emotional stress induced syncope in the first or second decade. Earlier or later occurrences have also been documented.
- It may be mistaken for epilepsy.
- Catecholaminergic polymorphic VT should be considered one of the causes of swimming-triggered cardiac events.
- RyR2 mutation is more common in males.

Differential diagnosis
- Exercise- or emotional stress-induced syncope with polymorphic VT should suggest the diagnosis of catecholaminergic polymorphic VT. Similar presentation may occur in some of the long-QT syndromes.
- Bidirectional VT, one of the hallmarks of catecholaminergic polymorphic VT, has also been described in Andersen–Tawil syndrome (LQT7).
- In catecholaminergic polymorphic VT, the ECG is normal and the QT interval is either normal or borderline.
- The heart is structurally normal.
- The arrhythmia can be induced by exercise or by isoproterenol infusion.
- Ambulatory monitoring may reveal exercise-induced arrhythmias.
- Electrophysiological studies are of limited value.

Electrocardiographic features
- The ECG during catecholaminergic polymorphic VT may demonstrate bidirectional VT.
- The resting ECG is usually normal. The frequency of ventricular premature beats increases with exercise, usually when the heart rate exceeds 120 bpm.
- The frequency and complexity of the PVCs increases as the heart rate increases and may result in bidirectional VT or polymorphic VT. Syncope may

occur. Arrhythmias resolve on discontinuation of exercise or on stopping of isoproterenol infusion.

- During exercise, atrial fibrillation may precede ventricular arrhythmias.
- The premature beats originate from the left ventricle and demonstrate right bundle branch block pattern with alternating right and left axis deviation.
- In ARVD2 premature beats arise from the right ventricle and have left bundle morphology.

Treatment[49]

- β-Blockers are the treatment of choice.
- IV propranolol can be used for terminating the tachycardia. Nadolol is effective prophylactically. Asymptomatic PVCs may persist in spite of β-blockers. Complete suppression of asymptomatic PVCs is not necessary.
- Amiodarone is not as effective.
- Calcium channel blocker verapamil is partially successful in suppressing arrhythmias.
- Catheter ablation was reported as unsuccessful.
- If the β-blocker dose is insufficient or missed it may lead to sudden death.
- An ICD implant provides protection against SCD.
- Potential problems of implanting an ICD in young patients include inappropriate shocks, regular ICD follow-up and replacement when the battery reaches depletion.
- A combination of β-blockers with an ICD appears to be the ideal therapy.
- The detection interval of the ICD should be extended to avoid shocks for nonsustained VTs. Maximally tolerated dosages of beta-blockers should be continued to minimize the number of ICD shocks.
- The use of volatile anesthetics or Succinylcholine may result in malignant hyperthermia in carriers of RyR1 mutations in skeletal muscle. Such complications have not been reported in carriers of cardiac RyR2 mutations or in patients with catecholaminergic polymorphic VT.

Prognosis

- Mortality in untreated patients is estimated to be 30–50% by the age of 20–30 years.
- Mortality may be reduced to 5–7% per year with the use of β-blockers; however, it is considered unacceptably high.
- Fifty percent of the patients may receive appropriate ICD shocks over 2 years.
- Early diagnosis of catecholaminergic polymorphic VT is essential. Undetected, it may lead to sudden death early in life. Family screening by genetic studies is useful to identify asymptomatic carriers who may develop symptoms during stress.

7.9 MISCELLANEOUS FORMS OF VENTRICULAR ARRHYTHMIAS

Bidirectional VT

- It is a fascicular tachycardia. The QRS complex is narrow with an RBBB pattern and alternating left and right axis deviation in the frontal plane giving rise to bidirectional appearance in the limb leads.
- Twelve lead electrocardiogram is required to make the diagnosis.
- It is a descriptive term where the causes and mechanism of the tachycardia may be different.
- It is often associated with digitalis toxicity in the presence of structural heart disease. It has also been observed in the presence of herbal aconite poisoning and familial hypokalemic periodic paralysis (Table 7.12).
- Aconitine results in persistent activation of the Na channel and may mimic LQT3.
- The mechanism of the digitalis-induced bidirectional VT appears to be triggered activity due to DAD.
- It carries poor prognosis.
- Digoxin-specific Fab fragment administration is the treatment of choice for digitalis-induced tachycardia.

Accelerated idioventricular rhythm (AIVR)[51]

- AIVR is characterized by more than three consecutive ventricular beats at less than 100 bpm but faster than the intrinsic ventricular escape rhythm.
- It may be associated with isorhythmic AV dissociation and fusion beats at onset and termination.
- Gradual onset and termination may occur depending on the intrinsic sinus rate.
- AIVR may occur in a normal heart or in the presence of structural heart disease such as myocardial ischemia and infarction, myocarditis, cardiomyopathy, digitalis, and cocaine toxicity.
- AIVR commonly occurs following myocardial reperfusion. QRS may be multiform.
- The mechanism of the AIVR appears to be abnormal automaticity.
- AIVR is generally benign. It does not require treatment.

Table 7.12 Causes of bidirectional VT

Causes of bidirectional VT	Therapeutic options
Catecholaminergic polymorphic ventricular tachycardia	β-blockers. ICD
Digoxin toxicity	Digoxin antibodies
Familial hypokalemic periodic paralysis[50]	Potassium replacement
Herbal aconite poisoning	IV lidocaine
Andersen–Tawil syndrome	ICD

- In patients with diminished cardiac function loss of atrial contribution may cause symptoms. Increasing sinus rate by atropine may resolve AIVR.
- Occurrence of AIVR in the presence of acute MI does not increase the incidence of VF or mortality.

Parasystole[52]

- Parasystole results from automatic and protected focus.
- Normal or abnormal automaticity, triggered activity due to EAD or DAD can cause parasystole.
- Parasystole is characterized by:
  i Varying coupled interval.
  ii Fusion beats.
  iii Mathematically related interectopic intervals that may vary due to autonomic influences.
- Parasystole is classified as:
  1 Continuous without exit block.
  2 Continuous with exit block.
  3 Intermittent.

References

1 Ideker RE. Walcott GP. Epstein AE. Plumb VJ. Kay N. Ventricular fibrillation and defibrillation – What are the major unresolved issues? *Heart Rhythm*. 2:555–8, 2005.

2 Stevenson WG. Khan H. Sager P. et al. Identification of reentry circuit sites during catheter mapping and radiofrequency ablation of ventricular tachycardia late after myocardial infarction. *Circulation*. 88:1164, 1993.

3 The Antiarrhythmics versus Implantable Defibrillator Investigators: A comparison of antiarrhythmic drug therapy with implantable defibrillators in patients resuscitated from near-fatal ventricular arrhythmias. *N Engl J Med*. 337:1576, 1997.

4 Bogun F. Kim HM. Han J. et al. Comparison of mapping criteria for hemodynamically tolerated, postinfarction ventricular tachycardia. *Heart Rhythm*. 3:20–6, 2006.

5 Kaplan SR. Gard JJ. Protonotarios N. et al. Remodeling of myocyte gap junctions in arrhythmogenic right ventricular cardiomyopathy due to a deletion in plakoglobin (Naxos disease). *Heart Rhythm*. 1:3–11, 2004.

6 Marcus FI. Fontaine GH. Guiraudon G. et al. Right ventricular dysplasia (a report of 24 adult cases). *Circulation*. 65:384–98, 1982.

7 Hulot JS. Jouven X. Empana JP. Frank R. Fontaine G. Natural history and risk stratification of arrhythmogenic right ventricular dysplasia/cardiomyopathy. *Circulation*. 110:1879–84, 2004.

8 Dalal D. James C. Tichnell C. Calkins H. Arrhythmogenic right ventricular dysplasia: A United States experience Heart Rhythm-2 (Supplement) S115, 2005.

9 Rampazzo A. Nava A. Malacrida S. et al. Mutation in human desmoplakin domain binding to plakoglobin causes a dominant form of arrhythmogenic right ventricular cardiomyopathy. *Am J Hum Genet*. 71:1200, 2002.

10 Kiès P. Bootsma M. Bax J. et al. Arrhythmogenic right ventricular dysplacia/ cardiomyopathy: Screening, diagnosis, and treatment. *Heart Rhythm*. 3:225–34, 2006.

11 Hodgkinson KA. Parfrey PS. Bassett AS. et al. The impact of implantable cardioverter-defibrillator therapy on survival, in autosomal-dominant arrhythmogenic right ventricular cardiomyopathy (ARVD5). *J Am Coll Cardiol*. 45:400–8, 2005.

12 Watkins H. McKenna WJ. Thierfelder L. et al. Mutations in genes for cardiac troponin T and α-tropomyosin in hypertrophic cardiomyopathy. *N Engl J Med*. 332:1058–64, 1995.

13 Maron BJ. Shen WK. Link MS. Epstein AE. Efficacy of implantable cardioverter-defibrillators for the prevention of sudden death in patients with hypertrophic cardiomyopathy. *NEJM*. 342:365–73, 2000.

14 Priori SG. Inherited arrhythmogenic diseases: The complexity beyond monogenic disorders. *Circulation Res*. 94:140–5, 2004.

15 Keating MT. The long QT syndrome. A review of recent molecular genetic and physiologic discoveries. *Medicine*. 75:1–5, 1996.

16 Rubart M. Congenital long QT syndrome: Looking beyond the heart. *Heart Rhythm*. 1:65–6, 2004.

17 Vincent MG. Risk assessment in long QT syndrome: The Achilles heel of appropriate treatment. *Heart Rhythm*. 2:505–6, 2005.

18 Shimizu W. Noda T. Takaki H. et al. Diagnostic value of epinephrine test for genotyping LQT1, LQT2, and LQT3 forms of congenital long QT syndrome. *Heart Rhythm*. 3:276–83, 2004.

19 Vincent GM. Role of DNA testing for diagnosis, management, and genetic screening in long QT syndrome, hypertrophic cardiomyopathy, and Marfan syndrome. *Heart*. 86:12–14, 2001.

20 Priori SG. From genes to cell therapy: molecular medicine meets clinical EP. *J Cardiovasc Electrophysiol*. 16:552, 2005.

21 Priori SG. Napolitano C. Schwartz PJ. et al. Association of long QT syndrome loci and cardiac events among patients treated with beta-blockers. *JAMA*. 292:1341–4, 2004.

22 Mönnig G, Köbe J, Löher A, Eckardt A. Implantable cardioverter-defibrillator therapy in patients with congenital long-QT syndrome: A long-term follow-up. *Heart Rhythm*. 2:497–504, 2005.

23 Fenichel RR. Malik M. Antzelevitch C. et al. Drug-induced torsades de pointes and implications for drug development. *J Cardiovasc Electrophysiol*. 15:475–95, 2004.

24 Gross GJ. IK1: The long and the short QT of it. *Heart Rhythm*. 3:336–8, 2006.

25 Brugada P. Brugada J. Right bundle branch block, persistent ST segment elevation and sudden cardiac death: A distinct clinical and electrocardiographic syndrome. A multicenter report. *J Am Coll Cardiol*. 20:1391–6, 1992.

26 Wilde AA. Antzelevitch C. Borggrefe M. Study group on the molecular basis of arrhythmias of the European Society of cardiology. Proposed diagnostic criteria for the Brugada syndrome. *Eur Heart J*. 23:1648–54, 2002.

27 Nogami A. Nakao M. Kubota S. et al. Enhancement of J-ST-segment elevation by the glucose and insulin test in Brugada syndrome. *Pacing Clin Electrophysiol*. 26:332–7, 2003.

28 Antzelevitch C. Brugada R. Fever and Brugada syndrome. *Pacing Clin Electrophysiol*. 25:1537–9, 2002.

29 Brugada R. Brugada J. Antzelevitch C. Sodium channel blockers identify risk for sudden death in patients with ST-segment elevation and right bundle branch block but structurally normal hearts. *Circulation*. 101:510–15, 2000.

30 Fish JM. Antzelevitch C. Role of sodium and calcium channel block in unmasking the Brugada syndrome. *Heart Rhythm*. 1:210–17, 2004.

31 Wang K. Asinger RW. Marriott HJ. ST-segment elevation in conditions other than acute myocardial infarction. *N Engl J Med*. 349:2128–35, 2003.

32 Noda T. Shimizu W. Tanaka K. Chayama K. Prominent J wave and ST segment elevation: serial electrocardiographic changes in accidental hypothermia. *J Cardiovasc Electrophysiol*. 14:223, 2003.

33 Goldgran-Toledano D. Sideris G. Kevorkian JP. Overdose of cyclic antidepressants and the Brugada syndrome. *N Engl J Med*. 346:1591–2, 2002.

34 Morita H. Takenaka-Morita S. Fukushima-Kusano K. et al. Risk stratification for asymptomatic patients with Brugada syndrome. *Circ J*. 67:312–16, 2003.

35 Viskin S. Inducible ventricular fibrillation in the Brugada syndrome: Diagnostic and prognostic implications. *J Cardiovasc Electrophysiol*. 14:458–60, 2003.

36 Hermida JS. Denjoy I. Clerc J. et al. Hydroquinidine therapy in Brugada syndrome. *J Am Coll Cardiol*. 43:1853–60, 2004.

37 Josephson ME. Callans DJ. Using the twelve-lead electrocardiogram to localize the site of origin of ventricular tachycardia. *Heart Rhythm*. 2:443–6, 2005.

38 Dixit S. Gerstenfeld EP. Callans DJ. Marchlinski FE. Electrocardiographic patterns of superior right ventricular outflow tract tachycardias: Distinguishing septal and free-wall sites of origin. *J Cardiovasc Electrophysiol*. 14:1–7, 2003.

39 Tada H. Ito S. Naito S. Kurosaki K. Ueda M. et al. Prevalence and electrocardiographic characteristics of idiopathic ventricular arrhythmia originating in the free wall of the right ventricular outflow tract. *Circulation Journal*. 68:909–14, 2004.

40 Tandri H. Bluemke DA. Ferrari VA. Bomma C. Nasir K. Findings on magnetic resonance imaging of idiopathic right ventricular outflow tachycardia. *Am J Cardiol*. 94:1441–5, 2004.

41 Tanner H. Wolber T. Schwick N. Fuhrer J. Delacretaz E. Electrocardiographic pattern as a guide for management and radiofrequency ablation of idiopathic ventricular tachycardia. *Cardiology*. 103 (1):30–6, 2005.

42 Dixit S. Marchlinski FE. Clinical characteristics and catheter ablation of left ventricular outflow tract tachycardia. *Curr Cardiol Rep*. 3 (4):305–13, 2001.

43 Caceres J. Jazayeri M. McKinnie J. et al. Sustained bundle branch reentry as a mechanism of clinical tachycardia. *Circulation*. 79:256, 1989.

44 Akhtar M. Gilbert C. Wolf F. et al. Reentry within the His-Purkinje system. Elucidation of reentrant circuit using right bundle branch and His bundle potentials. *Circulation*. 58:295, 1978.

45 Tchou P. Jazayeri M. Denker S. et al. Transcatheter electrical ablation of the right bundle branch: A method of treating macro-reentrant ventricular tachycardia due to bundle branch reentry. *Circulation*. 78:246, 1988.

46 Priori SG. Napolitano C. Tiso N. Memmi M. et al. Mutations in the cardiac ryanodine receptor gene (hRyR2) underlie catecholaminergic polymorphic ventricular tachycardia. *Circulation*. 103:196–200, 2001.

47 Coumel P. Catecholaminergic polymorphic ventricular tachyarrhythmias in children. *Card Electrophysiol Rev*. 6:93–95, 2002.

48 Lehnart SE. Wehrens XH. Kushnir A. Marks AR. Cardiac ryanodine receptor function and regulation in heart disease. *Ann NY Acad Sci.* 1015:144–59, 2004.

49 Sumitomo N. Harada K. Nagashima M. Yasuda T. et al. Catecholaminergic polymorphic ventricular tachycardia (electrocardiographic characteristics and optimal therapeutic strategies to prevent sudden death). *Heart.* 89:66–70, 2003.

50 Ai T. Fujiwara Y. Tsuji K. et al. Novel KCNJ2 mutation in familial periodic paralysis with ventricular dysrhythmia. *Circulation.* 105:2592–4, 2002.

51 Grimm W. Accelerated idioventricular rhythm. *Card Electrophysiol Rev.* 5:328–31, 2001.

52 Castellanos A. Saoudi N. Moleiro F. Myerburg RJ. In Zipes DP, Jalife J (eds): Cardiac Electrophysiology: From Cell to Bedside, 4th ed. Philadelphia, WB Saunders, 2004, pp. 739–46.

8 Sudden Cardiac Death and Risk Stratification

Self-Assessment Question

1 A 57-year-old man developed chest pain while playing tennis. Five minutes later he collapsed. Cardiopulmonary resuscitation was provided by his tennis partners until an ambulance crew arrived 6 minutes later. Electrocardiogram showed ventricular fibrillation, and external defibrillation restored sinus rhythm. He was admitted to the hospital.

   The next day coronary angiogram revealed significant (>75%) stenosis of major epicardial coronary arteries. Left ventriculogram showed ejection fraction of 55% and no regional wall motion abnormalities. Serial electrocardiograms showed transient T-wave inversion. Serum troponin I level peaked at 2.
   Which of the following is most appropriate at this time?
   A Electrophysiologic study
   B Implantation of a cardioverter-defibrillator
   C Coronary artery bypass grafting and implantation of a cardioverter-defibrillator
   D Coronary artery bypass grafting without implantation of a cardioverter-defibrillator

Sudden cardiac death

- It is defined as death, due to cardiac arrhythmias, that occurs within 1 hour of symptoms.
- In patients presenting with out of hospital cardiac arrest the initial rhythm could be ventricular tachycardia (VT), ventricular fibrillation (VF), pulseless activity, or asystole depending on the duration from arrest.
- If the time elapsed is less than 4 minutes, 90% of the patients will show VF and 5% will have asystole. As the time interval increases, the proportion of asystole as the detected rhythm increases.
- Post cardiac arrest survival depends on the time elapsed since arrest.
  The presence of asystole or pulseless cardiac contractions indicates long duration since cardiac arrest and survival of less than 5%.
- In the presence of acute ischemia or myocardial infarction (MI) the cause of sudden cardiac death (SCD) is VF. Less than 30% of these patients with SCD have inducible monomorphic VT.
- Patients with previous MI, abnormal signal average ECG (SAEKG), and low ejection fraction (EF) tend to present with monomorphic VT.
- 10% of SCD patients may be discharged alive from the hospital.
- Early resuscitation and return of spontaneous circulation RSC is predictive of better survival.
- In patients with sever congestive heart failure (CHF). SCD may be due to bradyarrhythmias.
- Commonest cause of the autopsy negative sudden unexpected death in young may be due to channelopathies induced arrhythmias.[1]

Clinical presentation of SCD
- In 25% of patients with coronary artery disease (CAD), SCD may be the first manifestation.
- Causes of SCD are listed in Table 8.1.
- Left ventricular function is the most important predictor of SCD. EF of less than 30% is associated with 3- to 5- fold increase in SCD.
- Premature ventricular contractions (PVCs) and nonsustain VT (NSVT) are predictors of SCD but suppression of these arrhythmias may not improve survival.
- Abnormal results of the SAEKG, heart rate variability(HRV), baroreceptor sensitivity and electrophysiologic study have a low positive predictive value and therefore are not useful in making treatment decisions.

Mechanisms
- Lethal ventricular arrhythmias occur in the presence of a substrate such as scar or hypertrophy and initiating factors such as ischemia, autonomic dysfunction, hypoxia, acidosis, electrolyte, gene expression, and ion channel abnormalities.

Table 8.1 Causes of SCD

CAD	Cardiomyopathies	Repolarization abnormalities	Infiltrative disorders	Arrhythmia induced
Ischemia MI	Idiopathic Hypertrophic RV dysplasia Myocarditis Valvular heart disease Congenital heart disease	LQTS Proarrhythmia Electrolyte Brugada CPVT	Sarcoidosis Amyloidosis Tumors	WPW Idiopathic VF Torsades Bradycardia asystole

CPVT, Catecholaminergic polymorphic VT.

- Increase in sympathetic activity, in patients with ischemic heart disease and CHF, is associated with an increased risk of SCD.
- Denervation of the sympathetic nerve may occur due to MI, which may result in supersensitivity to circulating catecholamines distal to MI. This may shorten the refractory period and cause arrhythmias.
- A decrease in parasympathetic activity may also lower the threshold for occurrence of ventricular arrhythmias.
- The onset of acute ischemia in the setting of prior MI may result in VF.
- Thromboxane A2 and serotonin may cause coronary artery spasm and ischemia.

Clinical evaluation and treatment
- Following an episode of SCD, an evaluation should be performed to determine extent of the underlying heart disease and assessment of reversible factors such as severe hypokalemia and use of proarrhythmic drugs, and cocaine.
- The risk of reoccurrence of SCD is 20% in the first year.
- If the VF occurs in the setting of acute ischemia or MI and subsequent evaluation shows normal EF, the reoccurrence rate of VF is approximately 2%.
- The treatment of choice is implantable cardioverter defibrillator (ICD) implant.
- In Antiarrhythmic Versus Implantable Defibrillator (AVID) trial, 2-year survival in patients treated with Amiodarone was 74.7% and it was 81.6% in patients randomized to ICD therapy.
- Ischemia should be identified and treated before an ICD implant.
- These patients should be treated with β blockers and ace inhibitors.
- Amiodarone and ablation can be considered for recurrent ICD shocks.

Risk stratification for SCD[1]
- 10% of all deaths, in western population are cardiac and 50% of all cardiac deaths are sudden.
- 75% of the arrhythmic deaths are due to VT or VF and 25% are due to brady-arrhythmias or asystole. The commonest terminal arrhythmia is VF and more

than 90% of the victims of SCD have CAD, although acute MI at the time of the SCD is uncommon.
- After the initial episode of VT or VF the possibility of reoccurrence is approximately 30% in the next 24 months. This risk is even higher in the presence of left ventricular dysfunction.
- Risk stratification is an attempt to identify specific and sensitive markers that could assess the probability of occurrence or reoccurrence of morbid ventricular arrhythmias and elimination of those risk factors will thus improve the outcome. This goal has not been achieved.
- Frequent PVCs in a post-MI patient are a well-established independent risk factor of mortality, yet suppression of this arrhythmia does not result in improved survival.
- Reduction in arrhythmic death does not imply reduction in total mortality.
- A combination of multiple risk predictors, each with low sensitivity or specificity, may not provide useful predictive information applicable to individual patients.
- Not all post-MI patients suffer from ventricular arrhythmias.
- Risk assessment provides probability association of risk factors and events. It does not, in absolute terms, distinguish between patients who will or will not suffer from arrhythmias.

PVC as risk factor[2]
- 5–10% of the post-MI patients have NSVT and 20% have greater than 10 PVC/h. Complex and frequent ectopy is an independent predictor of mortality and the presence of decreased EF of <30% is associated with a 4-fold increase in mortality within 2 years of MI.
- Suppression of PVC has not improved survival, it may even worsen the outcome.

Nonsustained VT
- NSVT may be detected in 5% of the general population with normal heart and those with CAD with normal LV function.
- It may occur during or after exercise. It does not signify an adverse prognosis under these circumstances.
- In the early post-MI period the occurrence of NSVT does not predict inducibility of sustained VT. However, if the EF is less than 40%, the 2-year mortality is 10%.
- In patients with NSVT, EF of less than 40% and inducible VT, the risk of sudden death is 50% in 2 years and 6% in whom VT is noninducible.
- The possibility of inducing VT in patients with CAD, EF of less than 40%, and asymptomatic NSVT is 30%.
- The number of episodes and the length of NSVT have no association with mortality.
- NSVT is not an independent predictor of SCD in patients with dilated cardiomyopathy (DCM), hypertrophic cardiomyopathy, or hypertension.

Signal average ECG[2]

- Late potentials are due to depolarization of the tissue within the MI region that outlast normal QRS due to slow conduction.
- Late potentials are likely to be detected more often in patients with inferior MI than anterior MI due to activation sequence of the ventricles where normally the base of the ventricle is the last to be depolarized.
- In the presence of bundle branch block and conduction delays the late potentials may be buried within the prolonged QRS duration.
- There are three parameters that are commonly used to characterize abnormal late potential:
  1 Total QRS duration is greater than 114 milliseconds.
  2 Root mean square voltage of terminal 40 milliseconds (RMS40) is less than 20 μv. This reflects the relative amplitude of late potential.
  3 The duration of low amplitude signal (signal whose initial valve is less than 40 μv) is greater than 38 milliseconds.
- The positive predictive value of SAECG is 20% and the negative predictive value is 97%.
- QRS duration is more sensitive than RMS or LAS (low amplitude signal).
- It is a useful tool in the assessment of the patient with syncope, where a negative SAEKG will make the diagnosis of VT as a cause of syncope less likely.

Heart rate variability[3]

- Variability of the individual cardiac cycle is measured.
- It is the measurement of the RR interval during normal sinus rhythm (NN interval).
- Premature beats and other rhythms are excluded using QRS morphology criteria. Variance of NN interval can be presented in time domain as follows:
  1 SDNN: standard deviation of the NN interval.
  2 SD ANN: standard deviation of the average NN interval.
  3 RMSSD: root mean square of differences between neighboring NN interval.
  4 pNN50: percentage of NN intervals differing by more than 50 milliseconds from the immediately preceeding NN interval.
- Length of ECG recording has a bearing on HRV measurement. Long-term recordings (Holter) provide more reliable information.
- Varying QRS voltage, tall T waves and recording artifacts may be mistaken for QRS and may affect interpretation.

Frequency domain

- Using frequency domain for HRV analysis requires identification of very low frequency (VLF) of less than 0.04 Hz, low frequency (LF) of 0.04–0.15 Hz, high frequency (HF) of 0.15–0.4 Hz and ultra low frequency (ULF) of below 0.0033 Hz.
- These frequency distributions provide information about the degree of autonomic modulation rather than autonomic tone.

- Long term (24 h) recording of ECG for HRV shows the responsiveness of autonomic tone to environment.
- Efferent vagal activity is a major contributor to the HF component.
- The LF component may be a marker of sympathetic modulation.
- A high value of LF during the day and a higher valve of HF at night have been recorded.
- HF and LF components account for 5% of the total power while ULF and VLF account for 95% of the power of spectral analysis.

Use of HRV in risk stratification post-MI

- HRV is depressed following MI due to increased sympathetic activity.
- Depressed HRV predicts increased mortality in post-MI patients.
- In post-MI patients, 24 hours SDNN of less than 50–70 milliseconds indicates high risk for arrhythmic death.
- Abnormal HRV has been observed in patients with diabetic neuropathy.
- In patients with CHF reduction of HRV is due to increased sympathetic tone rather than a decrease in vagal tone. In these patients SDNN of less than 100 milliseconds and peak O_2 consumption of less than 14 ml/kg/min is predictive of poor prognosis and 1 year mortality of 37%.
- A state of anxiety and anger decreases HRV.
- Sleep-related vagal activation is lost in post-MI patients.
- β Blockers increase HRV.

Baroreflex sensitivity (BRS)[4]

- Increased carotid pressure prolongs the the RR interval.
- BRS is decreased in patients following MI.
- Patients with decreased BRS do not tolerate VT and present with syncope and hypotension.
- Pressure sensitivity receptors are located in the carotid sinus and the wall of the aortic arch.
- Afferent impulses from the carotid sinus through the glossopharyngeal nerve and impulses from the aortic arch through the vagus nerve travel to the mid-brain.
- Increased systemic arterial pressure activates baroreceptors, resulting in decreased sympathetic and increased vagal activity, which decrease the heart rate, contractility, and vasoconstriction.
- A fall in blood pressure decreases baroreceptor firing and causes increased sympathetic and decreased vagal activity.
- Baroreceptors interact in concert with multiple inputs from mechanoreceptors, chemoreceptors, and cardiopulmonary receptors. Additional inputs come from posture, exercise, and respiration.
- Under normal circumstances, through baroreceptors, vagal tone in activated and sympathetic tone in inhibited.

- Monitoring of spontaneously occurring blood pressure and heart rate changes is a closed loop where in addition to baroreceptors all other reflexes are active.
- Open loop assessment of the BRS is performed by external pharmacological or mechanical stimulus such as an increase in blood pressure.
- When pharmacologic agents are used all baroreceptors are stimulated.
- Phenylephrine, an alpha agonist, is injected (as a bolus) at a dose of 1–4 μg/kg to increase blood pressure by 20–40 mm Hg. Changes in the RR interval (HR) are plotted against the preceding systole blood pressure and expressed as milliseconds of the increase in RR with a 1 mm Hg increase in BP.
- The test is repeated at least three times and the average slope of the correlation between the HR and the BP is obtained.
- In normal subjects the average value of BRS is 15 + 9 ms/mm Hg.
- Phenylephrine produces direct alpha adrenergic stimulation of the sinus node; however this does not interfere with the BRS assessment.
- The RR interval shortens with the lowering of BP with nitroglycerine or nitroprusside.
- BRS slopes tend to be higher with an increase in blood pressure than with a decrease in blood pressure. This indicates that the responses to rise and fall in blood pressure are asymmetrical.
- BRS decreases when sympathetic tone is dominant and increases when parasympathetic tone is dominant.
- The normal BRS slope suggests effective vagal reflex and normal sympathetic activity.
- A flat BRS response suggests decreased vagal response or increased sympathetic tone.
- BRS is altered in the presence of hypertension and is reduced with increasing age.

Neck chamber technique for assessment of BRS

- Increased neck chamber pressure is sensed as a decrease in arterial pressure by baroreceptors. This initiates vagal withdrawal and increased sympathetic activity.
- BRS slope by neck chamber and phenylephrine may differ because with the neck chamber technique the stimulus is localized to carotid baroreceptors only.
- In a neck suction technique negative pressure is applied for 10 seconds at −7 to −40 mm Hg. This stimulates an increase in BP and prolongs the RR interval.

Spontaneous BRS

- Continuous monitoring of blood pressure and heart rate in the time or frequency domain is determined. This provides information about autonomic tone on a continuous basis.
- A BRS value of 3 ms/mm Hg or less is suggestive of poor prognosis and increased cardiac mortality.

- There is a weak correlation between BRS and HRV suggesting that the two methods express different functions of the autonomic tone.
- Low EF and decreased BRS is associated with an increase in cardiac mortality.
- In patients with low EF and normal BRS or decreased BRS and normal EF, the mortality was the same but less than when both EF and BRS were decreased.
- Measures to increase vagal tone and restore autonomic balance may decrease mortality in patients with low EF.
- BRS declines more rapidly after age 65 whereas HRV is a more reliable indicator of autonomic tone in patients older than 65 years.

T wave alternans (TWA)[5-7]

- Electrical alternans observed on a surface ECG, in patients with pericardial effusion, can affect P, QRS, and T waves. It appears to be due to the rocking motion of the heart inside the pericardium that results in a change of electrical axis and QRS morphology in every other beat. This is a mechanical phenomenon without electrophysiologic changes. It does not increase the risk of ventricular arrhythmias.
- TWA is an electrical alternans involving the T waves. It is the result of myocardial repolarization changes.
- TWA visible on surface ECG is seen in the presence of ischemia, long QT syndrome (LQTS), and electrolyte abnormalities. It is associated with an increased risk of ventricular arrhythmia and SCD.
- Microvolt TWA is detected by computer using the spectral method.
- 128 beats are analyzed. The magnitude of alternans in even and odd beats is measured in microvolt compared with mean alternans.
- The average power spectrum of even and odd mean beats is computed.
- The Alternans ratio (K) is the ratio of the alternans amplitude to the standard deviation of the background noise.
- $K > 3$ is considered abnormal.
- Abnormal TWA correlates with inducibility of ventricular arrhythmia during electrophysiologic study with a sensitivity of 80% and specificity of 85%.
- Exercise-induced TWA increases with increasing heart rate.
- Sustained alternans is defined as 1.9 μV alternans with an alternans ratio of >3 that lasts for at least 1 minute during a threshold heart rate.
- Ectopy, noise, pedaling, respiration, and heart rate variation may produce artifacts and affect TWA.
- Patients who develop TWA at a very high heart rate are at low risk of developing ventricular arrhythmias.
- Occurrence of TWA at a threshold heart rate of less than 110 b.p.m. identifies high-risk patients with a high degree of predictability.
- The mechanism of TWA appears to be dispersion of refractoriness. In some regions of the myocardium refractoriness may exceed the cycle length. Recovery from refractoriness may occur in every other beat, resulting in alternans.
- AP alternans may create areas of refractoriness and cause TWA.

Left ventricular EF (LVEF)[8-10]

- LVEF is a strong independent predictor of SCD, arrhythmia reoccurrence and total mortality.
- Each 5% decrease in EF increases the risk of SCD or arrhythmic death by 15%.

Programmed electrical stimulation (PES)[8]

- In patients with low EF (30%) the survival rate in the inducible group is similar to that of those who are not inducible. The positive predictive value of low EF for arrhythmic death is low (11%) but for total cardiac mortality it is superior.
- In patients with previous MI, low EF, and NSVT, PES may identify the high-risk group.[8]
- Noninducibility in patients with CAD and EF of >40% identifies the low-risk group.
- Mechanism of monomorphic VT tends to be scar related reentry. It is often inducible and demonstrates late potential.
- Cardiac arrest survivors may have inducible polymorphic VT.
- In AVID study patients who presented with asymptomatic VT had same prognosis as those with symptomatic or syncopal VT.
- Myocardial ischemia may result in PMVT (Polymorphic VT) and VF.
- Revascularization reduces the risk of SCD but does not affect the occurrence or inducibility of monomorphic VT (MVT).
- Normal SAEKG provides a strong negative predictive value.
- Abnormal HRV may identify the high-risk group.
- In the presence of heart disease low EF is a determinant of arrhythmic death, SCD, and total mortality.
- The positive predictive value of Holter monitoring for life-threatening arrhythmias is low.
- Exercise test may precipitate ischemia it may also provoke ventricular arrhythmias.
- If PES is performed in all post-MI patients, 20% will demonstrate inducible VT and 11% inducible VF.
- A low incidence of events may indicate falsely high negative predictive accuracy for PES. Low positive predictive accuracy means a large number of patients will have to be treated for the protection of a few.
- The negative predictive value of SAEKG is 95% even in patients with a low EF and NSVT. This observation makes it an excellent tool for evaluating patients with syncope where the arrhythmic cause is low probability. When the arrhythmic cause is strongly suspected negative SAEKG is not sufficient to exclude VT as the cause of syncope.
- High sympathetic tone decreases the VF threshold and increases coronary vaso-constriction and platelet aggregation. β Blockers provide protection from these deleterious effects.
- In post-MI patients with normal EF the incidence of SCD is 1.5% in 1 year.

- If EF is less than 40% and VT VF is noninducible then the incidence of SCD is 5%. It increases to 40% if the arrhythmia is inducible.[8]
- A combination of the predictors of the risk may improve the positive predictive value.
- Micro TWA may be an independent predictor for spontaneous and inducible arrhythmias.
- In MADIT, 2 year mortality was 14% in spite of defibrillator implant, indicating that treatment of arrhythmia alone may not prolong life.[8–10]
- In 5% of SCD victims due to VF, the heart is normal. There is a high incidence of reoccurrence.
- In AVID the absolute benefit of risk reduction in the defibrillator group was 7%, resulting in prolongation of life by 3.2 months over a period of 3 years.[11]

Syncope as risk factor for SCD
- In patients with DCM, syncope is a strong predictor of SCD.
- NSVT, SAEKG, and PES do not reliably predict future arrhythmic events or SCD. The degree of LV dysfunction is a strong predictor of mortality in DCM.
- Patients with DCM, who present with NYHA II, have an annual mortality of 10%. Half of those are due to SCD. In patients with functional class IV, the annual mortality is 50%, and 15–20% is due to SCD, the rest are due to bradyarrhythmias or pulseless cardiac activity.
- In asymptomatic patients with hypertrophic cardiomyopathy the presence of NSVT does not denote increased risk of SCD. However history ofprevious cardiac arrest, syncope, presyncope, and NSVT indicates an increased risk of SCD.
- Following a repair of Fallot tetralogy SCD may occur in 5% of patients. PES does not provide predictive information.
- The presence of LVH increases the incidence of SCD by 3-fold.
- In patients with ventricular arrhythmia the substrate and triggers may change.

Substrate	Triggers	Electrical stimulus
Scar	Autonomic imbalance	PVC
Long QT	Ischemia	
	Electrolyte abnormality	
	Repolarization abnormality	

Primary prevention of SCD[8–10]
- Ace inhibitor and β-blockers may reduce the mortality by 30–35% in patients with decreased EF.
- In patients who meet the MADIT I criteria (previous MI, EF less than 35%, NSVT, and inducible VT) ICD implant reduced the mortality.
- In the MADIT II study (previous MI, EF < 30%) ICD implant reduced the mortality from 19 to 14%.

SCD following repair of congenital heart disease
- Sudden death could be due to AV block, atrial flutter with 1:1 conduction or VT.
- Atrial arrhythmias are very common after Mustard, Senning, or Fontan procedure.
- In children who have suffered from cardiac arrest, the commonest associated condition is surgically repaired Fallot's tetralogy.
- Patients with Fallot's tetralogy have VSD and infundibular pulmonary stenosis. Surgical repair requires closure of the VSD by a patch, resection of muscle from the right ventricular outflow tract, and repair of the pulmonary annulus. This procedure is performed through ventriculotomy.
- This approach leaves a scar in the right ventricle and results in pulmonary insufficiency and right ventricular dysfunction. This may lead to reentrant VT arising at the site of the ventriculotomy or VSD patch.
- PVCs and complex ventricular arrhythmias are common after surgical repair of Fallot.

Factors influencing occurrence of ventricular arrhythmias
- The Incidence of mortality is 0.25–1.6% after a successful repair.
- *Age at initial repair*: If the initial repair was performed after the age of 10 years the likelihood of ventricular arrhythmia occurrence is very high.
- *Time since repair*: As more time elapses since repair the incidence of arrhythmia increases.
- The presence of residual RVOT obstruction, pulmonary insufficiency, right ventricular hypertension, and dysfunction are associated with an increased tendency for arrhythmias.
- Patients with a QRS width of more than 180 milliseconds have an increased risk of spontaneous and inducible VT or SCD.
- A stress test might identify patients with exercise-induced arrhythmias.

Treatment
- Radiofrequency ablation can be considered for atrial arrhythmias and well-tolerated VT.
- ICD is the treatment of choice for patients with sustained VT or resuscitated cardiac arrest.
- Patients with right to left shunt may have an increased tendency for thromboembolic complications. These patients should not undergo transverse lead ICD or pacemaker implant without consideration for anticoagulation.
- Following a repair of the congenital heart defect there is a higher incidence of sinus node dysfunction, AV block, and atrial flutter.
- Prophylactic ICD could be considered for patients who following a repair of Fallot's tetralogy demonstrate pulmonary insufficiency, abnormal right ventricular hemodynamics, frequent nonsustained ventricular arrhythmias, and syncope even if the electrophysiologic study is negative.
- For asymptomatic patients electrophysiologic study, antiarrhythmic drug therapy, or insertion of ICD is not recommended.

References

1 Puranik R. Chow CK. Duflou JA. Sudden death in young. *Heart Rhythm*. 2:1277–82, 2006.

2 Steinbigler P. Haberl R. Bruggemann T. et al. Postinfarction risk assessment for sudden cardiac death using late potential analysis of the digital Holter electrocardiogram. *J Cardiovasc Electrophysiol*. 13:1227–32, 2002.

3 Bilchick KC. Fetics B. Djoukeng R. et al. Prognostic value of heart rate variability in chronic congestive heart failure (Veterans Affairs' Survival Trial of Antiarrhythmic Therapy in Congestive Heart Failure). *Am J Cardiol*. 90:24–8, 2002.

4 Zipes DP. Rubart M. Neural modulation of cardiac arrhythmias and sudden cardiac death. *Heart Rhythm*. 3:108–13, 2006.

5 Rashba EJ. Osman AF. MacMurdy K. et al. Exercise is superior to pacing for T waves alternans measurements in subjects with chronic coronary artery disease and left ventricular dysfunction. *J Cardiovasc Electrophysiol*. 13:845–80, 2002.

6 Bloomfield DM. Hohnloser SH. Cohen RJ. Interpretation and classification of microvolt T wave alternans test. *J Cardiovasc Electrophysiol*. 13:502–12, 2002.

7 Ikeda T. Saito H. Tanno K. et al. T-waves alternans as a predictor for sudden cardiac death after myocardial infarction. *Am J Cardiol*. 89:79–82, 2002.

8 Moss AJ. Hall WJ. Cannom DS. et al. Improved survival with an implanted defibrillator in patients with coronary disease at high risk for ventricular arrhythmia. *N Engl J Med*. 335:1933–40, 1996.

9 Moss AJ. Zareba W. Hall WJ. et al. Prophylactic implantation of a defibrillator in patients with myocardial infarction and reduced ejection fraction. *N Engl J Med*. 346:877–83, 2002.

10 Bardy GH. Lee KL. Mark DB. et al. Amiodarone or an implantable cardioverter-defibrillator for congestive heart failure. *N Engl J Med*. 352:225–37, 2005.

11 The AVID Investigators (prepared by the AVID Executive Committee: Zipes DP. Wyse DG. Friedman PL. et al.): A comparison of antiarrhythmic drug therapy with implantable defibrillators inpatients resuscitated from near-fatal sustained ventricular arrhythmias. *N Engl J Med*. 337:1576, 1997.

9 Cardiac Arrhythmias in Patients with Neuro-muscular Disorders

Self-Assessment Questions

1 Which one of the following conditions is least likely to present with prominent R wave in lead V1?
   A Posterior MI
   B RBBB
   C Duchenne muscular dystrophy
   D Friedreich ataxia

2 Which one of the following is likely to present with bidirectional VT?
   A Emery–Dreifuss muscular dystrophy
   B Hypokalemic periodic paralysis
   C Kugelberg–Welander syndrome
   D Friedreich ataxia

3 Which one of the following conditions is unlikely to present with BBR-VT?
   A Myotonic dystrophy
   B Hypertrophic cardiomyopathy
   C Ebstein anomaly
   D Anderson–Tawil syndrome

Muscular dystrophies

Duchenne and Becker dystrophies
- Both are X-linked recessive disorders, due to an abnormality in the dystrophin gene[1].
- In Duchenne dystrophy dystrophin is absent, which results in fibrosis due to loss of myocytes.
- In Becker's dystrophy dystrophin is present in reduced amount, leading to a more benign course.
- Heart muscle is involved in both dystrophies.
- Isolated X-linked cardiac muscle dystrophin abnormality may lead to dilated cardiomyopathy without skeletal muscle involvement.
- Duchenne dystrophy becomes symptomatic before the age of 5 years. Cardiac involvement becomes evident by the age of 10.
- It involves the posterobasal and posterolateral wall of the left ventricle. This results in prominent R wave in V1 and Q wave in lateral precordial leads. Similar EKG changes may occur in Becker dystrophy.
- The severity of cardiac involvement does not correlate with the degree of skeletal muscle involvement.
- Cardiac arrhythmias such as persistent and labile sinus tachycardia, atrial arrhythmia and short PR interval are common.
- Abnormal signal average ECG (SAEKG) is recorded in one-third of the patients.
- Mortality is high: 25% of the deaths are due to arrhythmias sudden cardiac death (SCD) or congestive heart failure (CHF).

Myotonic dystrophy[2,3]
- It is an autosomal dominant disease. The gene abnormality is found in chromosome 19. Gene abnormality is due to unstable trinucleotide (CTG) repeat.
- Impaired glucose utilization may be related to abnormal protein kinase function.
- It is characterized by reflex myotonia, weakness, atrophy of distal muscles, early balding, gonadal atrophy, cataract, mental retardation and cardiac involvement.
- Cardiac involvement in muscular dystrophy is manifested by degeneration of the conduction system including the SA, AV node and His Purkinje system.
- Slowing of conduction results in abnormal SAEKG.
- The heart may be involved before skeletal muscle.
- It is common in French Canadians and rare in African blacks.
- Symptoms appear at 20–25 years of age and are due to weakness of the muscles of the face, neck, and distal extremities. Death occurs at 45–50 years of age.
- Myotonia (delayed relaxation of muscle) is the hallmark of the disease. It can be demonstrated in the thenar muscles and the tongue.
- In an asymptomatic person EMG or genetic testing can make the diagnosis.
- In successive generations the symptoms occur earlier and with increasing severity. This may be related to amplification of CTG repeat.
- Cardiac involvement is manifested by arrhythmias, cardiomyopathy, and PMV.

- ECG shows conduction abnormalities and AV blocks.
- Atrial arrhythmias occur in 10% of the patients.
- Sudden death may occur due to asystole (complete AV block) or ventricular arrhythmias such as bundle branch reentry ventricular tachycardia (VT).

Clinical and genetic characteristics of other dystrophies are described in Table 9.1.

Treatment

- Permanent pacemaker is indicated for patients presenting with syncope.
- PR interval of greater than 240 milliseconds was predictive of future cardiac events such as atrial fibrillation, complete AV block, syncope, and SCD. In these high-risk patients prophylactic permanent pacemakers should be considered.

Table 9.1 Clinical characteristics of Dystrophies

Dystrophy	Genetics	Clinical presentation	Arrhythmia manifestation	Treatment
Emery–Dreifuss	X linked abnormality in STA gene codes for protein Emerin	Contractures of elbow Achilles tendon, posterior cervical muscles	Atrial fibrillation, flutter, atrial stand still, junctional bradycardia, AV block	Permanent pacemaker
Limb girdle	Autosomal recessive	Cardiomyopathy limb girdle weakness	In Dominant form atrial and ventricular arrhythmia	
Facioscapulohumeral	Autosomal dominant chromosome 4q35	Muscle weakness	Sinus bradycardia, prolonged QRS duration Significant arrhythmias rare	
Periodic paralysis[4] hypo or hyperkalemic	Mutation in alpha1 unit of dihydropyridine sensitive Ca channel for HypoK and in alpha subunit of SCN4A for HyperK	Episodic weakness, triggered by cold, post-exercise or carbohydrate ingestion	Bidirectional VT VT may occur independently of muscle weakness LQTS may be seen	Normalize K Mexiletine for HyperK, β-blockers Imipramine for bidirectional VT
Mitochondrial encephlomyopathy	Mutation Mitochondrial DNA Maternally transmitted	Ophthalmoplagia (Kearna–Sayer, KS), myopathy, encephalopathy epilepsy, acidosis	KS AV block, short PR and prolonged HV Leber optic neuropathy short PR and preexcitation	Pacemaker
Kugelberg-Welander syndrome	Autosomal recessive. Chromosome 5q	Atrophy weakness proximal muscles	AF. Atrial standstill, AV block.	Pacemaker symptomatic treatment

- Ablation should be considered for bundle branch reentry VT.
- Anesthesia may increase the risk of AV block and other arrhythmias.

Friedreich ataxia

- It is a progressive spinocerebellar degeneration manifested by ataxia, dysarthria, sensory loss, and skeletal deformities.
- It is an autosomal recessive disorder. Gene codes for the amino acid protein Frataxin and is located on chromosome 9.
- It is associated with concentric left ventricular hypertrophy (LVH) rarely asymmetric septal hypertrophy without myocardial fiber disarray. A deposit of calcium salts and iron has been noted.
- Degeneration and fibrosis of cardiac nerve, ganglia, and conduction system may occur.
- Symptoms appear between the ages of 15 and 25 years.
- Electrocardiogram and echocardiogram confirm the presence of LVH.
- Atrial arrhythmias are common. Conduction abnormalities are rare.

Guillain–Barre syndrome

- It is an acute inflammatory demyelinating neuropathy.
- It occurs 5–7 days following a viral infection, immunization, or surgery.
- Arrhythmias are due to autonomic neuropathy and characterized by sinus tachycardia. AV block and ventricular arrhythmias may occur.
- Plasmapheresis, IV immunoglobulin, and temporary pacing for AV block should be considered.

Subarachnoid hemorrhage

- Acute cerebrovascular diseases such as subarachnoid hemorrhage are associated with marked ECG repolarization changes. These are characterized by peak inverted T waves and prolonged QT interval.
- Ventricular fibrillation may occur.
- β-blockers and ganglion blockers can be used for the treatment of ventricular arrhythmias.

References

1 Kaprielian RR. Stevenson S. Rothery SM. et al. Distinct patterns of dystrophin organization in myocyte sarcolemma and transverse tubules of normal and diseased human myocardium. *Circulation*. 101:2586–94, 2000.
2 Groh WJ. Lowe MR. Zipes DP. Severity of cardiac conduction involvement and arrhythmias in myotonic dystrophy type 1 correlates with age and CTG repeat length. *J Cardiovasc Electrophysiol*. 13:444–8, 2002.
3 Merino JL. Peinado R. Sobrino JA. Sudden death in myotonic dystrophy: The potential role of bundle-branch reentry. *Circulation*. 101:E73, 2000.
4 Ai T. Fujiwara Y. Tsuji K. et al. Novel KCNJ2 mutation in familial periodic paralysis with ventricular dysrhythmia. *Circulation*. 105:2592–94, 2002.

10 Syncope

Self-Assessment Questions

1 A 70-year-old woman is referred to you because of an episode of syncope that occured last week while sitting at the dining table. She did not have any nausea, sweating or other prodromal symptoms. Following the episode she did not have any residual symptoms. Physical examination is unremarkable. ECG shows LBBB. Echocardiogram showed LVH and EF of 45%.
Which of the following is the most appropriate recommendation?
   A Head up tilt test
   B Electrophysiologic study
   C 24-hour Holter monitor
   D EEG and carotid duplex examination

2 Visual prodromal symptom (gray out feeling) prior to syncope is the result of
   A Hypoperfusion of the visual cortex
   B Vasoconstriction in the brain stem
   C Collapse of the retinal blood vessels
   D Lack of perfusion to posture maintaining skeletal muscles

3 A 37-year-old woman has been aware of fatigue, lightheadedness, precordial pain, and aching sensation in "coat hanger" distribution on assuming an upright posture. She does not have any nausea or sweating. On physical examination supine blood pressure is 106/60 mm Hg. Heart rate is 85 b.p.m. These symptoms are most likely due to which one of the following?
   A Orthostatic hypotension
   B Prodromal symptoms of vasovagal syncope
   C Prodromal symptoms of cardiac syncope
   D Fainting lark phenomenon

4 Which of the following factors predict the likelihood of recurrence of syncope during follow-up after a positive tilt test?

A Occurrence of syncope within 5 minutes of 80° tilt

B History of injury during clinical syncope

C Hypotension and bradycardia during head up tilt test without syncope

D Frequency and the number of syncopal spells preceding positive tilt tests

5 A 19-year-old army recruit fainted while running. The heart rate or blood pressure was not recorded during that episode. During exercise test the patient exercised for 11 minutes and achieved a heart rate of 180 b.p.m. Syncope did not occur either during or right after the exercise test. Does this exclude the possibility of exercise-induced neurocardiogenic syncope?

A True

B False

6 You are asked to see a 21-year-old male who has had two episodes of rapid palpitations associated with near-syncope in the past 8 weeks. He underwent repair of tetralogy of Fallot at age 3.

Which of the following is the most likely mechanism of this patient's near-syncope?

A Ventricular tachycardia from the left ventricular outflow tract

B Ventricular tachycardia from the right ventricular outflow tract

C Ventricular tachycardia from the left ventricular septum

D Ventricular tachycardia from the right ventricular apex

Syncope is characterized by transient loss of consciousness (LOC) and postural tone followed by spontaneous recovery.

Pathophysiology[1,2]

- LOC is due to a global reversible reduction of blood flow to the reticular activating area located in the brain stem. It results in syncope within 10 seconds.
- It can be provoked by reflex (vasovagal) responses, cardiac arrhythmias, autonomic failure, or any condition that reduces cerebral blood flow (CBF) and cerebral oxygenation.
- Many of the premonitory symptoms of a vasovagal syncope are indicative of cerebral hypoperfusion.
- Vagal stimulation during vasovagal syncope may be responsible for the release of pancreatic polypeptide, which could be responsible for gastrointestinal symptoms associated with syncope.
- The visual prodromal symptoms are due to reduction in blood flow to the retina through the ophthalmic arteries.
- The brain and the brain stem are protected by the pressure-equalizing effects provided by the cerebrospinal fluid (CSF). The absence of such pressure equalizing mechanisms and the presence of intraocular pressure result in a collapse of retinal blood vessels and perfusion. This occurs before the LOC (gray out feeling).[2]
- Syncope often occurs during upright posture.
- On passive or active assumption of the upright position, a gravitational displacement of blood to the dependent area of the body occurs. This results in a fall of venous return. Orthostatic stress (active standing, or passive standing during tilt test), may result in 0.5–1 liter of blood pooling into the abdomen and lower extremities. Orthostatic pooling of venous blood begins immediately and is completed within 3–5 minutes.
- The Bezold–Jarisch reflex is initiated by excessive venous pooling, resulting in a decrease in ventricular volume and an increase in ventricular contractility. This activates receptors located in the inferoposterior portions of the left ventricle, leading to paradoxical withdrawal of sympathetic output to the vasculature and the heart and an increase in parasympathetic activity. Marked vasodilatation, hypotension, bradycardia, and the LOC occur.
- Other triggers that may result in hypotension and bradycardia include serotonin and adenosine.
- On standing upright there is a 25–30 mm Hg drop in MAP within 30 seconds to 1 minute.
- This transient fall in MAP explains the feeling of lightheadedness that even healthy humans sometimes experience shortly after standing up. This may result in syncope.
- The rapid short-term adjustments to orthostatic stress are mediated by the autonomic nervous system.

- Muscle activity ("the muscle pump") prevents reduction in the central blood volume and prevents hypotension. Lack of "pump" activity, during the upright position may result in syncope.
- During vasovagal syncope there is a withdrawal of muscle sympathetic activity resulting in loss of vasomotor tone leading to hypotension and syncope.

The fainting lark

- It is a voluntary self-induced instantaneous syncope. It is a result of gravitational acute arterial hypotension, raised intrathoracic pressure by valsalva and cerebral vasoconstriction in response to hypocapnia due to hyperventilation.

Cardiac syncope

- It is due to bradycardia or tachy-arrhythmias that result in hypotension and cerebral hypo-perfusion.
- Onset is often sudden and there are no prodromal symptoms of autonomic activation. The syncopal episode may develop either in the erect or in the supine position. There is no pulse.
- Prolonged asystole may provoke myoclonic movements and urinary and fecal incontinence.
- Recovery is rapid with a return of the pulse, flushing of the face, and usually full orientation.

Syncope due to orthostatic hypotension in patients with autonomic failure

- Autonomic failure results in symptomatic orthostatic hypotension.
- Orthostatic hypotension is characterized by a 20 mm Hg drop in systolic blood pressure within 3 minutes of assuming an erect posture.
- Postural orthostatic hypotension is defined as an increase in HR by 28 b.p.m. and hypotension within 5 minutes of standing.
- Symptoms include lightheadedness and blurring of vision. A neck ache radiating to the occipital region of the skull and to the shoulders ("coat hanger" distribution) often precedes LOC. The mechanism of this unique symptom of postural hypotension may be ischemia of the postural muscles.
- Impaired muscle perfusion may result in lower back and buttock ache.
- A decrease in myocardial perfusion may result in angina pectoris.
- Symptoms develop within minutes on standing or walking and resolve on lying down. These symptoms are prodromal and may alert the patient to lie down to restore cerebral perfusion. If the erect posture is maintained, consciousness gradually fades and the patient falls slowly. Sudden postural attacks may occur. Patients with autonomic failure do not exhibit symptoms and signs of autonomic activation such as sweating or a vagally induced bradycardia.

Prognosis and natural history

- Vasovagal syncope often presents in clusters. Multiple events occur in a relatively short period of time and are followed by long periods of quiescence.
- The frequency of syncopal events may also decrease after head-up tilt-table testing.
- Syncope due to cardiac causes is associated with high (30%) 1 year mortality.
- In 35% of patients with syncope, the etiology remains unclear.

Causes of syncope (also see Table 10.1)

- In young people syncope is likely to be due to neurocardiogenic origin and in elderly persons, sick sinus, hypersensitive carotid, heart block, medication, and hypotension may be responsible.
- History of cardiac disease, family history of sudden death, and medication may help identify the cause of syncope.
- Prodromal symptoms are likely to precede vasovagal syncope.
- Disorientation, LOC of more than 5 minutes, tongue biting, nystagmus, and headache after syncope are likely to be due to seizure.

Diagnostic tests

Electrocardiogram (ECG)

- ECG identifies a direct cause of syncope in only 5% of patients.
- ECG may help identify long QT syndrome (LQTS), WPW, atrio-ventricular (AV) block, myocardial infarction (MI), Brugada syndrome, left ventricular hypertrophy, T wave inversion in right precordial leads, and incomplete RBBB pattern suggestive of right ventricle (RV) dysplasia as a cause of syncope.
- In the presence of normal ECG cardiac cause of syncope is unlikely.
- Signal average ECG, Holter monitor, and event recorders have a low yield in determining the cause of the syncope (less than 20%).

Table 10.1 Causes of syncope

Cardiac	Vascular	Neurologic	Metabolic
AV block	Subclavian steal	Seizures	Hyperventilation
Sick sinus syndrome	Autonomic neuropathy	Migraine	Hypoglycemia
Pacemaker failure	Drug-induced hypotension	TIA/CVA	Hypoxia
SVT	Hypovolemia	Hysteria/panic	Alcohol
VT	Carotid sinus sensitivity		
Aortic stenosis	Vasovagal		
Aortic dissection	Situational (cough,		
Cardiac tamponade	micturition, and swallow)		
IHSS			
Mitral stenosis			
Pulmonary emboli			

Echocardiogram
- It should be obtained in patients with abnormal physical examination and ECG. Echocardiogram may help identify Myxoma or aortic stenosis as a cause of syncope.
- In the absence of heart disease by history, physical examination, and ECG, the diagnostic yield of echocardiography is low.
- The yield from neurologic imaging studies is low.

Exercise stress testing
- It should be considered if ischemic heart disease is suspected or if there is a history of exertional syncope and echocardiography excludes significant obstructive valvular cardiac lesion.

Electrophysiologic testing
- The diagnostic yield of electrophysiology studies in patients with a structurally normal heart and a normal ECG is low (1% ventricular tachycardia (VT), 10% bradycardia) whereas in patients with organic heart disease, the yield is over 50% (21% ventricular tachycardia, 34% bradycardia). Patients with an abnormal ECG also have a significant diagnostic yield (17% ventricular tachycardia, 19% bradycardia).
- A negative electrophysiology study does not necessarily exclude an arrhythmic, cause of syncope, and has a poor predictive value in nonischemic cardiomyopathy and LQTS.
- EP testing should be considered in patients with structural heart disease and unexplained syncope.
- It may identify patients with sick sinus syndrome, abnormal AV node conduction (HV of >100 ms, infra Hisian block), SVT, and VT.
- Predictors of abnormal EPS include abnormal LV function, prior MI, bundle branch block (BBB), non-sustained VT, male sex, and injury during syncope.
- In patients with severe impairment of left ventricular function EPS may have less predictive value. Three year mortality is 50% irrespective of EPS findings.

Neurocardiogenic syncope[1–4]
- It is the most common cause of syncope. It is reflex mediated.
- Other designations include "vasovagal" or "neurally mediated" syncope.
- It typically occurs in the upright position but may occur in a supine or seated position.
- Neurally mediated syncope (NMS) is characterized by premonitory symptoms of nausea, sweating, and pallor.

Types of neurally (vagally) mediated syncope:

1 Vasovagal faint (common faint)
2 Carotid sinus sensitivity
3 Gastrointestinal stimulation
4 Glossopharyngeal neuralgia
5 Airway stimulation, Cough
6 Micturation syncope
7 Increased intrathoracic pressure as in wind instrument playing, valsalva.

- The mortality rate is low.

History and physical examination

- Primary diagnosis of syncope can be made in 45% of patients by clinical history, physical examination, and electrocardiography.
- Vasovagal syncope may be precipitated by the sight of blood, loss of blood, sudden stressful or painful experiences, surgical manipulation, or trauma. History of childhood neurocardiogenic syncope may provide a clue to the cause of vasovagal syncope in adults.
- Prodromal symptoms and signs are usually present.
- Symptoms of epigastric discomfort, nausea, sweating, and a desire to sit down or to leave the room, lightheadedness, fatigue, blurring or fading of vision, palpitations, and tingling of the ears are reported.
- Signs include facial pallor, sweating, restlessness, yawning, sighing and hyperventilation, and pupillary dilatation. The prodromal phase is often associated with a rapid heart rate. Continuing hypotension and bradycardia results in difficulty in concentrating, lack of awareness of the surroundings, loss of postural tone, and then LOC and fall occurs.
- Myoclonic jerks are uncommon in a spontaneous vasovagal syncope.
- The duration of unconsciousness is usually brief, lasting less than 5 minutes.
- Immediately following the recovery from syncope there is profound fatigue, a persistence of pallor, nausea, weakness, sweating, and oliguria. The patient is usually not confused. Syncope may reoccur if the individual is returned to the upright position prior to resolution of hypotension and bradycardia. If the patient sits or lies down promptly, frank syncope may be aborted.

Tilt test[4]

- It is not warranted in the evaluation of a single syncopal episode with clear vasovagal features.
- Tilt table testing is indicated when there is recurrent syncope, or a single episode accompanied by injury or a motor vehicle accident, or syncope in a high-risk

setting, or recurrent exercise-induced syncope after exclusion of organic heart disease, or syncope due to another established cause whose treatment might be affected by the diagnosis of vasovagal syncope.

- Patient is tilted head-up on a table, with straps and a footplate, at an angle between 60° and 80° for 30–45 minutes.
- A duration of 45 minutes is considered two standard deviations from the mean time to syncope and captures 95% of patients who will faint. The mean time to syncope during a tilt test is ~25 minutes.
- If the passive stage of the test is negative, the use of provocative agents, such as isoproterenol, epinephrine, or nitroglycerin may increase the diagnostic yield by 20–25%.
- An 80° tilt provides 92% specificity, which remains unchanged with a low dose of Isoproterenol.
- The tilt test may be reproducible in 60–70% of patients.
- The average likelihood of recurrent syncope in the first 2 years after a positive tilt test is ~30% in unselected and untreated patients.
- Factors that predict the likelihood of recurrence of syncope include the frequency and the number of syncopal spells preceding positive tilt tests.
- Age, sex, tilt test outcome, bradycardia, hypotension during tilt test without syncope and injury during clinical syncope are not useful predictors of the reoccurrence.
- Sensitivity is ~50%. Specificity, a measure of how often a head-up tilt-table test does not induce vasovagal syncope in asymptomatic controls is ~90%.
- It is not proven to be useful in follow-up evaluation of therapy to prevent recurrence of vasovagal syncope because of the difficulties associated with reproducibility.
- Vasovagal responses can be divided into mixed, cardio-inhibitory, and vasodepressor.
- Two additional responses may occur.
- Dysautonomic response in autonomic neuropathy, where the blood pressure gradually falls without a significant increase in the heart rate.
- Postural orthostatic tachycardia syndrome, where there is excessive sinus tachycardia in response to orthostatic stress.

Contraindications
- Head-up tilt-table testing is contraindicated in patients with critical obstructive cardiac disease (for example, critical proximal coronary artery stenosis, critical mitral stenosis, or severe left ventricular outflow obstruction) or critical cerebrovascular stenosis.

Treatment
- Results of the tilt test (cardio-inhibitory or vasodepressor) may influence the choice of pharmacologic agent in the treatment of NMS. However, it cannot be used to assess the efficacy of the treatment.

Table 10.2 Long-term therapy for vasovagal syncope

Agents to augment central blood volume	Increase fluids and salt intake, compression hose, mineral corticoids
Agents that increase peripheral vascular resistance	α1-Adrenergic agonist (ephedrine, midodrine)
Parasympatholytic agents	Scopolamine, propantheline, disopyramide
Adenosine blockers	Theophylline, caffeine
Contractility suppressants	β1-Adrenergic blocker, disopyramide
Centrally active agents	Serotonin reuptake inhibitors (Fluoxetine Proxetine, sertraline), α2-adrenergic agonist (clonidine), and central stimulants (phentermine, methylphenidate)
Device therapy	Pacemaker

- Simple measures such as adequate hydration and salt intake, and avoidance of precipitating stimuli may prevent the reoccurrence of syncope. Medications causing vasodilatation or volume depletion may need to be replaced with alternative agents.
- Leg tensing can also abort an imminent faint.
- Medical therapy is indicated in a minority of patients, those with recurrent syncope or injury during syncope Table 10.2.
- β Blockers may be useful in vasovagal syncope, especially if sinus tachycardia precedes the onset syncope.
- Serotonin reuptake inhibitors, Proxetine and Fluoxetine, have been shown to eliminate or decrease the frequency of syncope.
- Expansion of the intravascular volume with fludrocortisone and use of the α agonist (vasoconstrictor) midodrine can be helpful for vasodepressor vasovagal syncope and orthostatic hypotension.
- Implantation of dual chamber pacemaker with a "rate drop response" algorithm is indicated in patients with hypersensitive carotid sinus syndrome and a cardio-inhibitory type of vasovagal syncope.
- Infrequent episodes of vasovagal syncope that are preceded by prodromal symptoms may only require counseling and observation.
- β-Adrenergic blockers are the most widely prescribed first choice therapy for vasovagal syncope. Its use is logical but not proven by trials.
- Patients did not report any difference between disopyramide and β-blockers. β-Blockers may be safer due to lack of pro arrhythmias.
- American College of Cardiology and the American Heart Association guidelines suggest a class IIb indication for pacing in patients who experience cardio-inhibitory vasovagal syncope unresponsive to drug therapy and reproduced by a head-up tilt with or without isoproterenol or other provocative maneuvers.

- Complete resolution of symptoms is not possible and a satisfactory end point may be reduced frequency or severity of the episodes.
- Patients should be advised to avoid pro-syncopal situations such as prolonged static standing, and volume depletion. Drugs that produce volume depletion peripheral vasodilation and hypotension should be discontinued.
- Patients with low blood pressure that is aggravated by orthostatic changes may benefit from fludrocortisone, midodrine, and compression hose.
  Symptomatic resting bradycardia may respond to anticholinergic agents, such as propantheline.
- The duration of pharmacologic therapy should be determined on an individual basis.
- Syncope in the setting of ischemic cardiomyopathy predicts a high risk of sudden death. These patients benefit from ICD therapy.

Carotid sinus hypersensitivity
- Carotid sinus hypersensitivity is diagnosed when carotid sinus pressure for 5 seconds results in a pause of >3 seconds. It may be produced in 40% of asymptomatic patients.
- Carotid sinus massage has its greatest utility in elderly patients.
- Carotid sinus massage should be avoided in patients with:
   i Transient ischemic attacks.
   ii Strike in the last 3 months.
   iii Carotid bruits.
- CSH may be the cause of syncope in the elderly.
- A dual chamber pacemaker is recommended for patients with syncope due to CSH.

Syncope and driving privileges
- Patients with syncope should refrain from driving if:
   i there is potential for reoccurrence.
   ii presence and duration of warning symptoms.
   iii posture during syncope.
- Noncommercial drivers should not drive for several months.

Causes of exercise-induced syncope
- It includes vasovagal syncope, hypertrophic cardiomyopathy, anomalous origin of coronary arteries, RV dysplasia, myocarditis, WPW syndrome, aortic stenosis, and LQTS.
- Neurally mediated syncope may occur during or immediately after exercise.
- NMS during exercise may not be reproduced during an exercise test.

References

1 Sheldon R. Rose S. Components of clinical trials for vasovagal syncope. *Europace* 3:233–40, 2001.
2 Van Lieshout JJ. Wieling W. Karemaker JM. Secher NH. Syncope, cerebral perfusion, and oxygenation. *J Appl Physiol.* 94:833–48, 2003.
3 Heaven DJ. Sutton R. Syncope. *Crit Care Med.* 28(Suppl.):116–20, 2000.
4 Fenton AM. Hammill SC. Rea RF. Low PA. Shen W. Vasovagal Syncope. *Ann Intern Med.* 133:714–25, 2000.

11 Pharmacologic Therapy of Arrhythmias

Self-Assessment Questions

1 Intravenous administration of which of the following agents will result in the greatest increase in conduction time?
   A Amiodarone
   B Bretylium
   C Lidocaine
   D Procainamide

2 A 37-year-old African American man was told that he had CYP2D6 deficiency. Which one of the following accurately reflects the pharmacologic effects of this deficiency?
   A If propafenone is administered he is likely to demonstrate excessive β blocking effects
   B Analgesic effect of the codeine will be enhanced
   C There will be an increased level of 5-hydroxy propafenone
   D Likely to develop lidocaine toxicity when administered with Ca channel blockers and erythromycin

11.1 PHARMACOLOGIC PRINCIPLES AS APPLIED TO ANTIARRHYTHMIC DRUGS

Antiarrhythmic drugs

- Pharmacokinetics is the study of drug concentration, pharmacodynamics relates to variability in response after administration.
- The term bioavailability describes the amount of drug detected in systemic circulation following oral administration.
- Availability of the drug can be reduced by lack of absorption or rapid metabolism in the liver or intestine before reaching circulation.
- Drugs that have poor bioavailability after oral administration require smaller doses when administered intravenously.
- During steady state the amount of drug entering and leaving the plasma or tissues is the same.

Elimination half life (EHL)

- In a "first-order kinetics" drug elimination is dependent on the plasma concentration. If the drug elimination per unit time is constant irrespective of plasma concentration it is called "zero-order kinetics."
- An example of zero-order kinetics is ethanol.
- When first-order mechanisms are saturated, at high plasma levels of the drug, the mode may switch to zero-order kinetics. Thus, doubling of the dose may raise the plasma concentration by more than 2-fold.
- EHL is the time required for plasma concentration to fall 50%.
- Drug elimination will be complete in 4–5 half lives. Following a change in the dose of the drug it takes 4–5 half lives to reach a new steady state. This applies to initiation, termination, or dosage change of the drug.
- Loading dose may result in early attainment of therapeutic concentration but the time to steady state is still dependent on half life. When the steady state is achieved the plasma level may not be therapeutic. It means that at that dose and plasma level the drug entering and leaving the plasma and tissues is the same.
- Following a loading dose, drug concentration may be high but by steady state it may become subtherapeutic if the maintenance dose is inadequate.
- Loading dose is desirable for rapid results or when the drug's half life is long.

Clearance

- Clearance is defined as the amount of plasma cleared of a drug in a unit time by elimination or metabolism. Its unit is volume/time or ml/min.
- Half life determines the time to steady state while the clearance and dose of the drug determine the actual level of the drug when steady state is achieved. Decreased clearance will result in increased steady-state levels of the drug.
- Steady-state concentration = dose/clearance.

- Organ specific such as renal or hepatic clearance can be measured.
- A drug can clear the plasma by elimination, metabolism, or intracellular uptake (adenosine).

Volume of distribution
- The central volume of distribution is where an IV administered drug distributes.
- Steady-state-volume of distribution is the total volume into which drug distributes at a steady state.
- In congestive heart failure (CHF) the central volume of distribution is reduced.
- EHL varies directly with the volume of distribution and inversely with clearance.
- In CHF, lidocaine volume of distribution and clearance is reduced requiring reduced loading and maintenance dose. The EHL remains unchanged at 2 hours and the time to steady state at 8–10 hours.

Distribution half life
- The time it takes for distribution of the drug from the central compartment to the peripheral sites. For example lidocaine distribution half life is 8 minutes and EHL is 120 minutes. This may be responsible for the precipitous drop in drug concentration shortly after IV administration.

Protein binding
- Most drugs bind to circulating plasma proteins. The unbound fraction of the drug exerts a pharmacologic effect. Change in protein binding can affect the amount of free drug available. Drugs bind to plasma albumin.
- Drugs with a high affinity for plasma protein (such as warfarin, which is 99% bound) may result in large variations in free drug concentration with a slight change in protein binding.
- Drugs may bind to acute phase reactants such as alpha1 acid glycoprotein (AAG). The levels of AAG increase with acute illness, such as myocardial infarction (MI). This may result in lower free drug concentration during acute illness.
- In acute MI higher plasma levels of lidocaine may be well tolerated and required to suppress arrhythmias. In these situations the level of unbound drug concentration will be more reliable than total drug concentration.
- In general, the loading dose should be avoided and the dose should be reduced if clearance is reduced.
- Clearance can be reduced by:
  i Dysfunction of the eliminating organ.
  ii Concomitant drug therapy that inhibits (Erythromycin and Cisapride) or induces (Rifampin and Quinidine) metabolic/transport pathway.
  iii Defective function of drug eliminating proteins and channels.
- Therapeutic margin is a plasma concentration of the drug above which toxicity occurs and at lower levels effectiveness is lost.

- Drugs dosing is determined by the elimination rate and lower and upper therapeutic levels. A wide therapeutic margin allows infrequent dosing even if the drug is eliminated rapidly. Propranolol is administered twice daily even though half life is 4–6 hours.
- With narrow therapeutic margin the drug should be administered according to EHL.
- To measure the steady-state level the drug should be administered with a frequency of EHL. If the frequency of administration is more or less often than the EHL then the plasma level of the drug may not reflect steady-state levels.
- If the drug produces active metabolites then the level of parent drug and metabolite should be measured and expressed individually. Drugs may have multiple pharmacologic effects at different plasma levels.

CYP2D6 (Table 11.1)
- It is an enzyme that belongs to the cytochrome P450 (CYP) family and is expressed in liver. It is responsible for metabolism of β-blockers (Timolol, Metoprolol), antiarrhythmics (Propafenone), and non-cardiovascular drugs (phenformin, codeine).
- It is absent in 7% of Caucasians and African Americans. These patients are poor metabolizers.
- In poor metabolizers the parent drug will accumulate. In the case of propafenone excessive beta blocking effect will be evident. In the case of codeine, which is metabolized to morphine, lack of CYP2D6 will result in ineffective analgesia.
- In ultra rapid metabolizers (increase CYP2D6) there will be accumulation of metabolites.

N-acetyltransferase (NAT)
- Procainamide, Hydralazine and Isoniazide are metabolized by conjugation with the acetyl group of NAT. 50% of Caucasians and African Americans are slow acetylators.
- Procainamide is eliminated by the kidney and by N acetylation to N-acetylprocainamide (NAPA), which is eliminated by the kidney.
- Rapid acetylators will be at increased risk of developing NAPA-induced torsades de pointes (TDP) in the presence of renal failure. Slow acetylators are at a higher risk of developing lupus.
- NAT1 is present in everyone; however, NAT2 is absent in slow acetylators.

CYP3A4
- It is expressed in the liver (Table 11.1).
- Inhibitor of CYP3A4 will allow the substrate level to increase, for example, high levels of terfenadine or cisapride when given with erythromycin or ketoconazole or increased risk of rhabdomyolysis with simvastatin and mibefradil or increased levels of cyclosporine with ketoconazole and calcium channel blockers.

Table 11.1 Enzymes and Drug interactions

Enzyme	Substrate	Inducer	Inhibitor	Effect
CYP2D6	Codeine Debrisoquine Flecainide Mexiletine Phenformin Propafenone Propranolol Thioridazine Timolol		Flecainide Fluoxetine Mibefradil Propafenone Proxetine Quinidine	Deficiency results in poor metabolizers
CYP2C19	Mephenytoin Omeprazole		Omeprazole Ticlopidine	
CYP3A4	Astemizole Cisapride Cortisol Cyclosporine HMG-CoA reductase inhibitors HN protease inhibitors Lidocaine Nifedipine Quinidine Terfenadine	Phenytoin Rifampin	Ca channel blockers diltiazem mibefradil Cimetidine Erythromycin and macrolide antibiotics Grapefruit juice Ketoconazole and azole antifungal	Drug toxicity with inhibition
N-acetyltransferase	Hydralazine Isoniazid Procainamide			Increase drug levels in slow acetylators
P-glycoprotein	Cortisol Cyclosporine Digoxin HN protease inhibitors Quinidine Verapamil		Cyclosporine Quinidine Verapamil	Inhibition affects blood brain barrier
Thiopurine methyltransferase	6mercaptopurine Azathioprine		Sulfasalazine	Marrow aplasia paralysis
Pseudocholinesterase	Succinylcholine			

P-glycoprotein (PG)

- PG acts as a drug efflux pump. Its expression in cancer cells may be responsible for multi-drug resistance (MDR).
- PG is also expressed normally at multiple sites important for drug distribution such as intestinal epithelium, hepatocytes, renal tubular cells, and capillaries of the blood brain barrier.
- In the intestine PG eliminates the drug by efflux back into the intestinal lumen.
- In the liver and kidney PG eliminates drugs into bile and urine. In the blood brain barrier it removes the drug from capillary endothelium. PG is an integral

part of the blood brain barrier. Inhibition of PG in the brain capillaries results in higher levels of the drugs in cerebral tissues.
- Cells that express PG also express CYP3A4.
- Administration of digoxin with quinidine results in doubling of the serum digoxin levels. Digoxin is a substrate for PG and quinidine is an inhibitor of PG.

Pharmacodynamics
- The effect of a drug represents a net effect of its action on different receptors and channels. For example β blocking effects of Sotalol occur at a lower dose than the QT prolonging effects. The direct effect of Ca channel blockers may be nullified by vasodilator-induced increased sympathetic tone, which increases the Ca current.
- Spontaneous and drug-induced I_{Kr} blocked results in prolongation of the QT interval and reactivation of the inward calcium channel, resulting in arrhythmias. The effect of I_{Kr} blocked is variable in different cells of the ventricle, resulting in dispersion of refractoriness.
- External factors can modulate the effect of a drug on target channels, for instance, a minor decrease in extracellular potassium can potentiate the I_{Kr} block and an increase in extracellular potassium reverses this effect.
- Catecholamine stimulation increases I_{Ks} and blunts the effects of I_{Ks} blockers.
- Expression of a target molecule may be modified in a disease.
- Aberrant responses to drug therapy may be due to mutation in target protein. For example, patients with drug associated long QT, in fact, may have mutation in gene expression which becomes manifest after drug challenge. These are aberrant responses to therapeutic drug levels due to mutation in target protein and are not due to high level or toxicity.

11.2 ANTIARRHYTHMIC DRUGS
Class 1A

- CLASS I antiarrhythmics are subdivided into
  - IA Prolongs conduction and repolarizatiom
  - IB No effect on conduction shortens repolarization
  - IC Prolongs conduction no effect on repolarization

Quinidine
- It binds to alpha1 acid glycoprotein.
- It is metabolized in the liver through oxidation by the cytochrome P450 system. Its active metabolite is 3-hydroxy-quinidine.
- 20% is excreted unchanged in the urine.
- It crosses the placenta and is excreted in breast milk.
- It blocks the sodium and potassium channels, thus affecting depolarization and repolarization. It produces greater depression of upstroke velocity in ischemic

tissue. It produces use dependent block of the Na channel during the activated state. This results in suppression of automaticity.

- It also blocks I_{K1} (inward rectifier), I_K (delayed rectifier), steady state sodium current, I_{Ca}, I_{Katp}, I_{to}, and I_{Kach}.
- Quinidine blocks alpha 1 and alpha 2 adrenergic receptors. Its vagolytic effect is produced by M2 receptor blocked.
- Prolongation of QRS duration is directly related to the plasma level of quinidine while QT interval is not. It may produce prominent U waves.
- Alpha blocking effect may cause orthostatic hypotension. It does not cause negative inotropy.
- Vagolytic effect may enhance atrio-ventricular node (AVN) conduction and may increase ventricular response in atrial fibrillation (AF)/Atrial Flutter.
- Side effects include diarrhea, loss of hearing tinnitus, blurred vision, thrombocytopenia, coombs positive hemolytic anemia, QRS widening, and ventricular arrhythmias, which may respond to sodium lactate or sodium bicarbonate infusion.
- Proarrhythmias include TDP, which is due to prolongation of the QT interval. The plasma level does not predict the occurrence of arrhythmia. Hypokalemia facilitates quinidine-induced early after depolarization (EAD) and arrhythmias. These arrhythmias are treated by IV infusion of magnesium and pacing.
- It is 50% effective in controlling AF. It blocks conduction in accessory pathways. It is not very effective in controlling ventricular arrhythmias.
- Oral dose is 300–600 mg every 6 hours.

Procainamide

- 60% is excreted by the kidney, 40% by the liver. Protein binding is weak.
- NAPA is an active metabolite.
- NAPA has a half life of 6 hours; 90% is excreted by the kidney.
- Procainamide therapeutic level is 4–12 μg/ml and for NAPA it is 9–20 μg/ml. Both are removed by hemodialysis.
- It crosses the placenta and is excreted in breast milk.
- Pharmacologic effects are similar to quinidine.
- Neuromuscular side effects may occur when given with amnioglycosides.
- It may cause hypotension when given IV. Other side effects include hemolytic anemia. Antinuclear antibodies may develop in 80% of the patients in the first 6 months of therapy. Lupus syndrome occurs in 30%. Antibodies to DNA do not occur commonly.
- Slow acetylators are more likely to develop lupus.
- It may cause TDP.
- It is useful in the treatment of AF in the presence of Wolf Parkinson white (WPW) syndrome.
- IV bolus administration should not exceed 50 mg/min and infusion rate of 1–6 mg/min. Oral dose is 3–6 gm/day.

Disopyramide

- It is metabolized by N-dealkylation to desisopropyldisopyramide, which is electrophysiologically active.
- It binds to AAG.
- 50% of the drug is excreted unchanged in urine.
- Plasma half life is 4–8 hours. Dose reduction is warranted in hepatic and renal failure.
- It passes through the placenta and is excreted in breast milk.
- It causes use dependent block of I_{Na}. It may also block I_K, I_{K1}, I_{Ca} and I_{to}.
- The time to recovery from the block is 700 milliseconds to 15 seconds.
- It prolongs the QT interval and may cause TDP.
- Its anticholinergic effects are due to block of M2 cardiac, M4 intestinal, and M3 exocrine gland muscarinic receptors.
- It produces a significant negative inotropic effect.
- Anticholinergic side effects include dry mouth, constipation, and urinary retention.
- Hypoglycemia may occur due to enhanced insulin secretion.
- It may cause cholestatic jaundice and agranulocytosis.
- It is effective in the treatment of atrial arrhythmias.
  It may also suppress digitalis-induced arrhythmias.
- It has been effectively used in the treatment of neurocardiogenic syncope and hypertrophic cardiomyopathy.
- The usual dosing is 100–150 mg every 6 hours or 200–300 mg every 12 hours of slow release preparation. The dose should be reduced in the presence of hepatic and renal insufficiency.

Class 1B

Lidocaine

- Lidocaine blocks I_{Na} by shifting voltage for inactivation to more negative. It binds to activated and inactivated state of the sodium channel.
- Lidocaine, Quinidine, and Flecainide exert use dependent block with fast intermediate and slow kinetics, respectively.
- Continuous activation of I_{Na} may cause an increase in action potential duration (APD) (LQT3). This current is blocked by Lidocaine and Mexiletine, which may result in correction of long QT interval.
- It is metabolized in the liver to glycinexylidide and monoethylglycinxylidide, which are less active than the parent compound.
- It binds to AAG, which is elevated in cute MI and CHF. This protein binding results in a decreased level of free unbound drug.
- Its clearance is equal to hepatic blood flow. A decrease in the blood flow due to propranolol or CHF will result in decreased clearance.
- The half life of rapid distribution is 8–10 minutes after IV bolus. EHL is 1–2 hours.

- In CHF because of a decrease in the volume of distribution and clearance the EHL remains unchanged.
- It crosses the placenta.
- Its antiarrhythmic effects are the result of sodium channel blocked in its inactivated state.
- Because of rapid binding and unbinding of the drug the conduction slowing occurs during rapid heart rates or in tissue with partially depolarized membrane such as in the presence of ischemia, hyperkalemia, and acidosis. In ischemic ventricular muscle cells lidocaine depresses excitability and conduction velocity.
- It suppresses normal and abnormal automaticity in Purkinje fibers. This may result in asystole in the presence of complete AV block.
- EAD and delayed after depolarization (DAD) are also suppressed.
- It does not alter hemodynamics.
- Central nervous system (CNS) side effects include perioral numbness, paresthesias, diplopia, slurred speech, and seizures. It does not cause proarrhythmias.
- In acute MI lidocaine reduces ventricular tachycardia (VT) ventricular fibrillation (VF) but does not alter mortality.
- Prophylactic use of lidocaine in post-acute MI showed an increase in the death rate in the treated group.
- The bolus dose is 1.5 mg/kg. The continuous IV infusion rate is 1–4 mg/minutes.
- Because of rapid distribution plasma levels fall in 8–10 minutes. Three additional boluses of half of the amount of the initial dose can be given every 10 minutes.
- The bolus and the infusion dose should be reduced in the presence of CHF and liver disease.
- Renal dysfunction does not affect dosing.

Mexiletine
- It is an oral congener of lidocaine. It is eliminated by the liver utilizing the P450 system.
- Side effects include tremor, blurred vision, dysarthria, ataxia, confusion, nausea, and thrombocytopenia.
- The usual oral dose is 150–200 mg every 8 hours.

Class 1C

Flecainide
- It is a fluorinated analogue of procainamide.
- It is metabolized in the liver to meta-*O*-dealkylated-flecainide.
- 30% is excreted by the kidneys.
- It is a potent sodium channel blocker. The time constant for recovery from the block is 21 seconds. It causes use dependent block.

- It also blocks I_K and slow inward calcium currents. It prolongs the atrial refractory period.
- It has a negative inotropic effect. Its use is not recommended in CHF. It may be useful in patients with diastolic dysfunction and arrhythmias.
- Its side effects include blurred vision, headache, ataxia, and CHF.
- Flecainide-induced proarrhythmias occur in patients with ischemic heart disease, VT, and/or left ventricular dysfunction.
- Because of use dependent block proarrhythmias may occur during exertion. An exercise test is recommended after achieving a steady state.
- Use of β blockers and hypertonic sodium bicarbonate has been successful in the treatment of proarrhythmias.
- It is useful in controlling paroxysmal AF.
- The initial dose is 100 mg every 12 hours and it could be increased to 200 mg every 12 hours. A single dose of 300 mg can be used for converting recent onset AF.
- QRS duration should be monitored and it should not be allowed to exceed more than 20% of the baseline interval.

Propafenone
- High first pass metabolism results in low bioavailability.
- It is metabolized in the liver to 5-hydroxypropafenone, which is an active metabolite.
- 5-Hydroxylation but not N-dealkylation uses cytochrome P450.
- N-dealkylation produces a weak metabolite N-dealkyl propafenone.
- 7% of the Caucasians are poor metabolizers. They have high levels of propafenone and low levels of 5-hydroxypropafenone.
- Hepatic dysfunction decreases clearance. In renal failure the propafenone level remains unchanged, however, 5-hydroxypropafenone levels double.
- Propafenone and its metabolites are excreted in milk.
- It is an effective Na channel blocker in a use dependent manner. It demonstrates slow binding unbinding.
- 5-hydroxy and N-dealkyl propafenone also blocks I_{Na}. However, 5-hydroxy compound is as potent as the parent drug.
- It is a weak I_K and I_{Ca} channel blocker.
- It is a nonselective β blocker. This effect is enhanced in slow metabolizers.
- It has a negative inotropic effect. Blood pressure may decrease.
- Side effects include nausea, metallic taste, dizziness, blurred vision, exacerbation of asthma, and abnormal liver function test.
- Proarrhythmias occur in 5% of the patients. Sodium lactate can be used to reverse arrhythmogenic effects. It may cause atrial flutter.
- QRS duration monitoring and exercise test is recommended.
- The initial dose is 150–300 mg every 8 hours. Dose adjustment may be necessary in hepatic and renal failure. A single dose of 600 mg can be used in patients with PAF.

11.3 BETA BLOCKERS

β Blockers as antiarrhythmic drugs

- β Blockers are most effective on tissues under intense stimulation by adrenergic agents.
- β Agonists enhance I_{CaL} and I_f current. This respectively increases inotropy and heart rate. Both these effects are negated by β blockers.
- β Blockers decrease the slope of phase 4 depolarization and decrease conduction velocity in sinoatrial node (SAN) and AVN.
- Prolongation of the AH interval and the AVN effective refractory period may cause Wenckebach block.
- Shortening of corrected QT (QT_c) in post-MI patients and increase in refractoriness in ischemic tissues by counteracting the arrhythmogenic effects of adrenergic agonists has been observed.
- β Blockers with ISA may not benefit post-MI patients.
- Most β blockers competitively block β1 receptors.
- In post-MI patients there may be loss of autonomic receptors and sympathetic denervation, which may result in supersensitivity to circulating catecholamines predisposing to heterogeneity of refractoriness and arrhythmias. β blockers may improve survival in post-MI patients.
- Some of the beneficial effects of the β blockers may be due to alleviation of ischemia.
- β Blockers increase survival in post-MI, LQTS patients. Reduction in mortality in post-MI patients appears to be due to reduction in the incidence of VF sudden death. This beneficial effect was observed irrespective of age, sex, race, and site of MI. It correlates positively with the degree of bradycardia produced. β Blockers should be given routinely to post-MI patients.
- β Blockers complement the antiarrhythmic effects of amiodarone.
- Patients with CHF tend to have elevated adrenergic activity. β Blockers significantly reduce total mortality in patients with heart failure of ischemic and nonischemic etiology.
- Carvedilol, Labetalol, and Bucindolol also have vasodilator activity (Table 11.2).
- β Blockers complement device therapy in survivors of cardiac arrest.
- Patients with LQTS who develop arrhythmias due to sympathetic activation respond to β blockers. Bradycardia and pause dependent Torsade does not respond to β blockers.
- In LQTS the mortality is 25% in the first 3 years after initial syncope and it is reduced to 6% after β blockade.
- ICD is the treatment of choice after syncope in patients with LQTS.
- Premature ventricular contractions (PVCs) and nonsustained VT in the setting of left ventricular dysfunction increase the incidence of arrhythmic deaths. Suppression of arrhythmias by antiarrhythmic drugs does not improve survival.

Table 11.2 Pharmacological properties of β blockers

Name	Plasma half life (hrs)	Site of clearance	Lipid solubility	ISA	β_1 blocked potency ratio
Non selective					
Propranolol	6	Liver	+++	None	1.0
Nadolol	20	Kidney	None	None	1.0
Sotalol	12	Kidney	None	None	0.3
Timolol	5	Liver and Kidney	None	None	6.0
β_1 Selective					
Acebutolol	10	Liver and Kidney	+	++	0.3
Atenolol	6	Kidney	None	None	1.0
Betaxolol	18	Liver and Kidney	None	None	1.0
Bisoprolol	10	Liver and Kidney	None	None	10.0
Metoprolol	6	Liver	None	None	1.0
Vasodilator α_1 nonselective					
Labetalol	6	Liver	None	++	0.3
Pindolol	4	Liver and Kidney	++	+++	6.0
Carvedilol	6	Liver	+	None	10.0
Vasodilator α_1 selective β_1					
Celiprolol	6	Kidney	None	$+\beta_2$	

- β Blockers improve survival by exerting anti-ischemic effects, reducing the effects of adrenergic stimulation, improving electrical homogeneity, and increasing heart rate variability.
- β Blockers may be effective in controlling catecholamine sensitive VT but they do not prevent the induction of ischemic VT.
- In patients who survived cardiac arrest and subsequently were found to have an ejection fraction of 45–47%, β blockers were as effective as amiodarone in reducing mortality.
- Exercise-induced VT and PVCs respond well to β blockers.
- β Blockers are effective in the treatment of narrow complex supraventricular tachycardia, inappropriate sinus tachycardia, rate control in atrial fibrillation, and prevention of post cardiac surgery AF. They should not be used in the presence of preexcitation.

11.4 CLASS III ANTIARRHYTHMIC DRUGS[1,2]

Class III antiarrhythmic drugs
- Balance between conduction velocity and refractoriness of the tissue determines the properties of the reentrant circuit.

- APD influences the refractory period. A short refractory period favors reentrant arrhythmias and a long refractory period abolishes reentry.
- Class III drugs prolong APD and increase the refractory period without affecting the conduction velocity (Table 11.5). They tend to prolong the QT interval and may cause torsades.
- An increase in inward currents (sodium and calcium currents) or a reduction in outward currents (potassium or chloride) during the plateau phase will increase APD.
- Class III agents prolong APD by inhibiting potassium current.
- Dofetilide and Sotalol are selective I_{Kr} blockers. Their actions are more prominent at a slow heart rate (reverse use dependence). This limits their efficacy and increases the tendency for induction of proarrhythmias.
- Amiodarone, Ambasilide, and Azimilide are nonselective potassium channel blockers.
- Class III agents delay cardiac repolarization and increase refractoriness. This will manifest as prolongation of the QT interval without affecting the PR or QRS duration. Increased refractoriness without slowing conduction makes these agents very effective in terminating reentrant arrhythmias.
- These agents tend to be less effective in terminating AF due to reverse use dependent effect.
- An adverse effect is prolongation of the QT interval and TDP. It is a dose-related effect likely to occur when drug elimination is impaired. Other factors such as hypokalemia, bradycardia, and female gender predispose to drug-induced acquired long QTS.
- Agents with I_{Kr} blocking properties mimic mutation of HERG that encodes I_{Kr} and causes congenital LQTS.
- Subclinical abnormality in the ion channel may be brought to the surface by APD prolonging agents.

Factors predisposing to TDP in the presence of Class III agents

Female gender
History of sustained ventricular arrhythmias LV hypertrophy and heart failure
Use of diuretics
Recent conversion from atrial fibrillation
↑ Sympathetic activity and calcium loading
Hypokalemia
Hypomagnesemia
High drug doses
Factors affecting metabolism and/or excretion, e.g., renal failure
Bradycardia
Short–long–short coupling interval
Prolong baseline QT_c interval or excessive on-treatment QT_c interval prolongation

Amiodarone

- It contains two iodine molecules. It is lipid soluble.
- It demonstrates antiarrhythmic actions of all four classes.
- It blocks I_{Na} in its inactivated state. This results in slowing of conduction and prolongation of the QRS duration in a rate-dependent fashion.
- It noncompetitively antagonizes adrenergic effects, which may be due to adrenergic receptor blocked, hypothyroidism, or Ca channel blocked.
  This results in a blunted heart rate response to adrenergic stimulation.
- It prolongs APD by blocking I_{Kr}, I_{Ks}, and I_{K1}. It inhibits thyroid hormone binding to the nuclear receptors, which results in I_{Ks} block.
- It blocks I_{Ca}, which accounts for its depressant effect on AVN.
- Ca-dependent effects of amiodarone appear early and effects on repolarization appear more slowly. This may be due to time-dependent accumulation of the metabolite desethylamiodarone (DEA).
- All electrocardiographic intervals are prolonged with chronic administration of the amiodarone. This is a reflection of its electrophysiologic effect across all four classes.
- In CASCAD trial amiodarone was found to be more effective than conventional antiarrhythmic drugs.
- In AVID trial ICD was found to be superior to amiodarone.
- Prophylactic administration of amiodarone in patients with CHF did not demonstrate a significant reduction in mortality. In post-MI patients, prophylactic administration of amiodarone resulted in a reduction of arrhythmic deaths but not in total mortality (Table 11.3).
- In ARREST trial administration of IV amiodarone in VF cardiac arrest patients resulted in an increase in successful resuscitation.
- It is 60% effective in maintaining sinus rhythm in patients with AF. Given 7 days prior to surgery it has been shown to be effective in preventing post cardiac surgery AF.
- Amiodarone is the drug of choice in patients with ventricular arrhythmias in whom ICD cannot be implanted. It is also effective in the treatment of AF.
- Because of its lipid solubility it accumulates in fatty tissues; consequently its volume of distribution is ~5000 liters.
- Its EHL is 50 days. It is metabolized in the liver to active metabolite DEA. Dose adjustments are not necessary in renal failure.
- The loading dose is 1–1.6 g/day, the maintenance dose is 200–300 mg/day. IV administration should be through the central line to avoid phlebitis. The IV infusion rate should not exceed 30 mg/min. Infusion should be prepared in glass containers because of the drug's tendency to absorb into polyvinyl chloride surfaces.
- 20–30% of the patients may discontinue the drug due to side effects.
- It causes bradycardia and hypotension, especially with IV infusion. It is less likely to cause TDP (0.3%) in spite of prolonging the QT interval.

Table 11.3 Prophylactic use of class III agents in the prevention of SCD

Trial	Drug	Inclusion criteria	Results
Post-MI class III primary prevention trials			
BASIS	Amiodarone vs placebo	Asymptomatic ventricular ectopy	Total mortality: amiodarone 5% placebo 13%
SWORD	D-Sotalol vs placebo	LVEF $\leq$ 0.40	Total mortality: sotalol 5.0%; placebo 3.1%
EMIAT	Amiodarone vs placebo	LVEF $\leq$ 0.40	Total mortality: amiodarone 13.9%; placebo 13.7%
CAMIAT	Amiodarone vs placebo	$\geq$10 PVCs/h or non-sustained VT	Total mortality: amiodarone 6.1%; placebo 8.4%
DIAMOND-MI	Dofetilide vs placebo	LVEF $\leq$0.35	Total mortality: dofetilide 30.7%; placebo 31.9%
ALIVE	Azimilide vs placebo	15% $\leq$ LVEF $\leq$ 35% plus low heart rate variability	Total mortality: azimilide 11.6%; placebo 11.6%
Post-CHF class III primary prevention trials			
GESICA	Amiodarone vs control	LVEF $\leq$ 0.35; NYHA class II–IV	Total mortality: amiodarone 33.5%; controls 41.4%
CHF-STAT	Amiodarone vs placebo	LVEF $\leq$ 0.40;NYHA class I–IV	Total mortality: amiodarone 30.6%; placebo 29.2%
DIAMOND-CHF	Dofetilide vs placebo	LVEF $\leq$ 0.35; NYHA class III–IV	Total mortality: dofetilide 41%; placebo 42%
CASCADE	Empiric amiodarone	Cardiac arrest or sustained VT	Combined endpoint of cardiac mortality, resuscitated VT or syncopal ICD discharge: amiodarone 47%; other drugs 60%
CASH	ICD vs empiric drug treatment (propafenone, amiodarone, or metoprolol)	Cardiac arrest with documented VT/VF	Total mortality ($p = 0.08$): ICD 36%; amiodarone or metoprolol 44%
AVID	ICD vs amiodarone or EP-guided antiarrhythmic treatment	Cardiac arrest; sustained VT + syncope; sustained VT + LVEF < 0.40	Total mortality: ICD 16%; drugs 24%

(Continued)

Table 11.3 (Continued)

Trial	Drug	Inclusion criteria	Results
CIDS	ICD vs amiodarone	Cardiac arrest; sustained VT + LVEF ≤ 0.35; syncope + sustained VT/inducible VT	Yearly mortality rate: ICD 8.3%; amiodarone 10.2%

ALIVE, Azimilide Post-Infarct Survival Evaluation; BASIS, Basel Antiarrhythmic Study of Infarct Survival; CAMIAT, Canadian Amiodarone Myocardial Infarction Arrhythmia Trial; CHF-STAT, Congestive Heart Failure: Survival Trial of Antiarrhythmic Therapy; DIAMOND-CHF, Danish Investigators of Arrhythmia and Mortality on Dofetilide in Congestive Heart Failure; DIAMOND-MI, Danish Investigators of Arrhythmia and Mortality on Dofetilide in Myocardial Infarction; EMIAT, European Myocardial Infarct Amiodarone Trial; GESICA, Grupo de Estudio de la Sobrevida en la Insuficiencia Cardiaca en Argentina; SWORD, Survival with Oral D-Sotalol; AVID, Antiarrhythmics Versus Implantable Defibrillators; CASCADE, Cardiac Arrest in Seattle: Conventional versus Amiodarone Drug Evaluation; CASH, Cardiac Arrest Study Hamburg; CIDS, Canadian Implantable Defibrillator Study.

- Other side effects include interstitial pneumonitis and pulmonary fibrosis.
- Neurologic side effects include anxiety, tremor, headache, myoclonic jerks, and neuropathy. It may also cause corneal micro deposits, ophthalmic neuritis, photophobia, nausea abnormal liver function test, photosensitivity, and bluish-gray discoloration of the sun-exposed parts of the skin.
- Amiodarone may cause hypo or hyperthyroidism. It affects thyroid production, peripheral deiodenation to triiodothyronine, entry of the hormone to the tissue, and triiodothyronine binding to nuclear receptors.
- Amiodarone may interact with digoxin, quinidine, warfarin, procainamide, and phenytoin.

Bretylium

- It prolongs APD and refractory period without affecting conduction velocity.
- It causes initial release of norepinephrine followed by inhibition of release and uptake from the sympathetic nerve terminal. This may result in initial aggravation of arrhythmia and hypertension followed by hypotension.
- It increases the VF threshold. It is available for intravenous infusion for refractory ventricular tachyarrhythmias at a dose of 5–10 mg/kg bolus administered slowly.
- It is excreted unchanged in the urine. Its half life is 10 hours.
- Adverse effects include hypotension, nausea, vomiting, and parotid pain.

Ibutilide

- It is a methanesulfonamide derivative. It is a potent I_{Kr} blocker. It is effective in termination of AF (30% efficacy) and atrial flutter (60% efficacy). It prolongs QT QT_c intervals.
- It is administered as 1 mg infusion over a period of 10 minute followed by 0.5–1 mg if necessary. It is eliminated by the liver. Its EHL is 6 hours.
- Adverse effects include QT prolongation and polymorphic ventricular tachycardia in 8% of the patients. The patient should be monitored for ventricular arrhythmias 4–6 hours after administration of Ibutilide.
- Presence of CHF, female gender, bradycardia, and hypokalemia are associated with increased risk of TDP.

Sotalol

- d and l Isomers have class III and β blocking activity.
- It is a competitive nonselective β blocker without intrinsic sympathomimetic activity. Its β blocking activity resides in L isomer. Both isomers are I_{Kr} blockers. This action confers class III properties to Sotalol. D Isomer prolongs APD and it is a pure class III compound. At a lower dose of 80 mg/day it produces β blocking effect with little class III effect. At higher doses of greater than 160 mg/day class III effects become prominent.
- It causes bradycardia, prolongs AH and PR intervals, and increases atrial ventricular and AV nodal refractory periods. It does not affect QRS duration and HV interval.
- It produces reverse use dependent effects on atrial and ventricular repolarization. This limits its efficacy in terminating AF.
- D-Sotalol worsens mortality in post-MI patients with left ventricle (LV) dysfunction.
- It is eliminated unchanged in the urine. The dose should be reduced in the presence of renal dysfunction but not if liver disease is present.
- Plasma half life is 15 hours. The dose is from 40 to 460 mg/day. Larger doses are likely to produce TDP.
- Adverse effects include AV block, TDP, LV dysfunction, sinus node dysfunction, and bronchospasm. The incidence of TDP varies from 3 to 7% depending on the dose and associated factors such as hypokalemia and renal failure.

Dofetilide

- It is a methanesulfonamide compound.
- It selectively blocks I_{Kr} current. It prolongs the QT interval. There is a close relation between plasma level of dofetilide and the QT interval.
- It has no effect on conduction interval or cycle length. It lengthens the effective refractory period of the atrium, ventricle, and AP.
- It is eliminated by hepatic and renal clearance. Its EHL is 8 hours.

- It is metabolized by CYP3A4 and is thus likely to interact with drugs using the cytochrome P450 such as erythromycin and ketoconazole, resulting in a higher concentration of dofetilide.
- It is more effective in terminating atrial flutter than AF.
- It is administered orally at a dose of 500 μg twice daily.
- In Diamond study there was no adverse effect on mortality in patients with CHF and post-MI who received dofetilide.
- Incidence of Torsade is 3–5%.

Azimilide

- It blocks both I_{Kr} and I_{Ks} currents.
- It prolongs the refractory period and increases APD, and the QT interval.
- It does not affect conduction or hemodynamics.
- Its therapeutic effects are rate independent and are maintained during ischemia and hypoxia.
- It is 90% bound to plasma proteins. It can be administered once daily. Dose adjustments may not be required for age, gender, hepatic, or renal function.
- It is administered orally as 100 mg/day.
- Alive trial included post-MI patients with low ejection fraction who were at high risk of sudden death.

11.5 CALCIUM CHANNEL BLOCKERS

Calcium channel blockers

- Six classes of calcium channels have been identified; only L and T types are found in the heart.
- Dihydropyridines do not affect AVN conduction. Their depressant effects are overridden by reflex action from vasodilatation (Table 11.4).
- In spite of anti-ischemic anti-hypertensive properties, there is no effect on mortality in post-MI patients.
- Calcium channel blockers increase the refractory period and slow AVN conduction velocity by slowing phase 4-depolarization in SAN and AVN. This property may be useful in controlling the heart rate during AF.
- Bepridil blocks the fast sodium channel and prolongs repolarization.
- Ca channel blockers may be beneficial for coronary spasm inducted ventricular arrhythmias and may also be effective in exercise-induced idiopathic LV VT. There is no effect on ischemic VT.
- There is marked prolongation of the QT_c interval in hypothyroidism, chronic amiodarone therapy, and hypocalcemia, yet Torsade is rare perhaps due to depressed I_{Ca} activity.
- Ca channel blockers are effective in the treatment of SVT, where one of the limbs of the reentrant circuit is AVN. Verapamil at a dose of 7.5 mg IV was effective

Table 11.4 Hemodynamic and electrophysiologic effects of calcium antagonists

	Nifedipine*	Diltiazem	Verapamil
Coronary dilation	++	++	+
Peripheral dilation	++++	++	+++
Negative inotropic	+	++	+++
AV conduction↓	↔	+++	++++
Heart rate	↑↔	↓↔	↓↔
Blood pressure↓	++++	++	+++
Sinus node depression	↔	++	++
Cardiac output↑	++	↔	↔

+, minimal effect; ++++, maximal effect; ↔, no significant change; ↑, increase; ↓, decrease.

in terminating 90% of the AVN dependent SVT. Reinitiation is less likely with verapamil.

- The use of Ca channel blockers should be avoided in the presence of preexcitation.

11.6 ADENOSINE

Adenosine

- Adenosine is produced in the heart by two different pathways:
  - i Adenosine monophosphate (AMP) can undergo dephosphorylation by enzyme 5-nucleotidase to adenosine. Reverse reaction is mediated by adenosine kinase.
  - ii Reversible conversion of S-adenosylhomocysteine to adenosine by enzyme S-adenosylhomocysteine hydrolase.
- Metabolism of the adenosine occurs by deamination to inosine.
- Myocardial ischemia or hypoxia increases the production of adenosine using both pathways.
- Adenosine receptors have been classified into A1, A2A, A2B, and A3.
- A1 receptors are responsible for electrophysiologic and inotropic effects on the heart.
- Adenosine acts on the A1 receptor via guanine nucleotide binding protein complex.
- The direct effect of A1 stimulation is enhancement of $I_{K\text{-}Ado}$ outward potassium current.
- $I_{K\text{-}Ado}$ is present in the atrium, SA and AVN but not in ventricular myocytes.
- Activation of $I_{K\text{-}Ado}$ results in shortening of atrial APD, hyperpolarization of membrane, and prolongation of APD in AVN.
- Other direct effects include inhibition of I_f in SA and AV node and inhibition of I_{Ca}.

- The indirect effect of adenosine is produced by a decrease in intracellular cAMP due to inhibition of adenylyl cyclase. Additional indirect effects include inhibition of catecholamine stimulated I_{Ca}.
- Adenosine suppresses catecholamine stimulated DAD and EAD.
- Adenosine and acetylcholine produce a similar G protein mediated effect on the heart but through different receptors. Acetylcholine effects are mediated by the M2 receptor.
- Methylxanthines block the A1 receptor and nullify the effects of adenosine. Increased activity of adenosine deminase will also decrease the effectiveness of adenosine.
- Dipyridamole enhances the effects of adenosine by blocking its reuptake.
- AV block in inferior MI may be adenosine mediated and could be reversed by aminophylline.
- Adenosine prolongs the AH interval. It has no effect on the HV interval. It slows or blocks antegrade conduction over slow and fast pathways.
- Adenosine has minor effects on junctional and ventricular escape pacemaker.
- In the atrium it shortens effective refractory period (ERP) and may induce AF.
- It does not affect conduction over accessory pathways. Preexcitation becomes prominent due to delay in AV conduction.
- Slowly conducting accessory pathways may respond to adenosine.
- Continuous infusion causes sinus tachycardia and lowers diastolic pressure.
- Sinus tachycardia is mediated by adrenergic reflex by activation of aortic arch chemoreceptors. Pulmonary and systemic vascular resistance decreases.

Pharmacology

- Once injected it is rapidly cleared by cellular uptake and enzyme metabolism. Its half life is 0.5–5 seconds.
- Site and speed of injection and circulation time determine the response to bolus injection.
- It is effective in termination of SVT by inducing a block at the AVN. If ATP is used it degrades to adenosine before being effective.
- Adenosine produces atrial and ventricular extra systole.
- Its effect occurs within 15–30 seconds after injection.
- Adenosine does not accumulate between injections. A 12 mg dose is effective in terminating 90% of the AVN dependent SVT. Following a bolus injection frequent PACs, PVCs, AF, and reinitiation of tachycardia may occur.
- It is also effective in the pediatric age group at a dose of 37.5–300 μg/kg.
- Verapamil could be used when adenosine is contraindicated in patients with bronchial asthma.
- Adenosine is preferable in patients with LV dysfunction, who recently received β blockers, in neonates and in patients where electrocardiographic diagnosis is uncertain.
- Adverse effects from adenosine infusion include flushing, dyspnea, and chest pain.

- Chest pain is not prevented by acetylcholine or β blockers. It is aggravated by dipyridamole. It is relieved by theophylline. These observations suggest that the chest pain is due to the direct effect of adenosine on adenosine receptors.
- Adenosine increases the respiratory drive by chemoreceptor activation.
- Flushing is due to vasodilatation mediated by an increase in sympathetic activity.

Proarrhythmias
- Frequent PAC, PVC, sinus bradycardia, sinus arrest, AF, or AV block may occur.
- Bradycardia dependent polymorphic VT may occur especially in LQTS.
- It may cause AF by shortening the atrial refractory period. In patients with WPW syndrome this could be potentially dangerous.
- Acceleration of tachycardia may occur due to an increase in adrenergic tone.
- It may facilitate the induction of AVNRT.
- Adenosine has no direct effect on ventricular myocardium.
- Exercise-induced ventricular tachycardia, in structurally normal hearts with right bundle branch block and inferior axis QRS morphology, which are induced by isoproterenol and terminated by Verapamil and Vagal maneuver are mediated by catecholamine-induced cAMP-dependent triggered activity.
  These arrhythmias can be terminated by adenosine.
- Adenosine inhibits catecholamine-stimulated calcium current. It inhibits isoproterenol-induced EAD and DAD.
- It does not inhibit Quinidine-induced EAD or Ouabain-induced DAD.
- Adenosine is useful in the differential diagnosis of wide complex tachycardia.
- Infusion may help in the diagnosis of Sick Sinus Syndrome and during tilt test.

11.7 DIGOXIN

Digoxin
- It is a combination of aglycon, related to sterols, and sugar molecules attached to a lactone ring. Pharmacologic actions are mediated by aglycon.
- At high blood levels digoxin increases intracellular calcium and causes DAD.
- Digoxin inhibits NA/K ATPases. It increases intracellular calcium concentration by inhibiting sodium/calcium exchange. These actions contribute to a positive inotropic effect.

Pharmacologic effects (Table 11.5)
- The pharmacologic effects of digoxin result from an increase in vagal tone. It slows AVN conduction and increases the refractory period.
- In the atrium it shortens the refractory period and increases the conduction velocity due to the increase in vagal tone.
- At the toxic level automaticity is increased.

Table 11.5 Summary electrophysiologic properties of the antiarrhythmic drugs

Drug	APD	ERP	VFT	Contractility	Autonomic effects
Quinidine	↑	↑	↑	0	Vagolytic; alpha blocker
Procainamide	↑	↑	↑	0	Vagolytic
Disopyramide	↑	↑	↑	↓	Central: Vagolytic, Sympatholytic
Lidocaine	↓	↓	↑	0	0
Mexiletine	↓	↓	↑	↓	0
Phenytoin	↓	↓			0
Flecainide	0 ↑	↑		↓	0
Propafenone	0 ↑	↑	↑	↓	Sympatholytic
Moricizine	↓	↓	0		0
Propranolol	0 ↓	↓		↓	β Blocked
Amiodarone	↑	↑	↑	0 ↑	Sympatholytic
Bretylium	↑	↑	0 ↑	↓	Sympatholytic
Sotalol	↑	↑	0	↓	β Blocked
Ibutilide	↑	↑		0	0
Dofetilide	↑	↑		0	0
Azimilide	↑	↑		0	0
Verapamil	↓	0	0	↓	0
Adenosine	↑	↑	0	0	Vagomimetic

APD, action potential duration; ERP, effective refractory period; VFT, ventricular fibrillation threshold.

- Digoxin shortens the refractory period of accessory pathways; therefore, its use in preexcitation is not advisable.
- It may cause ST and T changes.

Pharmacokinetics
- After an oral dose 60–80% is absorbed.
- Eubacterium lentum in the intestine metabolizes digoxin to inactive dihydrodigoxin. Use of antibiotic may change the bacterial flora and make more digoxin available.
- Cholestyramine, colestipol, antacids, kaolin, and sucralfate decrease digoxin absorption.
- It takes 6–12 hours after an oral dose to achieve adequate serum concentration.
- It is excreted by the kidneys. Its half life is 30 hours. Its desired therapeutic level is between 0.8 and 2 mg/ml.
- Quinidine displaces digoxin from the binding site and reduces renal excretion.
- Amiodarone, Propafenone, and Verapamil decrease renal and nonrenal clearance.
- Cyclosporine and Benzodiazepine raise the serum digoxin level.

Clinical uses

- Digoxin is used for rate control during atrial arrhythmias, however, increased sympathetic tone nullifies this effect.
- Digoxin alone may be effective in controlling the rate in sedentary patients.
- Calcium channel blockers and β blockers provide more efficient rate control.
- There could be marked fluctuations in the heart rate in a 24-hour period. Pauses of 2.8 seconds during the day and 4 seconds during sleep could be considered normal.
- Digoxin could be added if left ventricular dysfunction is present.
- Magnesium deficiency reduces the effectiveness of digoxin.

Toxicity

- In the presence of sick sinus syndrome, digoxin causes bradycardia and exit blocks.
- Electrolyte abnormality, renal failure, thyroid disease, and hypoxia increase the risk of digoxin toxicity.
- Digoxin toxicity is manifested by anorexia, headaches, hyperkalemia, and visual changes.
- Cardiac toxicity of digoxin includes bradycardia, DAD due to calcium overload, AV block, and bidirectional VT.
- Digoxin may inhibit sodium/potassium exchange, resulting in hyperkalemia.
- Treatment of digoxin toxicity includes discontinuation of digoxin, correction of hypokalemia and hypomagnesemia.
- Lidocaine and phenytoin have been used in controlling digoxin-induced ventricular arrhythmias.
- Cardioversion during high digoxin levels may result in VF.
- In the presence of hyperkalemia avoid calcium administration. It may potentiate calcium overload and arrhythmia.
- Digoxin specific Fab antibodies should be used to reverse severe digoxin toxicity.
- It binds to digoxin and is excreted in the urine. In the presence of renal failure this complex may not be excreted.
- A dose of Fab antibodies can be calculated by

(digoxin level $\times$ body weight in Kg)/100.

Antiarrhythmic drugs and pregnancy

- Maternal and fetal arrhythmias occurring during pregnancy may jeopardize the life of the mother and the fetus.
- Well-tolerated minimally symptomatic arrhythmias should be treated conservatively by observation, rest, or vagal maneuvers.
- Arrhythmias causing debilitating symptoms or hemodynamic compromise can be treated with antiarrhythmic drugs.

Table 11.6 Definitions of US Food and Drug Administration (FDA) classifications (use in pregnancy ratings)

Category A: No risk to pregnant women or fetus.
Category B: No evidence of risk in humans. Animal studies show risk, but human.
studies do not; **or**, if no adequate human studies have been done, animal findings are negative.
Category C: Risk cannot be ruled out. Human studies are lacking, and animal studies are either positive for fetal risk, or are lacking as well.
Category D: Positive evidence of risk. Investigational or post-marketing data show risk to the fetus.
Category X: Contraindicated in pregnancy.

- Although no antiarrhythmic drug is completely safe during pregnancy, most are well tolerated and can be given with relatively low risk (using FDA labeling guidelines) (Table 11.6).
- Drug therapy should be avoided, if possible, during the first trimester of pregnancy, and drugs with the longest and strongest safety record should be used first (Table 11.7).
- Quinidine has the longest record of safety during pregnancy and is generally well tolerated. Procainamide is also well tolerated and can be used for acute treatment of undiagnosed wide complex tachycardia.
- All IA agents should be administered in the hospital under cardiac monitoring due to the potential risk of ventricular arrhythmias (TDP).
- Lidocaine is well tolerated as an antiarrhythmic agent.
- Phenytoin should be avoided.
- Flecainide has been shown to be very effective in treating fetal supraventricular tachycardia complicated by hydrops.
- β Blockers are well tolerated and can be used. They may cause intrauterine growth retardation if administered during the first trimester.
- Amiodarone should be avoided during the first trimester and used only to treat life-threatening arrhythmias.
- Adenosine is the drug of choice for acute termination of maternal supraventricular tachycardia.
- Digoxin can be safely used during pregnancy.
- Direct current cardioversion to terminate maternal arrhythmias is well tolerated and effective, and should not be delayed if indicated.
- The use of an implantable cardioverter-defibrillator should be considered for women of childbearing potential with life-threatening ventricular arrhythmias.

Table 11.7 FDA class and pharmacodynamics of antiarrhythmic drugs

Drug	FDA class	Placental transfer	Excretion through breast milk	Adverse effects	Teratogenic	Injury to the fetus
Quinidine	C	Yes	Yes	Thrombocytopenia, rarely oxytocic	No	Minor
Procainamide	C	Yes	Yes	Fetal AV block, Lupus	No	Minor
Disopyramide	C	Yes	Yes	Uterine contraction	No	Minor
Lidocaine	B	Yes	Yes	Bradycardia, CNS adverse effects	No	Minor
Mexiletine	C	Yes	Yes	Bradycardia; low birth weight, low APGAR, low blood sugar	No	Minor
Phenytoin	D	Yes	Yes	Mental and growth retardation, fetal hydantoin syndrome	Yes	Significant
Flecainide	C	Yes	Yes	Rare	None	Minor
Propafenone	C	Yes	Unknown	Rare	No	Minor
Propranolol	C	Yes	Yes	Growth retardation, bradycardia, apnea hypoglycemia	No	Minor
Atenolol	C	Yes	Yes	Low birthweight	No	Minor
Sotalol	B	Yes	Yes	β Blocker effects, Torsade de pointes	No	Minor
Amiodarone	D	Yes	Yes	Hypothyroidism, growth retardation, premature birth, large fontanelle	Yes	Significant
Bretylium	C	Unknown	Unknown	Hypotension	Unknown	Unknown
Ibutilide	C	Unknown	Unknown	TDP	Unknown	Unknown
Verapamil	C	Yes	Yes	Bradycardia, AV block, hypotension	No	Unknown
Digoxin	C	Yes	Yes	Low birthweight	No	Minor
Adenosine	C	No	Unknown	None	No	Minor
Diltiazem	C	No	Yes	Bradycardia hypotension	Unknown	Moderate

References

1 Brendorp B. Pedersen OD. Torp-Pedersen C. Sahebzadah N. A Benefit-Risk Assessment of Class III Antiarrhythmic Agents. *Drug Safety*. 25(12):847–865, 2002.

2 Dorian P. Mechanisms of action of class III agents and their clinical relevance. *Europace*. 1(Suppl. C):C6–9, 2000.

12 Electrical Therapy for Cardiac Arrhythmias

Self-Assessment Questions

1 What is the likely cause of the absence of ventricular pacing at longer AV interval?

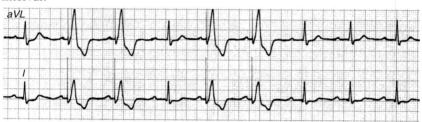

  A Lack of ventricular sensing
  B Inappropriate AVI programming
  C Lack of atrial sensing
  D Loss of pacemaker output

2 What is the correct interpretation of the following ECG tracing?

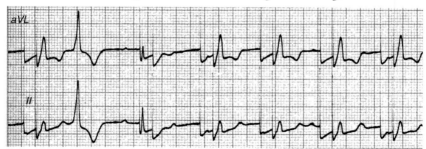

  A Pacemaker is functioning in asynchronous mode
  B Pacemaker is functioning normally in DDD mode
  C Pacemaker is functioning normally in VDD mode
  D Pacemaker is functioning normally in DVI mode

3 An ICD was implanted in a 57 year old male 4 years ago for ischemic cardiomyopathy. He was recently seen in the clinic because he had received 2 ICD shocks
in last 24 hours. Intracardiac electrograms from that episode are shown.

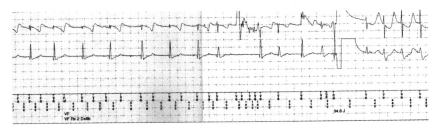

What will be your recommendations?
A A. Reprogram sensitivity to avoid T wave sensing
B B. Replace high voltage lead
C C. Replace pace sense lead
D D. Initiate amiodarone

4 A 54-year-old man is brought to the hospital after he lost consciousness while
walking near his home. Cardiac catheterization reveals normal coronary arteries
and left ventricular ejection fraction of 30%. Fifteen beat nonsustained ventricular tachycardia associated with palpitations was noted on telemetry monitor.
A dual chamber ICD was implanted. One day later following recording was
obtained.

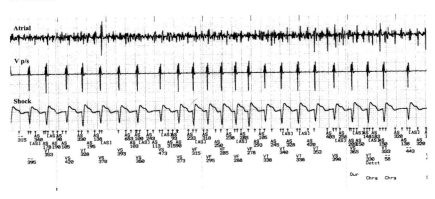

Which of the following is the most appropriate therapeutic maneuver?
A Replace atrial lead
B Reprogram the ICD to perform antitachycardia pacing prior to delivering a
shock
C Begin treatment with flecainide
D Begin treatment with sotalol

12.1 CARDIOVERSION DEFIBRILLATION

- The success of defibrillation depends on the waveform and the electrode characteristics.
- The waveform characteristics include – shape, duration, tilt, and number of phases.
- The electrode characteristics include – number, location, size, and material.

Shape of the waveform

- Damped sinusoidal (used for external defibrillators requires a large inductor).
- Straight capacitor discharge.
- Truncated capacitor discharge (used for internal defibrillators).

Waveform duration

- Rheobase is defined as the minimal amount of electrical energy that is required to produce a physiologic response; any stimulus of lower strength will not produce a response even if it is maintained for a long duration.
- Chronaxie is defined as the smallest amount of time that is required to produce stimulation (pulse width) when the electrical energy is maintained at twice the threshold.
- Monophasic waveform requires a larger current at a shorter duration. In biphasic waveform the duration of the second phase could be the same as the first phase or longer.

Waveform tilt

- It is defined as the percentage difference in the leading edge and trailing edge voltage of the waveform.
- A square waveform occurs with large capacitors, high resistance, or short duration of the pulse and tends to have a small tilt.
- In a defibrillation system with a fixed tilt the duration of the waveform changes with impedance.
- In a system with a fixed duration of the waveform the tilt is determined by impedance.
- Commonly, 50–65% tilt is used.

Waveform polarity

- Defibrillation thresholds (DFTs) are lower when the right ventricular electrode is an anode for a monophonic waveform of greater than 2 milliseconds in duration and for a biphasic waveform when the second phase is longer than the first phase.

Number of phases

- A biphasic waveform requires less energy to defibrillate. Which of the two phases results in defibrillation is unknown. One possibility is that the first phase results in defibrillation and the second phase removes the residual current from the cell membrane. This phenomenon is called burping of the cell membrane.

- The second possibility is that the first phase preconditions the cell membrane by activating Na channels and the second phase depolarizes the cell membrane.
- The amplitude of the second phase is more important than the duration of this phase.
- A defibrillating electric shock produces an electrical potential gradient throughout the heart. It tends to be greatest near the defibrillating electrode.
- For a successful defibrillation the minimal potential gradient has to be achieved throughout the heart.
- Subthreshold shocks produce multiple areas of activation and result in unsuccessful defibrillation.
- Stronger shocks produce more effective defibrillation.
- A biphasic waveform is superior to a monophasic waveform because it eliminates the conditions necessary for reentry.

Action potential
- When a shock is delivered to a cell that has recovered from previous depolarization it generates a new response. If the cell is refractory, when the shock is delivered, no response is elicited.
- A strong electric shock may depolarize partially refractory cells and produce extension of refractoriness.
- Cathodal stimuli depolarize tissue whereas an anodal stimulus hyperpolarizes the tissue.
- Myocardial discontinuities and anisotropic conduction may affect the depolarization of the tissue from the shock.

Detrimental effects of the shock
- High potential gradients created by shock may cause bradycardia, atrioventricular (AV) block, and ventricular fibrillation (VF).
- Potential gradients exceeding 100 V/cm can cause tissue necrosis.
- At transmembrane potential of greater than 200 mV, pores form in the cell membrane. This is called electroporation and results in ion leak and arrhythmias.

Defibrillation cardioversion
- The unit of energy for cardioversion defibrillation is joules or watts/seconds.
- The amount of energy selection depends on the type of arrhythmia being treated.
- The synchronized shock of 50 J may be sufficient for atrial flutter, 100–150 J for atrial fibrillation (AF) and ventricular tachycardia (VT). For VF 200–300 J of unsynchronized energy is delivered. For a pediatric age group the dose is 1 J per pound.
- The success of cardioversion and maintenance of sinus rhythm depends on the duration of arrhythmia and left atrium (LA) size.
- Prior to cardioversion for AF or atrial flutter the patient should be anticoagulated for three to four weeks maintaining the INR between 2 and 3 or a negative TEE.
- The flow of transthoracic current depends on the electrode position. The anteroposterior or apex to right infrascapular position provides satisfactory results.

- Only 4% of the current flows through the myocardium.
- The size of the electrodes determines the transthoracic impedance and current flow. For adults the size of the electrodes should be between 8 and 12 cm in diameter. The contact area should be at least 50 cm^2/electrode or 150 cm^2 for both electrodes.
- Two electrodes must remain apart without any water or gel between them to avoid short circuiting of the current.
- Current flow is influenced by the amount of energy and transthoracic impedance.
- Impedance depends on interelectrode distance (chest size), electrode size, electrode chest wall contact, couplant, and respiratory phase.
- Impedance decreases after repeat shock perhaps due to tissue hyperemia.
- The average transthoracic impedance in an adult is 75 Ω.
- The minimum current necessary to defibrillate is constant but the amount of energy required to achieve that current varies with impedance.
- Transthoracic impedance can be determined prior to shock by passing a low level of current between the electrodes. If impedance is determined to be high then a higher energy level or a longer pulse width should be used.
- Current-based defibrillation is independent of transthoracic impedance.
- Current and shock success relationship is parabolic. The highest success occurs with 30–40 A for defibrillation and 15–25 A for cardioversion. Lower current strengths were ineffective and higher currents produced toxicity.
- The biphasic waveform is superior and requires less energy for cardioversion defibrillation.
- Early defibrillation using external automated defibrillators in public places may improve survival after cardiac arrest.

12.2 PACEMAKERS

Permanent pacemakers[1,2]

NBG Code (developed by North American and British electrophysiology groups) for Pacemaker function designation (Table 12.1):

Table 12.1 NBG pacemaker function designation code

Chamber paced	Chamber sensed	Effect of sensing	Rate modulation	Multi-site pacing
0 = none	0 = none	0 = none	0 = none	0 = none
A = atrium	A = atrium	T = triggered	R = rate modulation	A = atrium
V = ventricle	V = ventricle	I = inhibited		V = ventricle
D = dual	D = dual	D = dual		D = any combination

Table 12.2 Guidelines for pacing indications

Class I	Class IIA	Class IIB	Class III

1 Third-degree AV block at any anatomic level
2 Symptomatic second degree AV block at any site
3 Chronic BFB with
  a Intermittent AV block
  b Type II AV block
4 Symptomatic SND
5 Syncope due to HCS
	1 Asymptomatic third-degree AV block
	2 Type II AVB narrow QRS
	3 Type I intra or infra His AVB
	4 Chronic BFB with
	  a Syncope (VT excluded)
	  b HV >100 milliseconds
	  c Infra His AV block not physiologic
	5 SND and HR <40
	6 Syncope and EP documented SND and abnormal AV conduction
	7 Cardio-inhibitory NCS symptomatic and recurrent
		1 Prolong PR interval >300 milliseconds
		2 Neuromuscular diseases with any degree of AV block with or without symptoms
		3 HR <40 awake
		4 IHSS with gradient
			1 Prolong PR
			2 Asymptomatic type I AVB
			3 Transient AVB due to correctable cause
			4 FB without AVB
			5 Asymptomatic SND, HCS
			6 Transient post op AV block

ACC AHA HRS guidelines for pacing indications (Table 12.2)

Class I = generally indicated.

Class IIA = possibly indicated but limited published data.

Class IIB = possibly indicated disagreement exists.

Class III = not indicated.

- Pacemaker syndrome may occur with any pacing mode if AV dissociation occurs.
- Symptoms include dyspnea, dizziness, fatigue, cough, pulsation in the neck and apprehension.
- If the AV conduction remains intact up to the heart rate of 120–140 beats per minute (bpm) then the incidence of AV block is less than 2%.

Factors influencing pacing mode selection

Underlying rhythm
Exercise capacity
Chronotropic response
Associated medical problems

Pacemaker timing cycle (Fig. 12.1)

- If the timing circuit is not reset it will result in the release of stimulus at its completion.
- Output is inhibited by sensed ventricular/atrial event.
- The refractory period is initiated after a sensed or paced atrial (ARP)/ventricular (VRP) event.
- Any event occurring during the refractory period is not sensed and does not reset the timing cycle.
- A blanking period is initiated during and immediately after the pacemaker stimulus is released and during which the opposite channel of the dual chamber pacemaker is blinded.
- With ventricular-based timing, the AEI is fixed. A ventricular sensed event occurring during the AEI resets this timer.
- In an atrial-based timing system the AA interval is fixed. A ventricular sensed event during the AEI will reset the AA interval as opposed to the AEI in a V-based timing system.
- The timing cycle in DDD consists of a lower rate (LR) limit, an atrioventricular interval (AVI), a post-ventricular atrial refractory period (PVARP), and an upper rate limit. The AVI and PVARP together constitute the total atrial refractory period (TARP). If intrinsic atrial and ventricular activity occurs before the LR times out, both channels are inhibited and no pacing occurs. If no intrinsic atrial or ventricular activity occurs, there is AV sequential pacing (complexes 1 and 2). If no atrial activity is sensed before the ventriculoatrial (VA) interval is completed, an atrial pacing artifact is delivered, which initiates the AVI. If intrinsic ventricular activity occurs before the termination of the AVI, the ventricular output from the pacemaker is inhibited, that is, atrial pacing (complex 4). If a P wave is sensed before the VA interval is completed, output from the atrial channel is inhibited. The AVI is initiated, and if no ventricular activity is sensed before the

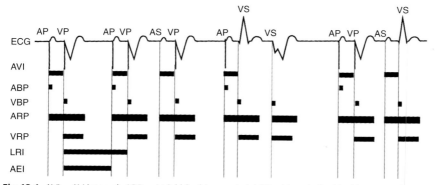

Fig 12.1 AVI = AV interval. ABP = Atrial blanking period. VBP = Ventricular blanking period. ARP = Atrial refractory period (includes AVI and PVARP). VRP = Ventricular refractory period. LRI = lower rate interval. AEI = Atrial escape interval.

Table 12.3 Pacing modes and indications

Mode of pacing	Indications	Pitfalls
VVI/VVIR	Chronic AF slow rate	Pacemaker syndrome if SR
AAI/AAIR	SSS bradycardia normal AV conduction	Ineffective if AV block develops. Does not recognize/respond to ventricular events. Far field sensing from ventricle may inhibit A pacing
DDI	A and V sensing no competitive A pacing. Inhibited, no P wave tracking V pace rate will not exceed the programmed base pacing rate. Useful for mode switches	Acts as VVI during high atrial rates
DVI	SSS bradycardia. Like atrial based pacemaker that responds to ventricular events	Competitive atrial pacing whenever V pacing is required
VDD	P tracking (Triggered), responds to ventricular events (Inhibition). Normal SA node and AVN disease. Single lead pacing system	Unable to pace in atrium if SAN dysfunction occurs. Acts as VVI in the absence of sensed atrial activity. May track Atrial signal in SVT
DDD	Normal sinus function and AV block	May track atrial signal during SVT

SR, sinus rhythm; SSS, sick sinus syndrome.

AVI terminates, a ventricular pacing artifact is delivered, that is, P-synchronous pacing (complex 3).

- In rate adaptive pacing AAIR/VVIR mode paced rate may vary and may reach the programmed upper limit for the sensor.
- Tracking rate refers to when the pacemaker is tracking the intrinsic atrial activity. MSR refers to the maximum rate allowed under sensor control.
- In patients with sinus node dysfunction, but normal AV conduction, as demonstrated by $1:1$ AV node (AVN) conduction to rates of 120–140 bpm, the occurrence of clinically significant AVN disease is $<2\%$ per year.
- Non P wave synchronous AV sequential pacing with dual chamber sensing (DDI) is like DDD pacing without atrial tracking. The DDI pacing mode could be considered for patients with intermittent atrial tachyarrhythmias (Table 12.3).
- In the VDD mode a sensed atrial signal initiates AVI. If intrinsic QRS occurs before the end of the AVI the ventricular output is inhibited and the lower rate timer (LRT) is reset. If a paced beat occurs at the end of AVI it will also reset LRT. In the absence of an atrial signal paced ventricular complex (VVI) occurs. VDD pacing may be appropriate for the patient with normal sinus node function and conduction disease of the AVN or if the intent is to pace in the atrium and have the backup ventricular pacing should AV conduction fail.

Table 12.4 Rate responsive sensors and mechanism of action

Type of sensor	Mechanism
Piezoelectric crystal	Senses vibration from up and down motion
Accelerometer	Also senses anterior posterior motion
Minute ventilation	Transthoracic impedance which varies with respiration is used to calculate minute volume
Stimulus-T (QT)	This interval shortens with ↑ sympathetic activity
Temperature	Depends on change in core venous temperature

- In the DDD mode during lower rate pacing the timing cycle is divided into the AVI and the VA interval. The AVI is initiated by a spontaneous or paced atrial event and terminates with a spontaneous or paced ventricular event. The maximum tracking rate (MTR) is limited by TARP which includes the AVI and the PVARP.
- In rate responsive DDD pacemakers an increase in the heart rate may be atrial or sensor driven.

Rate adaptive pacing sensors
- Rate responsive pacemakers use sensors to detect vibrations, motion, respiration or other parameters of physical activity (Table 12.4).
- Some pacemakers combine more than one sensor to smooth the effect of different type of physical activities.
- Complications may occur during pacemaker implant and include cardiac perforation, infection, and pneumothorax.

Pacemaker follow-up
Output programming
- The output must be high enough to allow an adequate safety margin for pacing; this will maximize pacemaker longevity.
- A strength–duration curve plots voltage and pulse width thresholds and allows determination of appropriate values to ensure an adequate safety margin.
- Output programming options include doubling the voltage amplitude at the threshold, tripling the pulse width at the threshold, or programming output parameters to achieve triple the threshold determined in microjoules.

AV interval
- In dual-chamber pacemakers it is the interval between a paced or sensed atrial event and a paced ventricular event. This corresponds to the intrinsic PR interval. It must be programmed to optimize the hemodynamic benefit from the pacemaker. It is desirable to maintain intrinsic ventricular activation by programming a longer AVI, thus avoiding the potential adverse effects of right ventricular apical pacing.

Lead impedance
- Lead impedances should be measured to assess the integrity of the pacing system.

Mode switch
- Mode switching is the ability of the dual chamber pacemaker to automatically switch from one mode to another in response to paroxysmal supraventricular tachyarrhythmias. In the DDD or DDDR pacing modes, supraventricular tachyarrhythmias may result in rapid ventricular pacing.
- Pacing modes such as DDI, DDIR, DVI, or DVIR eliminate tracking of atrial activity.
- Mode switching allows the DDD or DDDR mode during sinus rhythm to switch to a non-tracking mode, such as DDIR, during atrial tachyarrhythmias and than back to the DDD/R mode on termination of the arrhythmia.

Analysis of pacemaker ECG
- The following pacemaker functions should be evaluated:
  1 Which chamber(s) is/are paced?
  2 Which chamber(s) is/are sensed?
- If pacemaker spikes are present, which event follows the stimulus? Is it QRS complex, P wave, both or neither?
- Is QRS induced by pacemaker stimulus, or is pacemaker stimulus occurring coincidentally with spontaneous QRS?
- Is sensing of the P and QRS appropriate? Loss of sensing results in asynchronous pacing.
- Atrial or ventricular events that occur during the refractory or blanking period are not sensed.
- Analysis of the pacemaker ECG is facilitated by the assessment of the timing cycles, such as escape interval, lower rate interval (Fig. 12.1).
- In a dual chamber pacemaker a sensed P wave terminates the atrial escape interval and initiates AVI. This will allow AV sequential pacing up to the upper rate limit, referred to as the maximum tracking rate.
- MTR is defined by TARP. It is the sum of AVI and PVARP. When the atrial rate exceeds this limit every other P wave will fall in the refractory period and will not be sensed, resulting in 2 : 1 pacemaker AV block.
- Other upper rate responses include pacemaker AV Wenckebach, fall back, and rate smoothing.
  Sensing abnormalities could include (Table 12.5):
  1 Undersensing – failure to recognize normal cardiac activity.
  2 Oversensing – unexpected sensing of intrinsic or extrinsic signals. A normally functioning pacemaker may fail to sense premature beats.
  3 Functional undersensing occurs when an intrinsic cardiac event is not sensed because it falls in the refractory period. For instance, an atrial event falling in the PVARP will not be sensed.

Table 12.5 Causes of abnormal pacemaker EKG

Absence of pacer spikes	Lack of capture	Over/under sensing	Altered pacing rate
1 Battery depletion	**1** Inadequate output	**1** Over sensing P and	**1** Sensor rate
2 Conductor coil	**2** High threshold,	T wave	**2** Magnet rate
fracture	spontaneous, or	**2** Undersensing PVC	**3** Hysteresis
3 Loose set screw	drug and	**3** Lead dislodgment	**4** Cross talk
4 Oversensing	metabolic induced	**4** Insulation break	**5** Oversensing
noncardiac signal	**3** Insulation defect	**5** EMI	**6** Circuit failure
5 Lack of anodal	**4** Lead dislodgment	**6** Asynchronous	**7** Altered recording
contact	**5** Perforation	mode/magnet	speed
6 Circuit failure	**6** Functional	application	
	noncapture (stim	**7** Circuit failure	
	on refractory	**8** Functional	
	period)	undersensing	
	7 Battery depletion	(event during	
	8 Poor connection	refractory period)	

- Programming the pacemaker temporarily to the triggered mode may reveal the source of abnormal sensing.
- When a cardiac event has morphology between an intrinsic and a paced beat it is called a fusion beat.
- Pseudo fusion occurs when a pacer spike falls on an intrinsic event but does not contribute to or alter that event. This is due to insufficient cardiac voltage to inhibit the sensing circuit. Pseudo fusion may occur when there is intraventricular conduction delay.
- Class IC drugs may increase pacing thresholds and may also cause sensing abnormalities.
- Electrolyte and metabolic abnormalities such as hyperkalemia, acidosis, hypoxia hyperglycemia, and myxedema may affect pacing and sensing thresholds.
- Ventricular pacing may result in pacemaker syndrome manifested by shortness of breath, dizziness, fatigue, pulsations in the neck or abdomen, cough, and apprehension.

Pacemaker-related complications

- Subclavian puncture may be associated with traumatic pneumothorax and hemopneumothorax, inadvertent arterial puncture, air embolism, arteriovenous fistula, thoracic duct injury, subcutaneous emphysema, and brachial plexus injury.
- Hematoma, at the pulse generator site may occur with spontaneous or therapeutically induced coagulation abnormality. Aspiration is not advised.
- Cardiac perforation and tamponade may occur.
- Venous thrombosis of the subclavian vein may occur.

- Lead-related complications include lead dislodgment, loose connector pin, conductor coil (lead) fracture, and insulation break.
- Pocket erosion and infection may occur. Impending erosion should be dealt with as an emergency. Once any portion of the pacemaker has eroded through the skin, the pacemaker system should be removed and implanted at a different site.
- Infection may be present even without purulent material. Culture should be obtained and proven negative before pocket revision. Adherence of the pacemaker to the skin suggests an infection, and salvage of the site may not be possible.
- The incidence of infection after pacemaker implantation should be less than 2%. Prophylactic use of antibiotics before implantation and in the immediate postoperative period remains controversial. There appears to be no significant difference in the rate of infection between patients who received prophylactic antibiotics and those who did not.
- Irrigation of the pacemaker pocket with an antibiotic solution at the time of pacemaker implantation may help prevent infection.
- Septicemia is uncommon.
- Early infections are caused by *Staphylococcus aureus*. Late infections are caused by *Staphylococcus epidermidis*.

Electromagnetic interference (EMI)

- An intrinsic or extrinsic signal of such frequency that is detected by the sensing circuit may cause sensing abnormalities.
- Biological signals are T waves, myopotentials, after potentials, P wave, and extrasystole.
- Nonbiological signals include electrocautery, cardioversion, MRI, lithotripsy radiofrequency ablation, diathermy, electroshock, and radio frequency signal (cell phones).
- Welding equipment, degaussing equipment, cellular phone, and antitheft devices are potential sources of EMI.
- Patients should avoid placing the "activated" cellular phone directly over the pacemaker or implantable cardioverter defebrillator (ICD), either from random motion of the phone or by carrying the activated phone in a breast pocket over the device.
- Patients should avoid leaning on or lingering near electronic equipment for surveillance of articles. Passing through these kinds of equipment is unlikely to adversely affect the pacemakers/ICDs.

12.3 IMPLANTABLE DEFIBRILLATORS

Implantable cardioverter defibrillators design

- An ICD is housed in a stainless steel or titanium case that also serves as an active electrode. An ICD is implanted subcutaneously in the prepectoral region.

- Pace sense leads are connected to a generator header using an IS-1 connector, and defibrillation leads are connected using a DF-1 connector. The header is made of clear polymethylmethacrylate.
- Other components of an ICD include battery, capacitor, telemetry coil, and microprocessor.
- The battery is made of lithium silver vanadium oxide. It stores 18,000 J of energy. It generates 3.2. V Battery voltage of less than 2.2 V indicates that the elective replacement parameter has been reached.
- Aluminum electrolyte capacitors are used to store 30–40 J using a DC/DC converter. A capacitor is capable of charging and delivering 750 V to the heart in 10–15 milliseconds. Capacitor charging begins after tachycardia detection criteria are met. Capacitor charge time should be less than 15 seconds.
- Long charge time would result in a longer period of circulatory arrest. In addition to battery voltage longer charge time is also an indication for ICD replacement.
- A single ventricular lead incorporates pace sense and a defibrillation electrode.
- A defibrillation electrode consists of two coils, made of platinum–iridium alloy or carbon and is capable of delivering high voltages. A distal coil is located in the right ventricle (RV) and a proximal coil is located in superior vena cava (SVC).
- The pace sense component consists of bipolar electrodes. Some systems use intergraded bipolar electrodes that record between the tip and the distal coil. Other systems use true bipolar electrodes that record between the tip and the ring electrode.
- A dual chamber ICD uses a standard bipolar atrial lead. In addition to atrial pacing, an atrial lead provides intracardiac electrograms, which are helpful in differentiating VT from supra VT (SVT).
- Virtually all ICD systems are implanted transvenously and include antitachycardia pacing (ATP) and ventricular bradycardia pacing, dual-chamber pacing with rate-adaptive options. In addition, atrial defibrillation and CRT features are available.
- Defibrillating current is directly proportional to the voltage and inversely proportional to lead impedance. Polarization at lead tissue interface may occur.

Sensing

- Ventricular heart rate is the cornerstone of tachyarrhythmia detection by the ICD. Each and every electrogram must be detected and interval analyzed for proper sensing and detection of the tachycardia. Detection of the electrogram depends on the quality of the signal received from the ventricular myocardium. Assessment of far field signal detection by the ventricular lead should be performed at the time of implant. If far field signals are detected in spite of sensitivity reprogramming the lead should be repositioned.
- A band pass filter is utilized to filter out very low and very high frequency signals that are out of range of ventricular signals. However, ventricular repolarization, atrial events, post pacing, and post depolarization polarization, myopotentials

and external environmental signals may be detected by the ventricular lead, resulting in false detection of tachyarrhythmia and spurious shock or inhibition of the pacemaker.

- In addition to the amplitude of the signal the frequency contents of the signal (Slew rate V/s) are also important for better detection of the signal. A large signal improves the specificity of detection. A small signal (4–6 mV) but with good frequency contents as represented by a slew rate of >1 V/s is better than a larger signal with poor frequency content and a slew rate of <0.1 V/s.

- The device must quickly and accurately identify the amplitude variation that occurs between normal beat of 10 mV, pacing spike of >500 mV, VF with amplitudes of 0.2–10 mV and asystole where the amplitude of the electrogram may be 0–0.15 mV. Attempts have been made to overcome these limitations by using autogain or an auto sensing threshold function. The autogain technique uses fixed amplitude voltage threshold and amplifies it for better detection. In the autothreshold technique amplification is fixed and continuously varying amplitude voltage is detected.

- Adequate signals during sinus rhythm may be inadequate during VF, therefore, assessment of the adequacy of signal detection should be performed by inducing VF at the time of implant. Failure to detect <10% of the VF signals during the detection period would still result in proper detection and treatment of VF. A ventricular electrogram amplitude of 5 MV during sinus rhythm predicts reliable detection of VF.

Detection

- After the detection of the electrogram the algorithm to detect and classify the intervals between electrogram is activated. This algorithm differentiates between bradycardia that may require pacing, VT that may require antitachycardia pacing and VF requiring shock.

- The primary features for the detection of the ventricular arrhythmias are heart rate and the duration of the arrhythmia. For faster rhythm shorter detection intervals should be programmed. Rate detection alone does not describe the hemodynamic status of the patient. Algorithm, where X number of intervals out of the total Y number of intervals, that meet the detection criteria may improve the sensitivity of detection.

- Supraventricular tachycardias with overlapping rates with ventricular detection may result in inappropriate therapy. Attempts have been made to improve the specificity of detection by adding additional criteria such as suddenness of onset (to differentiate from sinus tachycardia), beat-to-beat variation in cycle length (to differentiate from AF) and use of the atrial electrogram and its relationship to ventricular electrogram.

- The presence of AV dissociation will confirm the diagnosis of VT. If there is a 1 : 1 relationship between a ventricular and an atrial electrogram then it could be due to VT with 1 : 1 retrograde conduction or SVT. The ratio of the AV to VA interval may help in differentiating these arrhythmias. These additional features may delay the detection and decrease the sensitivity of detection.

- Algorithms should be programmed to deliver shocks immediately for rapid arrhythmias irrespective of their origin. Sensitivity should not be sacrificed at the expense of specificity. A lower rate cutoff may result in inappropriate shocks.
- A reconfirmation feature reconfirms the presence of arrhythmia during the charging period. This may avoid unnecessary shocks in the presence of nonsustained arrhythmias which might terminate spontaneously during the charging period.
- A redetection feature redetects the occurrence of arrhythmia a few beats after its successful termination. This interval could be shortened by reducing the number of intervals required for redetection.

Indications for ICD implant (Tables 12.6 and 12.7)

1 Ejection fraction (EF) of <35% irrespective of etiology (ischemic or nonischemic).
2 Cardiac arrest due to VF or VT not due to a transient or reversible cause.
3 Spontaneous sustained VT associated with structural heart disease.

Table 12.6 Secondary prevention trials

Study	Inclusion criteria	Endpoint(s)	Treatment arms	Key results
AVID	Survivor of cardiac arrest VT with syncope Symptomatic sustained VT with LVEF ≤ 0.40	Total mortality Mode of death Quality of life Cost benefit	Amiodarone or sotalol or ICD	Significant improvement in overall survival with ICD
CASH	Survivor of cardiac arrest	Total mortality Recurrences of arrhythmias requiring CPR Recurrence of unstable VT	ICD amiodarone, propafenone, or metoprolol	Significant improvement in overall survival with ICD
CIDS	Survivor of cardiac arrest Syncope with sustained or inducible VT. EF ≤35	Total mortality	Amiodarone or ICD	No significant improvement in survival with ICD

AVID, Antiarrhythmics Versus Implantable Defibrillators; CASH, Cardiac Arrest Study Hamburg; CIDS, Canadian Implantable Defibrillator Study.

Table 12.7 Primary prevention trials

Study	Patient inclusion criteria	Endpoint(s)	Treatment arms	Key results
MADIT	Q wave MI ≥3 weeks Asymptomatic NSVT LVEF ≤35% Inducible VT during EPS and nonsuppressible with procainamide NYHA classes I–III	Overall mortality	ICD Conventional therapy	ICDs reduced overall mortality by 54%
CABG-PATCH	Scheduled for elective CABG surgery LVEF <36% Abnormal SAECG	Overall mortality	ICD versus Standard treatment	Survival not improved by prophylactic implantation of ICD at time of elective CABG
MUSTT	CAD EF ≤40% NSVT Inducible VT or VF	Sudden arrhythmic death or spontaneous sustained VT	ICD in nonsuppressible group	>70% risk reduction in arrhythmic death or cardiac arrest and >50% reduction in total mortality
BEST-ICD	Acute MI EF ≤0.40 SDRR <70 ms or ≥109 PVCs/h or abnormal SAECG	All-cause mortality	EPS: if inducible, ICD and BB; if noninducible, BB	No significant survival improvement with ICD too few patients enrolled
MADIT-II	Prior MI EF ≤0.30	All-cause mortality	Conventional therapy or ICD	With ICD, 31% reduction in mortality
SCD-HeFT	Ischemic or nonischemic cardiomyopathy EF ≤35% NYHA Class II or III No history of sustained VT/VF	All-cause mortality	Placebo, amiodarone or ICD	Significant survival improvement with ICD

BB, beta blocker; BEST-ICD, Beta-Blocker Strategy Plus Implantable Cardioverter-Defibrillator; CABG, coronary artery bypass graft; CABG-PATCH, Coronary Artery Bypass Graft Patch Trial. MADIT, Multicenter Automatic Defibrillator Implantation Trial; MI, myocardial infarction; MUSTT, Multicenter Unsustained Tachycardia Trial; SCD-HeFT, Sudden Cardiac Death in Heart Failure Trial.

4 Syncope, associated with structural heart disease, and clinically relevant, hemodynamically significant sustained VT or VF induced at EP study.

5 Nonsustained VT in patients with coronary disease, prior MI, EF 40–45%, and inducible VF or sustained VT at EP study.

6 Familial or inherited conditions with a high risk for life-threatening ventricular tachyarrhythmias such as long-QT syndrome or hypertrophic cardiomyopathy.

Exclusion criteria

- Terminal illnesses with projected life expectancy <6 months coronary bypass surgery.
- NYHA Class IV drug-refractory congestive heart failure in patients who are not candidates for cardiac transplantation.

Therapy

- The ICD functions by continuously monitoring the patient's cardiac rate and delivering therapy when the rate exceeds the programmed rate "cutoff".
- ICD provide separate bradycardia and post shock pacing. In dual chamber ICD routine bradycardia pacing could be programmed to AAI if AVN conduction is adequate. This will obviate the need for ventricular pacing with its possible detrimental effects on LV function.
- ATP consists of delivering a specified number of ventricular pacing impulses at a faster interval than the programmed ventricular detection interval. The number of sequences of ATP could be programmed. If the interval between pulses is constant the technique is called burst pacing, if the interval progressively decreases then it is termed ramp. If the pacing interval decreases from one sequence to the next, although it remains constant within that sequence, the technique is called scan. A combination of scan and ramp will result in more aggressive ATP protocol.
- ATP may be effective in terminating VT in 90% of the episodes.
- ATP may accelerate the tachycardia.
- Electrical shock is delivered by the device through the coils into the myocardium.
- Placement of the distal coil along the interventricular septum improves the efficacy of defibrillation. The speed with which the total output is delivered depends on the impedance of the electrodes and the duration and tilt of the pulse width.
- The device may contain two capacitors each capable of 250–300 μF capacitance maximum voltage of 350–375 volts. Capacitors are charged simultaneously in parallel, however, the shock is delivered in series, so the total voltage is doubled 700–750 V. This configuration reduces the capacitance by one-half to 120–150 μF. High voltage lead impedance is between 30 and 60 Ω.
  This combination of low capacitance and low impedance allows 60–90% of the stored energy delivered in <20 milliseconds.

Defibrillation threshold and safety margin

- VF is induced and a progressively lower amount of energy is delivered. The lowest amount of energy that successfully defibrillates is called the DFT. This may necessitate repeated induction of VF. Alternatively, two consecutive successful defibrillation using energy with a 10 J margin has been shown to provide a success rate of 98% during follow-up.
- Using biphasic shock a margin of twice the DFT provides 95% probability of successful defibrillation.
- The upper limit of vulnerability (ULV) can be used to assess the DFT. A test shock is delivered on the T wave. Normally, low energy shock delivered on the T wave will induce VF. If the test shock fails to induce VF it is believed to be above the DFT. The shock of the lowest energy that fails to induce VF is considered the DFT.
- One of the advantages of ULV is that the DFT can be determined without inducing VF.
- One of the disadvantages is the inability to determine the sensing from electrodes during VF.
- Both methods can be combined to achieve a high success rate without inducing VF repeatedly. First the VF is induced and 15 J of energy is delivered if successful; then ULV is determined by delivering 5 J on the T wave. If VF is not induced then DFT is greater than 5 J.

Biphasic wave form

- The capacitor discharge is divided into two phases with opposite polarity. After the first phase the polarity is reversed. The first phase is longer than the second phase. Switching the capacitor from series to parallel configuration in the second phase could double the second phase voltage.
- The magnitude of the wave form is characterized by its amplitude (peak voltage or current) and tilt. The percent change in amplitude of the wave form from its initial value to its terminal value is described as the tilt. If the amplitude is reduced by $\frac{1}{2}$ then the tilt for that wave form is 50%.
- Current is delivered from the cathode (negative) electrode located in the RV to a can and SVC coil configured as anode (positive electrode). Sometimes this configuration does not provide a satisfactory DFT and reversal of polarity (RV) as an anode is required.
- ICD provides defibrillation cardioversion and antitachycardia pacing for termination of sustained ventricular arrhythmias.
- Shocks are synchronized during VT (cardioversion) or are asynchronous during ventricular fibrillation (defibrillation).
- The device can be programmed into three zones depending on the rate cutoff. Slower rates are labeled as VT zone and faster rates are labeled as VF zone. Fast VT may fall into the VF zone and will be treated according to the programmed criteria for the VF zone.
- The DFT remains stable over the years, antiarrhythmic drugs do not significantly affect the biphasic DFT.

- Low energy cardioversion defibrillation has the advantage of short charge time, rapid conversion and less battery consumption.
- Acceleration of the VT may occur following a low energy cardioversion or ATP in 3–5% of patients. ATP has a success rate of 90% in terminating VT.
- Faster VT in patients with low EF is likely to accelerate if short coupling intervals are used.
- ATP can be programmed empirically in patients who did not have spontaneous or sustained VT.
- Follow-up ICD testing should be limited to patients in whom device malfunction is suspected or antiarrhythmic drugs have been added that might alter the DFT.

Device selection

- Patients who have bradycardia may benefit from dual chamber ICD programmed in a AAI mode to prevent ventricular pacing.
- As suggested by dual-chamber and VVIT implantable defibrillator (DAVID) trial, ventricular pacing may increase mortality and incidence of CHF.
- Devices that combine CRT and ICD therapy can be considered for patients who meet the CRT criteria.
- The survival benefit of ICD was noted in patients with an ejection fraction of <35%.

DFT

- DFT can be defined as the minimal energy that terminates ventricular fibrillation.
- An acceptable DFT is a value that ensures an adequate safety margin for defibrillation, usually being at least 10 J less than the maximum output of the ICD, which ranges from 30 to 41 J of stored energy.
- Generally, the preference is to implant the ICD in the left pectoral region because of a more favorable vector for delivery of the shock.

Complications associated with ICD implant

- These include infection, pneumothorax, cardiac tamponade, and dislodgement of the leads.
- Inappropriate shock may occur in 10% of the patients in the first year and up to 30% of the patients may receive inappropriate therapy within 4 years after implant.
- AF is the most common cause of inappropriate therapy. Stability and onset criteria may help prevent inappropriate shocks due to AF.
- In patients with advanced heart failure bradycardia and pulseless cardiac electrical activity are the commonest cause of death.

Management of the patient with a pacemaker or ICD during an operative procedure

- Prior to surgery the device should be interrogated and detection and therapy should be deactivated. After the procedure, the device should be reinterrogated and ICD therapy reinitiated. During the time ICD therapy is "off," the patient must be monitored.

- For pacemaker-dependent patients, the pacemaker could be programmed to an asynchronous pacing mode, VOO or DOO, or the same effect can be achieved by placing a magnet over the pacemaker throughout the procedure.
- The potential effects of electrocautery on the device include reprogramming; permanent damage to the pulse generator; pacemaker inhibition; reversion to a fall-back mode, noise reversion mode, or electrical reset; and myocardial thermal damage.
- If cardioversion and defibrillation is required in a patient with a pacemaker or ICD, place paddles in the anteroposterior position, keep the paddles at least 4 inches from the pulse generator, have the appropriate pacemaker programmer available, and interrogate the pacemaker after the procedure.

MRI and implanted devices

- MRI is still considered a relative contraindication in patients with a pacemaker or ICD given the potential for induction of rapid hemodynamically unstable ventricular rhythms and the theoretical possibility of heating of the conductor coil and thermal damage at the electrode–myocardial interface.
- Although there are reports of MRI being performed safely in non-pacemaker-dependent patients, there are also reports of deaths resulting from MRI-induced rhythm disturbances.

Effect of antiarrhythmic drugs and metabolic abnormalities on pacemaker/ICD

- Flecainide and propafenone have the potential to increase pacing/sensing thresholds and DFT.
- These agents may alter the detection of VT and produce proarrhythmic effects. Drug-induced slowing of the VT rate can result in inadequate detection of the arrhythmia. Amiodarone can cause an increase in the DFT.
- Electrolyte and metabolic abnormalities can also affect the pacing and sensing thresholds. Hyperkalemia, severe acidosis or alkalosis, hypercapnia, severe hyperglycemia, hypoxemia, and hypothyroidism can alter the thresholds.

Causes of multiple ICD shocks

- Frequent VT or VF (electrical storm).
- Unsuccessful ICD therapy due to inappropriately low-output shock or elevation of DFT.
- Lead fracture.
- Lead dislodgment.
- Detection of supraventricular rhythms.
- Oversensing separate pacing system, EMI or other intracardiac signals such as P or T waves.

Device follow-up

- Follow-up can be accomplished through office-based assessment; transtelephonic follow-up; or Internet-based device follow-up.
- Once a year, appropriateness of the rate-adaptive pacing mode should be assessed.
- The appropriateness of delivered therapy or other changes in the patient's medical status or drug regimen that could affect ICD therapy should be analyzed.
- The aspects of follow-up include history with specific emphasis on awareness of delivered therapy and any tachyarrhythmic events, device interrogation to assess battery status; charge time, lead impedances, pacing thresholds, and retrieval and assessment of stored diagnostic data.
- Periodic radiographic assessment of the leads should be performed.
- Arrhythmia induction in the electrophysiology laboratory to assess the DFTs and detection should be considered especially if there is a change in the patient's clinical or therapeutic status.

References

1 Bernstein AD. Daubert JC. Fletcher RD. et al. North American Society of Pacing and Electrophysiology/British Pacing and Electrophysiology Group: The revised NASPE/BPEG generic code for antibradycardia, adaptive-rate, and multisite pacing. *Pacing Clin Electrophysiol* 25:260, 2002.
2 Gregoratos G. Abrams J. Epstein AE. et al. ACC/AHA/NASPE 2002 guideline update for implantation of cardiac pacemakers and antiarrhythmia devices. Summary article: A report of the American College of Cardiology/American Heart Association Task Force on Practice Guidelines (ACC/AHA/NASPE Committee to Update the 1998 Pacemaker Guidelines). *Circulation.* 106:2145, 2002.

Self-Assessment Answers

1

1.1 POTASSIUM CHANNELS

1 A
2 B
3 C
4 A
5 B
6 A
7 B
8 C
9 C
10 A

1.2 SODIUM CHANNELS

1 A
2 B
3 C
4 D
5 A
6 B
7 A
8 D
9 A

1.3 CALCIUM CHANNELS

1 C
2 B
3 D
4 C
5 D
6 A

2 Cardiac Autonomic Activity

1 B
2 B
3 D
4 A
5 A
6 B
7 D
8 B

3 Mechanisms of Arrhythmias

1 D
2 C
3 C
4 D

4 SA Node and AV black

1 A
2 B
3 C
4 D
5 A
6 D
7 C
8 A

5

5.1 ATRIAL FLUTTER
1 C
2 C
3 B
4 A

5.2 ATRIAL TACHYCARDIA
1 B
2 C
3 A

5.3 ATRIAL FIBRILLATION
1 C
2 B
3 A
4 C
5 B
6 A
7 D

5.4 AUTOMATIC JUNCTIONAL TACHYCARDIA
1 A
2 C

5.5 AVNRT
1 B
2 C
3 B
4 A
5 C and D
6 A
7 C
8 D
9 C
10 A

5.6 AVRT
1 B
2 D

3 C
4 D
5 A
6 B
7 D
8 A
9 B
10 C
11 D
12 C
13 A
14 C
15 A
16 B
17 A
18 C
19 D
20 C

6 Wide Complex Tachycardia
1 C
2 B

7
1 A

7.1 VT IN THE PRESENCE OF CAD
1 B
2 C

7.2 ARVD/C
1 A. Not performed
   B. Negative
   C. Negative
   D. Negative
2 D
3 C
4 C

7.3 HYPERTROPHIC AND DILATED CARDIOMYOPATHY

1 C
2 A
3 D
4 C
5 D

7.4 LQTS

1 D
2 C
3 A
4 B
5 B
6 A

7.5 BRUGADA SYNDROME

1 B
2 B

7.6 VT NORMAL HEART

1 C
2 D
3 A
4 B

7.7 BBRVT

1 C
2 D
3 A

7.8 CPVT

1 B
2 A

7.9 MISCELLANEOUS VT

1 D

8 SCD

1 D

9 Cardiac Arrhythmias in Neuro-muscular Disorder

1 D
2 B
3 D

10 Syncope

1 B
2 C
3 A
4 D
5 B
6 B

11 Pharmacologic Therapy of Arrhythmias

1 D
2 A

12 Electrical Therapy for Cardiac Arrhythmias

1 C
2 D
3 C
4 D

Index

Page numbers in *italics* refer to figures; those in **bold** to tables or boxes. Abbreviations are listed in full at the beginning of the book.